Why The United States Healthcare System Should Be A Limited Human Right For All

Why The United States Healthcare System Should Be A Limited Human Right For All

Section One (2009) and Section Two (2010-2017)

Mark G. Tozzio, M-IHHS, Fache

WHY THE UNITED STATES HEALTHCARE SYSTEM *SHOULD* BE A LIMITED HUMAN RIGHT FOR ALL
Section One (2009) and Section Two (2010-2017)

©Copyright MARK G. TOZZIO, M-IHHS, FACHE
(Original) November 15, 2009 **Section One**
(Update) September 6, 2014 Section One with ***Postscript***;
(New) March 20, 2017 with **Section Two**

All Rights Reserved. No part of this book may be reproduced in any form or by any means without permission in writing from Mark G. Tozzio.

Library of Congress Cataloguing-in-Publication Data

Tozzio, Mark G., 1951-

Why the United States Healthcare System Should be a Limited Human Right for All --
Section One (2009) and Section Two (2010-2017)
/ by Mark G. Tozzio, M-IHHS, FACHE.

p. cm.

Includes bibliographical references and footnotes.

EAN-13: 9781544025216
ISBN-10: 1544025211

1. Healthcare in the United States. 2. Reform. 3. Healthcare Policy. 4. Morality and Healthcare. 5. Philosophy of Healthcare in the United States. 6. Health Care Issues. 7. Healthcare Ethics. 8. Health Access. 9. Healthcare and Human Rights. 10. Basic Healthcare Services in the US

Title ID 6975147 (new)

Cover photo by Emma Brown, *The Washington Post*.

Project sponsored by:
HPPD, Inc.
P.O. Box 2437
Broken Arrow, Oklahoma 74013
918-521-7468

Printed in the United States of America by:
CreateSpace, An Amazon.com Company (paperback and e-book versions).
eStore URL https://www.createspace.com/3408078

ISBN 1544025211

$19.95 US

SECTION ONE (2009)

Dedicated to Our Nation's Children

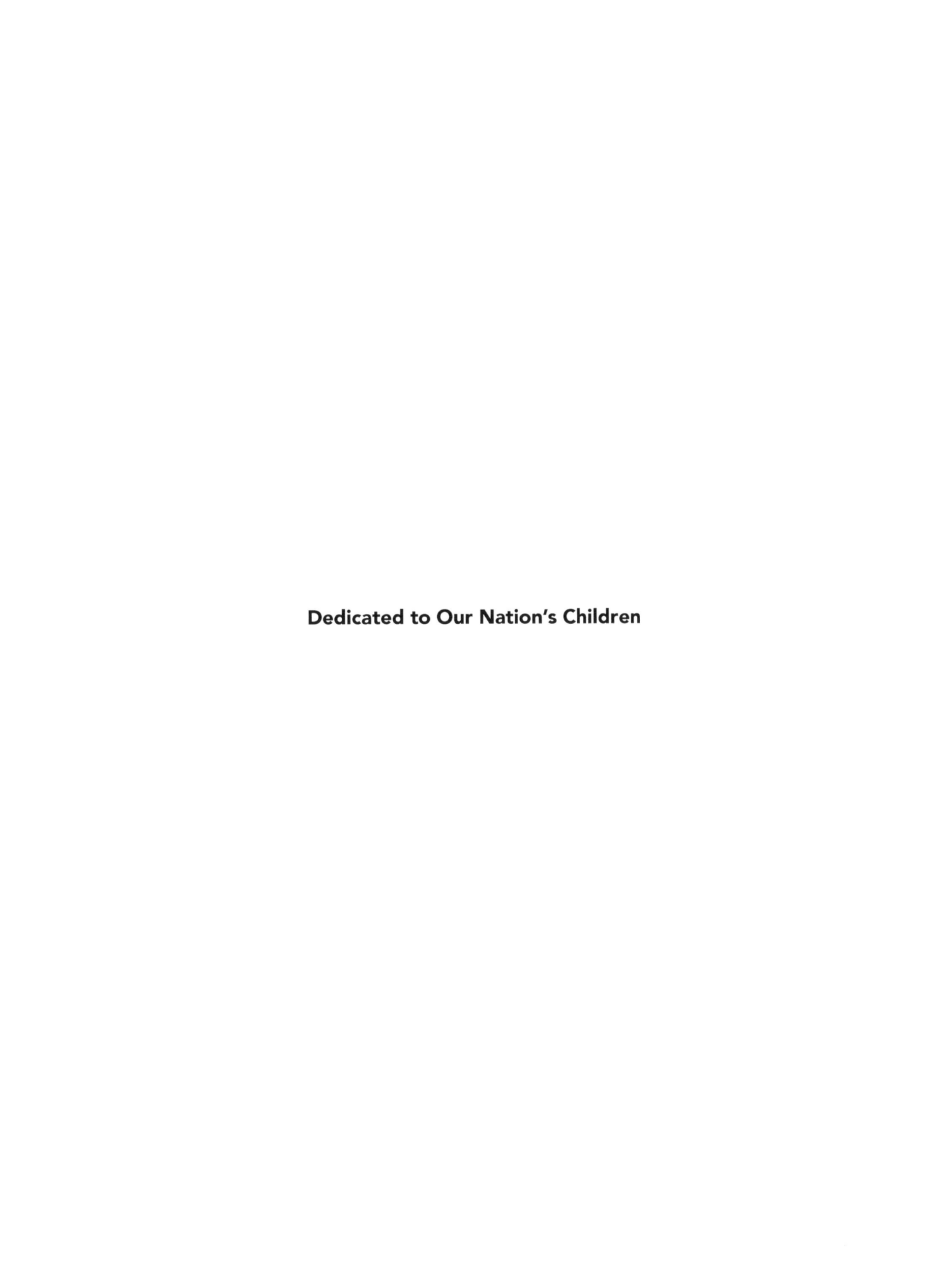

Foreword for Section One

The United States is a world leader in many areas, including human rights, and freedom of speech and expressions, to mention only two vitally important rights. As one of the wealthiest nations on this planet, we spend more on healthcare than all other economically and socially developed countries. However, many would argue that as a population we actually receive less quality services for the amount of money spent than other developed nations. A healthier population significantly increases the chances of being a highly productive nation, from an economic standpoint; therefore, if one accepts this premise, isn't there a significant advantage for United States to vigorously pursue having a healthier population?

Many years ago some countries, not necessarily the United States, made education available *only* to the wealthy and elite. The result of this shortsighted strategy was to create socially stratified societies, with the educated elite having privilege and power, and the less educated functioning as servants and laborers. For a considerable period of time this was an acceptable practice. However, these populations became more enlightened to the fact that a better educated society meant a more productive nation; thus, everyone within the society would benefit. Gradually education became an accepted human right within most developed countries.

Hopefully, within the United States we are on the threshold of similar enlightenment with regard to healthcare. Mark Tozzio makes a compelling and convincing argument that the American healthcare system *should* be a limited human right for all. This book explains *why* it is critical to develop a concise and coherent national policy surrounding the moral and ethical reasoning for reforming the healthcare system in a manner that offers basic health services to all citizens. This book points out that the United States' healthcare system should be changed to provide basic healthcare to all Americans regardless of socioeconomic conditions (according to the theory of distributive justice).

Mark's book is a must read for anyone who is interested in gaining an interdisciplinary understanding of the current conditions of the United States' healthcare system, and is open to rational discussion about *how* and *why* the system should be enhanced.

Willie V. Bryan, Ed.D.

WHY THE UNITED STATES HEALTHCARE SYSTEM *SHOULD* BE A LIMITED HUMAN RIGHT FOR ALL

Section One (2009)

MARK G. TOZZIO, M-IHHS, FACHE

REVIEW COMMITTEE FOR THE
UNIVERSITY OF OKLAHOMA,
COLLEGE OF LIBERAL STUDIES,
NORMAN, OKLAHOMA

Dr. John L. Duncan, Chair
Assistant Professor of Cultural Studies, College of Liberal Studies
Clinical Associate Professor, College of Medicine

Dr. Vicki L. Tall Chief
Adjunct Professor, College of Liberal Studies
Associate Professor of Health Promotion Sciences, College of Public Health

Dr. Willie V. Bryan
Professor Emeritus
Adjunct Professor, College of Liberal Studies
Adjunct Professor, Advanced Programs
Former Associate Professor of Health Promotion Sciences, College of Public Health
Former Vice Provost for Educational Services, Health Sciences Center

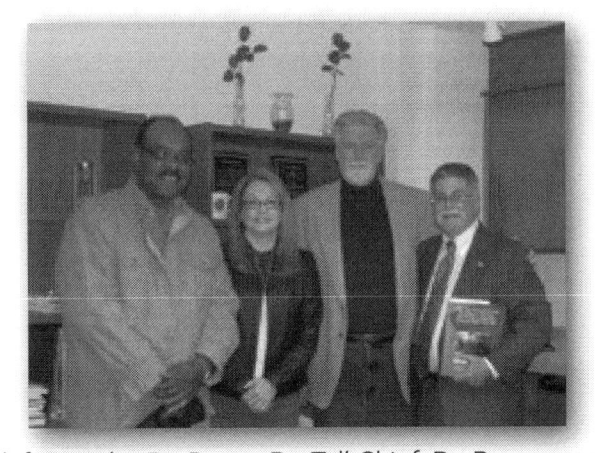

Pictured from left to right: Dr. Bryan, Dr. Tall Chief, Dr. Duncan, and Mark Tozzio

Table of Contents for Section One

Foreword for Section One ix
Table of Contents for Section One. xiii
List of Graphs and Tables. xvii
List of Charts, Figures, and Illustrations xix
Acknowledgements for Section One xxi
Overview xxiii
Research Approach xxx
Goals xxxi

Part 1: Background 1
One   Historical Perspective. 3
           1.1 -- US Health System during the 1900s to 1990s 3
           1.2 -- Clinton Healthcare Era 6
Two   Current State of Healthcare System 11
           2.1 -- Market-Based Healthcare 11
           2.2 -- Competition, Duplication of Services, and Spiraling Costs 13
Three   The Perfect Healthcare Storm 17
           3.1 -- Political Climate and Rhetoric 17
           3.2 -- Obama-Biden Health Reform Recipe 19

Part 2: Problem Statement 23
Four   Major Issues and Concerns. 25
           4.1 -- Physician-Hospital Evolution 28
           4.2 -- Lack of Commitment to Prevention and Public Health Initiatives. 29
           4.3 -- Complementary Medicine and Wellness Approach. 31
           4.4 -- Economic (Dis)Incentives of America's Health System 31
           4.5 -- Assuming Personal Responsibility for Health and Wellness 36
Five   The Hippocratic Oath. 38
           5.1 -- Patient-Physician Relationship 41
           5.2 -- Corporatization of Healthcare and the Oath 46

Six	Ethics and Modern Medicine	48
	6.1 -- Ethics, Fairness, Justice, and Healthcare in the United States	48
	6.2 -- Medicine for Profit	51
Seven	Two Contrasting Approaches for Providing Universal Health Coverage	64
	7.1 -- The Dutch Health System Experience	64
	7.2 -- The Oregon Health Program Experience	68
Eight	Sick Care vs. Preventive Health Measures	76
	8.1 -- Health Care Equals Sick Care	76
	8.2 -- Preventive Health Measures and ROI	80
	8.3 -- Can Rationing Be Rationalized?	87
Nine	Employer-Sponsored Health Insurance	91
	9.1 -- Will the Real Number of Uninsured Persons in the United States Please Come Forward	91
	9.2 -- Addressing the Health Insurance Conundrum	99
	9.3 -- Joe the Consultant	107
	9.4 -- Healthcare is an Economic Issue	109

Part 3: Foundational Elements of Healthcare ... 115

Ten	Health Care (Not Sick Care), a Limited Human Right for All	117
	10.1 -- Is Culture the Basis for Healthcare Ethics and Morality?	119
	10.2 -- John Stuart Mill – Utilitarian Theory	124
	10.3 -- Immanuel Kant – Principle of the Categorical Imperative	129
	10.4 -- John Rawls – Distributive Justice Theory	134
	10.5 -- Norman Daniels – Equality of Opportunity Theory	140
	10.6 -- Yroam Amiel and Frank Cowell – Income Inequality Theory	155
	10.7 -- Jonathan M. Mann, et al. – Health and Human Rights Theory	158
	10.8 -- Should Healthcare in the United States Be Considered a Right or a Commodity?	165
Eleven	The Push for Universal Healthcare Coverage	173
	11.1 -- Public Health Plan, a Realistic Part of Universal Healthcare Coverage?	173
	11.2 -- What Constitutes Basic Health Services?	176
	11.3 -- Transitioning to the Next Generation of Healthcare in the United States	185

Part 4: Critical Findings, Conclusions, and Epilogue ... 191

Twelve	Critical Findings	193
Thirteen	Conclusions	196
	13.1 -- Why Healthcare in the United States Should be a Limited Human Right for All	199

	13.2 -- Relevance of this Book to Current Healthcare Reform Efforts	205
	13.3 -- The Politics of Healthcare Reform	206
Fourteen	Epilogue	211
	14.1 -- Advice for Policymakers	211
	14.2 -- Advice for Providers	213
	14.3 --Advice for Consumers	214
	14.4 -- Next Steps for Reforming the US Healthcare System	216

Postscript - March 23, 2010	217
Postscript - June 28, 2012	219
References for Section One	223
Exhibit A – Community Forum on Healthcare Reform	235
Supplemental Bibliography for Section One	239

List of Graphs and Tables

GRAPHS
Graph 1 – Public Concerns about Healthcare in the US 8
Graph 2 – International Spending on Healthcare Services 12
Graph 3 – Expenditures on Health Insurance Administration 13
Graph 4 – Access Problems Because of Income: 2007 15
Graph 5 – Public Support for President Obama's Health Plan 20

TABLES
Table 1 A – Number of US Hospitals by Class: 2007 32
Table 1 B – Number of Hospitals Trended: 1987-2007 32
Table 1 C – 50th Percentile Total Operating Profit of Hospitals: 2002-2006 33
Table 2 – US Bed Supply Trend: 1987-2007 34
Table 3 – Physician-Patient Alignment 45
Table 4 – Number of US Hospitals by Class: 2007 52
Table 5 – Health Association's Executive Compensation: 2007 57
Table 6 – By the Numbers- How the US Compares with Other Developed Nations 67
Table 7 – Current Examples of Conditions-Treatment Pairs on the OHP Prioritized List 73
Table 8 – ROI Impact of Preventive Health Initiatives 82
Table 9 – Sampling of Healthcare Status Quo of US States 85
Table 10 – Health Insurance Providers' Performance: 2008 95
Table 11 – Definition of Key Terms 117
Table 12 – Federal Poverty Guidelines: 2009 157
Table 13 – Reasons Why Health and Healthcare Are Special Elements of Society 170
Table 14 – Potential Impact of a Proposed Public Health Plan on the Traditional Health Insurance Industry Utilization in the US 174
Table 15 – Oregon Evidence-Based and Community Driven Essential Benefits Package Proposal (Framework) 182
Table 16 – Causes of Death in the US: 2003-2004 186

List of Charts, Figures, and Illustrations

CHARTS

Chart 1 – US Healthcare Spending Trend: 1987-2007 xxiv
Chart 2 – Sick Care versus Healthcare Financial Impact xxvii
Chart 3 – Federal Budget Surplus and Deficit Trend 28
Chart 4 – Differential Inpatient Utilization Rates 78
Chart 5 – USA Today Headlines: Economic Collapse --September 2008 to 2009 113
Chart 6 – Population Growth in the US: 2000-2020 145
Chart 7 – Tozzio's Prescription for US Health Reform Based On Principles of Justice 198

FIGURES

Figure 1 – The Johnson Era. 3
Figure 2 – The Clinton Era. 6
Figure 3 – Hippocratic Oath for Physicians. 39
Figure 4 – Larry "Curly" Haubner at Age 107. 79
Figure 5 – National Healthcare Spending by Industry Sector: 2006-2007 86
Figure 6 – Percentage of Uninsured Adults 18-64 and Children 0-17 by State. 94
Figure 7 – Cycle of Healthcare Utilization by the Uninsured and Employer-Sponsored
          Health Insurance Coverage By State, Under 65: 2000/2001 to 2006/2007. 101
Figure 8 – Elements of a Balanced Democratic Social Structure. 138
Figure 9 – United Nation's Protection of the Right to Health. 160
Figure 10 – Foundational Dimensions for Human Dignity, Morality, and Rights. 165
Figure 11 – Cycle of Health and Healthcare 171
Figure 12 – Washington, D.C. Health Reform Demonstration. 176
Figure 13 – Health Insurance Coverage Schemes. 178

ILLUSTRATIONS

Illustration 1 – Congressional Bipartisanship and Healthcare Reform 209

Acknowledgements for Section One

Many friends and colleagues have contributed directly and indirectly to my thought processes during the four years it took to formalize the material for this book. The University of Oklahoma has provided an excellent interdisciplinary learning environment for expanding my knowledge of health, healthcare, and human services. Russ Tressner served as my advisor and was always willing to help and encourage me during my journey – I consider him a true friend.

I am especially grateful to Professor John Duncan for volunteering to chair the Review Committee and for encouraging and guiding me during my academic work at the University of Oklahoma, Norman. Professor Duncan introduced me to the discipline of philosophy and its importance to the subject of healthcare rights – the basis of this book. His unique blend of practical experience in drug law enforcement and academic knowledge of the philosophy of medicine was an inspiration to my work. Professor Vicki Tall Chief offered insightful suggestions about how to strengthen the content of the public health and wellness subject matter. Professor Willie Bryan provided the underlying theoretical framework for integrating the social and economic realities into the complex analysis of health and healthcare and its relevance to human rights issues. Professor Bryan's extensive knowledge and kind words of encouragement helped inspire me when the "light at the end of the tunnel" was distant and dim. Collectively, my Review Committee provided outstanding support for this work – above and beyond my expectations.

I am also indebted to Darren Coffman, Executive Director of the Oregon Health Services Commission, Office for Oregon Health Policy and Research, for spending extra time to share details about the Oregon Health Plan and his personal experience with this innovative program since its inception 20 years ago. The Oregon Health Plan is the only working example in the United States of a systematic and rational healthcare allocation program, which was extremely relevant to this work.

My friends Myrna and Bill Bailie were great listeners during my research and helped me refine the central arguments about healthcare reform and its moral ramifications into a coherent and understandable discussion. Lee Conroy, Phil Ronning, Webster Russell and James Whitmer also provided valuable assistance during the final editing stage of this book. I especially want to acknowledge the research assistance, editorial advice, patience, understanding, and love of my wife Darlina, and the support of our daughter Aungela and her family, which carried me to the successful conclusion of this daunting task – I could not have succeeded without them. Thanks to all!

Why the United States Healthcare System *Should* Be A Limited Human Right for All
Section One (2009)

Speaking to the American people at a multimedia event, the President called the healthcare reform initiative a "moral imperative," and asked Americans to pressure Congress to enact legislation by the end of 2009.

PRESIDENT BARACK OBAMA, AT A TOWN-HALL MEETING AT NORTHERN VIRGINIA COMMUNITY COLLEGE, ANNANDALE, VIRGINIA, JULY 1, 2009.

Overview

The debate over healthcare reform in the United States reached a two-year culmination in the summer of 2009 with the public and politicians sparring off in town hall meetings across the country. Although the majority of Americans agreed that the current US health system was *broken*, the public and stakeholders were divided over the best approach for change. A large group of Americans advocated that healthcare should remain a *market-driven commodity* and believed that the status quo could be tweaked to make the health insurance programs more affordable and responsive to the needs of a burgeoning uninsured and underinsured population estimated at over 70 million. An equally large constituency was ready for a major revamping of our healthcare system, claiming that healthcare services should be universally available to Americans, regardless of socioeconomic status. They generally agreed with President Barack Obama that healthcare reform is a moral imperative, a *human right*.

Americans are concerned about the mounting cost of healthcare in the US, which topped $2.3 trillion in 2008 – close to 18% of the Gross Domestic Product (GDP).[1] To put these figures into perspective and better understand the magnitude of the problem, consider that in 1960, overall expenditures for healthcare in the US amounted to $148 per capita, and 5.2% of the GDP. According to the Centers for Medicare and Medicaid Services (CMS), thirty years later (1990), the expenditures had exploded to $2,813 per capita, which consumed 12.3% of the GDP. Today, the per capita healthcare expenditures are approximating $8,000, and nearly 18% of the GDP (Chart 1).

The consensus of policymakers is that the current trend in escalating healthcare costs is simply not sustainable. The United States Congress was wrestling once again with this controversial issue

---

[1] Gross Domestic Product is a basic measure of a country's overall economic performance within the national boundaries. It is used to express the relative standard of living of a nation. The difference between GDP and the Gross National Product (GNP) is that the later is product produced by enterprises owned by a country's citizens and excludes foreign-owned enterprises. The United States switched from using the GNP to GDP as the primary means of determining production output.

during the remaining term of the 2009 fall session. Perhaps the most important decision to be made at this critical crossroad of US healthcare history is to resolve the century-long argument in a public and democratic fashion: is healthcare a commodity or a right? Once this determination is reached, then policymakers can proceed with the details about *how* to reform the system that will affect the structure of the American healthcare system in the 21st century and beyond.

If the consensus is that healthcare should continue to be a market-driven commodity, then the corporate practice of medicine probably will go the way of *Walmart* and *Nordstrom's* emphasizing a tiered health system for those who can afford to pay for it, with an additional tax-subsidized *safety net* for the least fortunate in our society. If, on the other hand, the general consensus is that healthcare should be a human right, then comprehensive reform will need to augment the existing employer-sponsored market-driven health insurance system with additional publically-sponsored solutions to ensure universal access to a reasonable array of quality health services. This book attempts to analyze and understand the complex dimensions of the healthcare predicament for Americans.

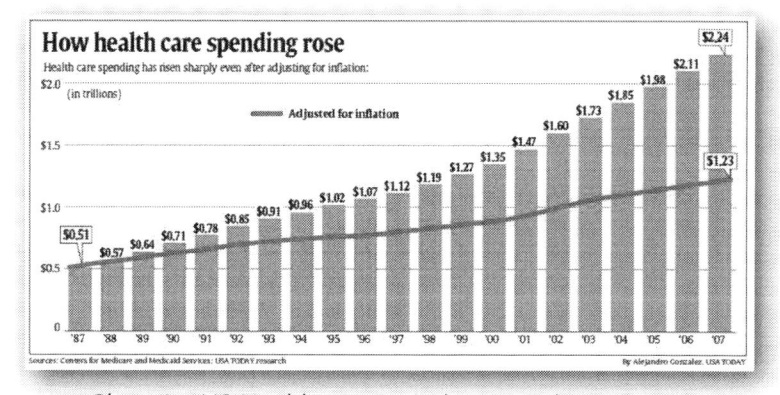

Chart 1 – US Healthcare Spending Trend: 1987-2007
Source: Alejandro Gonzales, USA Today, September 23, 2009, 8E; Centers for Medicare and Medicaid Services.

Numerous research studies reviewed during the course of writing this book point to the conclusion that the healthcare system in the United States *should* be a *limited* right for all Americans because it influences the moral and economic fabric of this nation. It should be limited because it is not possible for the national economy, measured by the GDP, to support unlimited consumption of health resources (defined primarily as sick care services) for all citizens. Development of a reformed healthcare system should be based on *rational* criteria in order to fairly allocate basic healthcare services that result in a process of *distributive justice* (Daniels, 2008).

The general findings imply that healthcare (a critical vehicle for promoting community health and wellbeing) does not bode well with the concept of a true market-based commodity. The system is focused on treating sickness rather than promoting wellness – America is in the sick care business. By insuring that basic *healthcare* services (primary care, prevention, and wellness education) are accessible to all members of society through national legislation, it would be possible to improve health and wellbeing and reduce the amount of sickness, pain, and suffering, including the most disadvantaged persons in our society in the long run.

Policymakers must be willing to move beyond the traditional "sick care" model and substantially commit to a *prevention and wellness model* that enhances the overall wellbeing of Americans. In order to substantially improve health status, we must commit an estimated 30% of all healthcare dollars to prevention and wellness services and initiatives. The challenge for Americans is to design a fair and affordable healthcare system that offers a reasonable array of basic services to meet health improvement goals for our nation without simultaneously bankrupting the country. The evidence discussed in this book suggests that the current dependency on the sick care model will *guarantee* that Americans will not be able to enjoy a viable healthcare system beyond the next twenty-year horizon.

Admittedly, there is no national healthcare model in today's world that offers the *best* example of an affordable array of healthcare services that promotes a *healthier* community (healthier, since *complete health* is an unattainable state). Several international examples have demonstrated what might work and what might not, in their particular circumstances. The question is how to adapt successful foreign models to the US healthcare philosophy and public expectations. As far as the United States is concerned, an innovative and bold plan was developed in Oregon about twenty years ago that applied a rational allocation methodology to healthcare services for Medicaid recipients in that state. Although it too has shortcomings, the Oregon Health Plan (OHP) is the only longstanding model in this country that attempts to balance *evidenced-based* medicine with an emphasis on wellbeing rather than simply funding sick care.

In June 2009, Oregon's Governor Ted Kulongoski signed legislation to expand the OHP beyond the Medicaid population to include all government employees and their families. The Essential Benefit Package (EBP) "emphasizes evidence-based care in the integrated health home" in such a manner that enrollees have little or no cost sharing for outpatient visits for certain chronic diseases and preventive services (Oregon Health Fund, 2009, June 20).

A reformed healthcare system in the United States must integrate multi-generational and multicultural solutions without infringing on the basic democratic beliefs that prevail in America. There is no single solution for the healthcare crisis, only multiple approaches based on a sound theoretical and practical framework. Before major structural changes are legislated by the US Congress, it is imperative to reach a political and public consensus about the *moral* and *ethical* dimensions of our healthcare system. A clear consensus must be reached by the American people about the morality of basic healthcare -- should it be a limited human right for all? Only then can a just healthcare system be implemented. Our national goal should be to promote a healthier society since it is the best way to foster personal and societal *happiness,* which forms the basis of our humanity (Mill, 1992 and 2005). Unfortunately, time is running out to implement a workable solution.

Why is it so difficult for Americans to embrace the concept of universal healthcare? One explanation is that Americans have a strong tendency to emphasize *individualism* rather than social solidarity. Brannigan and Boss (2001) termed this stance as the *individualist paradigm*. Other cultures that have adopted universal healthcare as part of their moral fabric have developed policies and government-run programs that ensure access to basic health services because they support the concept of *social solidarity* and *equity* for allocating finite health resources. In the United States, however, private healthcare coverage remains tethered to employer-sponsored plans and profit-oriented health insurance companies.

The philosophical justification for considering the US healthcare system a *foundational* element of American society is predicated on the conviction that (1) positive health status enhances overall human potentiality, which in turn (2) maximizes individuals' access to a fair *life-plan opportunity realization* suggested by Norman Daniels (1985) in *Just Health*. In essence, a *healthier* nation enables its citizens to achieve increasing social and economic progress that is the result of a rational methodology for promoting and restoring normal individual functioning relative to one's circumstances along the continuum of life (Fisk, 2000). This process of attaining maximum wellbeing should also entail a balanced public and personal *obligation* relating to the *human right* to healthcare. With every right (natural, moral / ethical, contractual, and legislative) there are associated individual and communal responsibilities (Baumrin, 2002). Therefore, *a fair healthcare system demands that the recipients of communal benefits contribute back to the welfare of society – not just take the entitlement for their personal benefit.*

This special consideration for classifying *basic* healthcare services as a limited *human right* of society, in conjunction with other key elements such as basic education, general safety, food and shelter, relates to our general beliefs about the value of human life. Americans value life and have a deep sense of compassion for those suffering and in need of care. Healthcare plays a crucial role in helping individuals to achieve their unique potentiality and opportunities in life (Daniels, 1985 and 2008).

Perhaps one of the most cost-effective and ethical approaches for rectifying the current shortcomings of the US healthcare system entails greater emphasis on universal access to affordable and basic primary care as well as preventive, public health and wellness services (defined here as true *healthcare*) in order to promote a healthier society. This in turn would help restrain the exponential growth in the national debt attributable to a disproportionate investment in the utilization of acute and ambulatory care services (defined here as traditional *sick care*). A workable healthcare solution should commit to an *outcomes-oriented* process with serious economic incentives that discourage wasteful and unnecessary consumption of limited healthcare resources in order to constrain present and future substantial investments.

My suggestion is that for every dollar spent on sick care in the US, participating healthcare providers -- the full range of organizations and health professionals -- should reinvest at least 30% of net revenues on *demonstrable* health maintenance and preventive initiatives within the communities they serve. This approach would be an innovative and radical change from our present dependency on sick care services. In this manner, we would move definitively into the healthcare business. Such a strategy could also replace the cumbersome and complex *community benefit* reporting that is required of tax-exempt organizations in order to meet the Internal Revenue Service guidelines for qualifying for income-tax exemptions. Since uncompensated and charity care would almost cease to exist under a universal healthcare model, it would be possible to redirect the current federal, state and local subsidies necessary to offset institutional operating losses (in the form of a higher reimbursement "bonus" payment for improved performance) to increase reimbursement for outcomes-oriented services to healthcare providers. Presently, public and private providers are subjected to continuous reimbursement cuts to offset budgetary shortfalls or to increase profitability of private insurance carriers.

Under this type of a reformed healthcare system, it is reasonable to anticipate that the total national healthcare bill would settle in at about 20% of the GDP within the next eight to ten years, or a budget of around $3.2 trillion annually (as contrasted with the projected $4.3 trillion figure by the federal government, representing a reduction of $1.1 trillion). A serious commitment to *healthcare* (prevention and wellness orientation) through public and private initiatives should yield close to $900 billion annually for primary and preventive care services. This is a far cry from today's miniscule investment in *wellcare* nationwide, amounting to approximately three percent of the national budget (Timmreck, 2003).

The anticipated financial savings resulting from the enactment of an aggressive national healthcare reform policy supporting greater commitment to fund *healthcare* initiatives is depicted in Chart 2 below:

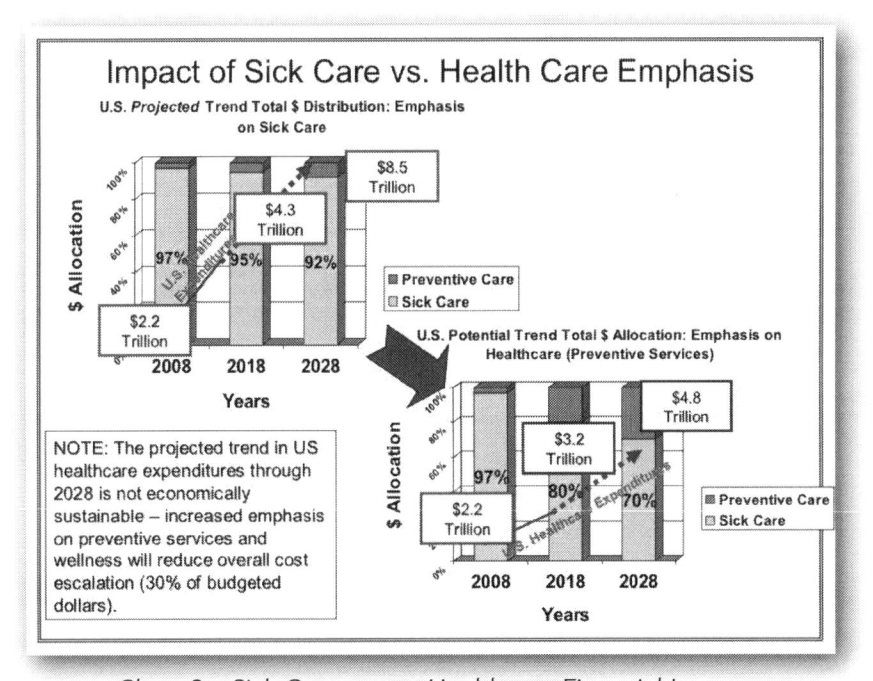

Chart 2 – Sick Care versus Healthcare Financial Impact

A substantial slowdown in the forecasted increase of overall healthcare costs (to about $4.8 trillion by 2028) should be possible based on the information gathered throughout this book. The anticipated figure is almost half of the $8.5 trillion spending trend currently projected by the Congressional Budget Office (CBO) twenty years into the future. These potential savings also take into consideration the increased healthcare utilization by an unprecedented number of older Americans which make up the *age wage* of Baby Boomers reaching age 65 over the next twenty years (Dychtwald & Flower, 1989**).**

The inherent benefits of a *paradigm shift* in healthcare funding and insurance coverage emphasizing *well-care* in the US include (1) creation of a healthier and more productive nation, and (2) lowering of the projected growth in healthcare expenditures and debt for future generations of Americans (Fisk, 2000). Several policy analysts working for Washington, DC healthcare think-tanks have suggested a combined public-private partnership with shared goals aimed at ensuring basic healthcare services for all citizens through a universal healthcare system.

Not everyone is convinced that healthcare should be a human right. A healthcare executive with 42 years of experience in hospital management and health service delivery offered his critique of the position that healthcare in the United States *should* be a limited human right for all.[2] He commented:

> *My belief is that by invoking the 'limited human right' point of view [in your book], you are leaving the philosophical arena and entering the legal arena. At this time, the American system is governed by the Constitution, and our rights as humans and citizens are elucidated in the Bill of Rights. I do not find anywhere in the Constitution a definition of a limited right, nor do I find an explicit or implicit reference to the right to receive healthcare. Secondarily, to create a right under our governing mechanism, it must be passed as an amendment to the Constitution. In this case the proposed right becomes a black and white issue; it is or it is not a right, and it is only limited by definition. One can only wonder if a right that is by its very nature one that rations, if it would be in conflict with the Civil Rights Act of 1964 and equal protection clause.*

These are reasonable criticisms. The US Constitution does not explicitly refer to healthcare as a Constitutional right. However, this book has attempted to develop the philosophical logic of *why* the US healthcare system *should* be considered a limited human right – not that it *is* presently a human right. The preamble to the Constitution does state that its purpose is to "promote the general welfare" of the people of the United States. The dictionary definition of welfare

---

2 WR is a retired healthcare executive who was gracious about reviewing the final draft of my book and provided valuable written comments and suggestions which have been incorporated throughout the text.

is "the state of doing well" (wellbeing), the attainment of health, prosperity, and happiness.[3] Furthermore, all human rights have inherent limitations within the confines of each diverse society in relationship to the abundance of resources available to its citizens. The major problem with the necessity of rationing limited resources is in developing a fair and equitable system that offers basic services to those with the greatest need and the greatest benefit from said services. Norman Daniels argues that *accountability for reasonableness* is the answer to this challenge.

This book seeks to demonstrate *why* healthcare should not be simply regarded as a market-driven commodity as has been the case for decades. The rationale presented herein supports the notion that healthcare should be considered a limited human right. It is predicated on the belief that healthcare is a *foundational* element of any successful society. The right to healthcare should serve as a fair and equitable aspect for achieving an individual's maximum potential while contributing to greater national prosperity. This is the core reason why basic universal healthcare, which cannot encompass *unrestricted* access to all types of sick care services, should be every citizen's right. Careful allocation of limited healthcare resources and an equitable reimbursement approach should be based on measurable health status improvement and quality outcomes (value), *instead of* the traditional market incentives for the volume-driven sick care system. A healthier community maximizes individual opportunities for success, which leads to increased national resources for socioeconomic growth and the ultimate reduction of healthcare inequalities. In summary:

- Healthcare should be considered a *foundational* element of society because all other needs depend on our society's wellbeing.
- Health and healthcare directly contribute to individual and social wellbeing and productivity.
- The current growth trend in healthcare spending on "sick care" rather than *healthcare* in the United States is unsustainable beyond 2016, when the projected annual budget is anticipated to top $4 trillion; systemic change is both an *economic* and *moral imperative*.
- Universal healthcare coverage should afford every citizen *basic* health services to enhance the individual's opportunity for life-plan fulfillment (Daniels, 1985; Daniels and Sabin, 2008).
- The US healthcare system should include a reasonable mechanism for allocating limited resources, involving scientific knowledge which is tempered by community standards and national principles of fairness and justice; the Oregon Health Plan is a valuable model to examine.
- The challenge today is how to effectively rank healthcare needs according to life-rescuing, life-sustaining, life-improving, and prevention. This will require a delicate balance between evidence-based medicine and community determined valuation.

---

[3] The *Merriam-Webster* dictionary.

- Immediate reform of the present employer-sponsored market-driven health insurance system is imperative! A tiered healthcare system including public and private options, or the so-called *Puritan Paradigm*, seems most compatible with America's future needs and belief system (Brannigan and Boss, 2001).
- Universal health insurance coverage, with ample freedom of choice, would ensure that basic health needs are met at the lowest per capita cost. This could also reduce inequities experienced by providers with higher indigent patient populations that cause them to struggle under the burden of uncompensated care.
- Healthcare *should* be a limited human right for all Americans and should offer a basic or core package of health services heavily weighted to prevention and wellness.

Research Approach

The research approach used to develop this book followed a *Qualitative Research Approach* described by Bruce L. Berg (2007, p. 24). The key developmental aspects of this project included:

1. A focus on reviewing the literature encompassing the historical, social, cultural and philosophical dimensions of the United States' healthcare system. It was important to evaluate major theoretical and applied contributions to the field of morality and healthcare ethics by notable scholars such as John Rawls, John Stuart Mill, Norman Daniels, Paul Starr, Clovis Semmes, Anthony R. Kovner, Stuart Altman, Uwe E. Reinhardt, Laurie Garrett, and several others (see list of references and supplemental bibliography attached). A synthesis of the collective knowledge base from an *interdisciplinary* perspective has shed a "bright light" on the topic of fairness and equity regarding delivery models of healthcare services in the United States as we progress into the 21st century. Major reform should result in the continuation of a first rate and financially viable health system in the United States that is universally accessible to Americans, regardless of economic status.
2. Most of the research material consulted for this book was gathered from university libraries, public libraries, Internet resources, and commercial sources. Limited structured interviews with healthcare leaders were also conducted during the research process.
3. Scholarly materials and reliable governmental resources were used in order to construct a realistic picture of the past and present state of healthcare in the United States. An interdisciplinary analytical approach of the foundational elements of healthcare helped discern the key issues and problems that exist with our system and postulate a theoretical and practical framework for guiding legislators in their deliberations about feasible solutions for the future of . . . healthcare in the US The timing of this investigation perfectly matched the growing momentum for healthcare reform that is culminating in historical legislation in Congress at this time.

Goals

This book explores the important and timely topic of the necessity for implementing radical reform of the United States healthcare system. It discusses alternative ways that this nation's consumers, regulators, providers, and payers can regard our essential healthcare resources. The overarching conclusions outlined in this book are that (1) healthcare is a foundational[4] element of the socioeconomic fabric of the US, and (2) it should not be regarded as a *commodity* to be traded according to ordinary economic considerations. Finally, it examines the basic philosophical reasons why healthcare should be considered a limited *human right* for all, according to the principles of distributive justice.

In order to substantiate the argument that healthcare in the United States should be a limited human right for all, the work from numerous philosophers, scientists, healthcare providers, and others devoted to the field of health and human rights have been studied. Collectively, these works served as guideposts for the philosophical, social, and economic considerations in support of the notion that the future healthcare system in the US should be a limited human right, as well as a moral commitment by society.

I have theorized that the underlying focus of healthcare reform in 2009 and beyond should be based on the premise that healthcare should be regarded as a *limited* human right, and that it should be recognized as a foundational[5] element of our social and political infrastructure. This infrastructure is necessary to enable *progressive* changes in the current health system in the United States (Altman, Stuart & Reinhardt, 1998). A national policy enacting meaningful healthcare reform and treating healthcare as a limited human right will be a major *paradigm shift* (Kuhn, 1996) in how future health services could be provided to the poor, middle class, and wealthy Americans. If our society accepts the foundational premise that healthcare is a limited human right, then US policymakers should address the problems faced by the healthcare system much differently than a market-based commodity where price and profit dominate "purchase and access" considerations (Daschle, 2008). Such a paradigm shift in how Americans view healthcare could result in a more equitable and viable model for universal healthcare for future generations in the United States.

---

4 The *Merriam-Webster* dictionary cites various meanings for the word *foundational*. In this thesis, the usage relates to the following context: "A basis (as a tenet, principle, or axiom) upon which something stands or is supported." Furthermore, *foundationalism* is any theory of justification (epistemology) that beliefs are justified based on what are referred to as *basic beliefs*, or foundational beliefs, that give justificatory support to other beliefs, but are not justified by other beliefs. Essentially a basic belief does not require justification because it is a different kind of belief than a non-foundational one (see also *Stanford Encyclopedia of Philosophy*).

5 The assumption herein is that healthcare services should be provided on the basis of a solid foundation of moral and ethical values that shape the development and implementation of the United States system as presented by Howard Brody in his essay "Ethics, Justice, and Health Reform," in the collection edited by Engstrom and Robison (2008), pp. 40-57. In this sense, I have used the term *foundational* to refer to healthcare as a self-evident human right for all throughout this book.

This book suggests that there is a rationale for limiting universal healthcare services and examines the ethical implication of developing a "minimum healthcare threshold," or package of "basic health services" available to all Americans. Due to space limitations and the complexity of these specific topics, this text has not addressed three important aspects of the healthcare delivery challenge: (1) the impact of illegal immigrants in the US, which is a sizeable portion of the uninsured and underinsured patient population; (2) the effects of healthcare malpractice reform initiatives; and (3) the positive implications of recent legislation mandating health insurance portability for employees who switch jobs. This analysis, has attempted to demonstrate *why and how* greater investment in prevention, primary care, and wellness services will ultimately result in a substantial reduction in the growth curve of sick care in the United States in the long term.[6] This book has four parts:

Part 1 – Background (Chapters 1-3)
Part 2 – Problem Statement (Chapters 4-9)
Part 3 – Foundational Elements of Healthcare (Chapters 10-11)
Part 4 – Critical Findings, Conclusions, and Epilogue (Chapters 12-14)

> *Vienna, VA. "When a dozen consumers gathered over the weekend to discuss health care at the behest of President-elect Barack Obama, they quickly agreed on one point: they despise health insurance companies. They also agreed that health care was a right; that insurance should cover 'everything,' not just some services; and that coverage should be readily available from the government, as well as from employers."*
>
> ROBERT PEAR, DECEMBER 23, 2008, THE NEW YORK TIMES.

---

[6] The United States spent an estimated $2.2 trillion on healthcare in 2008 according to the National Coalition on Health Care, and the group projects that the figure could reach $4 trillion by 2015, or 20% of the nation's Gross Domestic Product.

Part 1
Background

One

HISTORICAL PERSPECTIVE

1.1 -- US Health System during the 1900s to 1990s

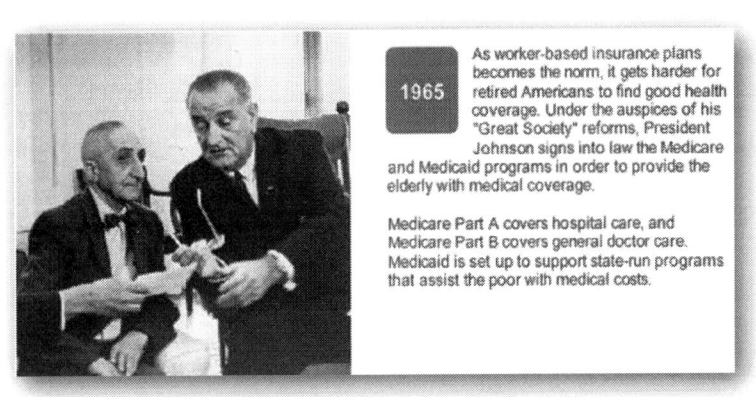

Figure 1 – The Johnson Era
Source: CNN.com Health Timeline.

An understanding of the general evolution of modern medicine in America is helpful to address the current dilemma we find ourselves in with regards to the unabated rise in the number of uninsured and underinsured individuals in the United States. While the traditional *sick care* system presently consumes approximately $2.3 trillion, minimal dollars are allocated for preventive and public health measures that have proven effective in reducing acute maladies and chronic diseases. With the projected percentage of seniors in America reaching over 20% by the year 2020 (presently around 13%), the dramatic growth of chronic illness, cardiovascular disease, and cancer will bring the current health system to its knees because of the economic burden resulting from unabated utilization of limited resources. There are two interrelated components to the healthcare delivery system: (1) curative and rehabilitative, and (2) primary and preventive care. A brief historical summary is presented below.

Paul Starr's *The Social Transformation of American Medicine* (1982) depicts the early grip that medical professionals maintained over the healthcare field and healing arts profession since the emergence of modern medicine in the 1760s (p. 30). Starr's book describes how physicians ascended to their current level of social and economic status as well as key factors that transformed the American healthcare delivery system into a multi-billion-dollar industry.

According to Starr, the authority vested in the medical profession was derived from three central characteristics: (1) specialized training and competency in medical care validated by peer review, (2) knowledge based on rational and scientific grounding, and (3) practice of a *valued social* discipline involving personal health and general wellbeing (p. 15). State and federal regulatory licensing requirements for physicians reinforced their authority to direct the care of patients, including the unique privilege of admitting patients to healthcare facilities and the power to *order* specific tests and treatments administered by technical staff and caregivers employed by hospitals and other medical institutions. This level of control granted to physicians makes them essential to the economic engine of hospitals and other healthcare facilities. In most cases, physicians have enjoyed wealth and higher social status as a result of the authority vested in the medical profession and its inherent control over the healthcare marketplace (pp. 18-29).

During the 1970s, the large-scale economics of modern medicine and rapid expansion of technology shifted the balance of traditional authority and power away from individual physicians, and into the hands of corporate managers of the health delivery systems. This was particularly true for health insurance companies who had access to vast amounts of capital and resources necessary to influence the success of large organizations (pp. 235-390). The escalating cost of medical care encouraged the development of the private health insurance industry, which further eroded the control physicians exercised over the health system. Eventually, the public and politicians demanded widespread accessibility to medical care, which also "meant that cost control had to be built into the medical system" (p. 393).

The complexity of medical care and increasing demand for health services by an aging society has forced government officials and politicians to find new ways to curtail the cost of healthcare through payment reform and tighter eligibility criteria for government-subsidized programs, including Medicaid and Medicare. Private insurance companies followed suit because of cost-shifting by providers to non-governmental payers. The growth of the *corporate practice of medicine* and inclination toward universal health insurance seems inevitable to Starr (pp. 420-430). Starr finishes his epic book with his views about the role of physicians in shaping the corporate, economic and political forces that impact today's healthcare delivery system. Considering the early timeframe in which Paul Starr wrote his book – back in 1982 – it is amazing that the contemporary trends are validating his most popular prediction: "Pressure for efficient, business-like management of health care has also contributed to the collapse of the barriers that traditionally prevented corporate control of health services" (p.428). Starr's vision was that America would have to undergo profound changes in the structure and culture of the practice of medicine, and that a "two-class system in medical care [was] likely to become only more conspicuous" as resources became scarcer, and the ranks of the uninsured population continued to swell (p. 448).

Laurie Garrett's (2000) classic chronicles of the evolution of the profession of public health in America and abroad, *Betrayal of Trust: The Collapse of Global Public Health*, also offers enlightening information about the perception of preventive health services. She describes how the welfare of mankind, more than ever, was at the mercy of an efficient public health infrastructure. Garrett cautions that our commitment to a basic public health infrastructure was poor at best, until the population is struck by an unpredicted and uninvited epidemic or disaster. Then suddenly there is a major (temporary) surge in funding to address the problem (pp. 1-14). Garrett states:

> The challenges of public health have never been greater, either in counties like Los Angeles, prosperous states such as Minnesota, or former superpowers like the Russian Federation. Each is now linked to the other. (p.13)

Essentially, the discipline of *public health* is concerned with maintaining the overall wellbeing of the community-at-large. It is concerned with the masses, and much less with an individual's acute medical ailments and debilities (curative medicine). *Curative medicine*, on the other hand, is focused on treating episodic illnesses and ameliorating physical limitations of individuals. As an example, Garrett's account of the haphazard evolution of public health services in the US graphically illustrates the serious public health problems of the 1980s and 1990s resulting from the indiscriminant usage of antibiotics by medical professionals used to combat hospital-acquired microbial infections throughout America.

The Institute of Medicine (IOM) issued a detailed report in 1998 concerning the catastrophic resistance to antibiotics in the US, declaring that both the scope and pace of resistance at which microbes were adapting and mutating was accelerating at an alarming rate. Nine out of ten staph infections in 1998 involved bacteria that were completely resistant to penicillin and related compounds. Just forty years earlier, staph infections were easily curable with moderate doses of inexpensive penicillin-class drugs (p. 488). To this date, Illinois is the only state in America that has adopted legislation to proactively fight public dangers of drug-resistant staph infections. On August 20, 2007, Governor Rod Blagojevich signed a healthcare bill into law requiring all hospitals in Illinois to test patients in the intensive-care units for methicillin-resistant staphylococcus aureus (MRSA) infections, and to isolate patients with this acquired bacteria to prevent infecting patients. Imagine, people getting sicker *because* of hospital care.

In addition to public health problems associated with communicable diseases, consider the health ramifications of disasters resulting from changing global weather conditions – hurricanes, landslides, floods, and droughts -- that cause massive destruction and leave an aftermath of disruption to housing, sanitation services, water purification, electricity, etc. that cause pestilence and diseases in affected citizens (for example, hurricane *Katrina* and New Orleans). Man-made bio-terrorism is perhaps the ultimate threat to mankind, with unimaginable consequences to vast populations in a relatively short period of time – anthrax, botulinum, smallpox and other deadly viruses – these are the ultimate weapons of mass destruction (WMD) that only strong public health measures can effectively control (pp. 502-508).

With so many vivid examples of recent public health failures depicted by Garrett in *Betrayal of Trust*, it is difficult to comprehend why the US public health infrastructure is so poorly supported at the local, state, and federal levels. Most all known common illnesses, diseases, and major injuries are preventable and manageable through strong public health initiatives. Yet Americans persist in pouring trillions of dollars into the traditional sick care system (curative medicine), and devote very limited resources to strengthening public health initiatives (preventive and wellness services) that have a proven track record of improving the human condition world-wide.

1.2 -- Clinton Healthcare Era

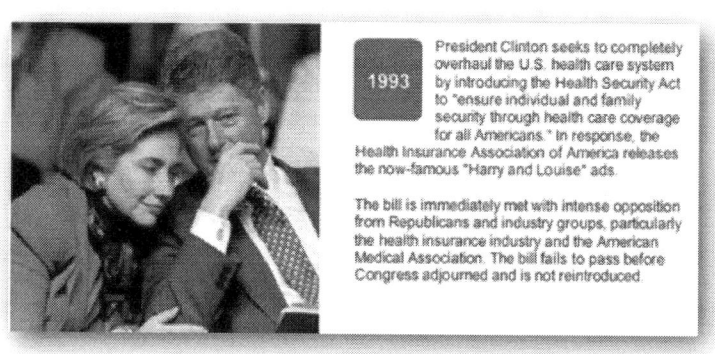

Figure 2- The Clinton Era
Source: CNN.com Health Timeline.

The topic of healthcare reform in the United States is not new to politicians, government officials, or policymakers. This controversial topic has been smoldering for decades. During Bill Clinton's presidential era in the early 1990s, there were several major initiatives in Congress aimed at radically transforming the American healthcare system; however, as in the past Administrations, the process came to a halt due to opposition from special interest groups (mostly healthcare providers and insurance companies). It was not until the 2008 Presidential campaign of Barack Obama that healthcare once again emerged as a top issue to change the basic structure of the system. Obama did not waiver from his campaign promise to make healthcare reform one of the highest priorities of his new presidential Administration. In fact, during the transition period after the election in December 2008, the president-elect gathered nearly 30,000 people from across the nation to meet in ad hoc community forums and develop *their* vision of a reformed healthcare system in the US, encouraging group facilitators to share the comments and recommendations with officials in the new Obama Administration.

I facilitated a community group discussion involving healthcare co-workers from a healthcare corporation headquartered in Houston Texas (see Exhibit A – General Staff Discussion on Healthcare Reform).[7] A summary of the group's comments and conclusions was submitted to the healthcare Presidential Transition Team headed by Secretary-designate of the United States Department of Health and Human Services (HHS) and Former Senator Tom Daschle, along with 3,276 other Health Care Community Discussion groups reporting in January 2009.[8]

HHS published a special report covering these grass roots sessions: *Americans Speak on Health Reform: Report on Health Care Community Discussions*, on March 5, 2009.[9] Daschle (2008) co-authored a book entitled *Critical: What We Can Do about the Health-Care Crisis* along with Scott Greenberger and Jeanne Lambrew, which presents a detailed account of the challenges that healthcare reform faced in the United States Congress during its 60-year history. They offer their own *prescription* for change. According to Daschle et al. (pp. 3-28), the healthcare crisis in the United States was being fueled by a combination of four main forces: (1) the present highest number of uninsured and underinsured Americans in this country's history (50 million, or 17% of the total population), (2) persistent run-away healthcare inflation consuming 16% of the nation's GDP, (3) runaway rising premiums for market-driven private health insurance paid by individual policy holders and small businesses that have little or no negotiating leverage, and (4) declining health insurance coverage by larger employers due to high medical expenses that are taking a large portion of company profit margins.

The authors noted that "the federal government's patchwork of health-care programs is just as irrational as the private 'system'" (p. 29). They urged immediate change from the traditional insurance industry-controlled system that rewards high utilization rather than the quality of patient care outcomes. Daschle et al. advocated the creation of a Health Board similar to the Federal Reserve Board to oversee the implementation of healthcare reform. The Health Board would develop a framework that establishes *evidence-based* medical care standards:

---

[7] A total of 14 Nexus Health Systems employees participated in a two-hour discussion session and addressed topics listed in the discussion guide provided by the Presidential Transition Team (see the attached Exhibit A).
[8] Former Senator Tom Daschle withdrew his nomination for Secretary of HHS on February 3, 2009 in the midst of Congressional confirmation hearings due to personal taxation issues.
[9] HHS Press Office, News Release, Thursday, March 5, 2009; the full report is available for public review on the new Web Site, http://www.healthreform.gov.

A Federal Health Board would have both political and practical benefits. It would help us break the legislative logjam that has blocked previous attempts at comprehensive reform, and it would establish a strong public framework for a high-performing, private health system. (p. 142)

The American public generally seemed to agree with Daschle and his colleagues that radical reform is necessary. Graph 1 presents the priorities listed in the 2009 HHS special report of the healthcare community discussion groups:

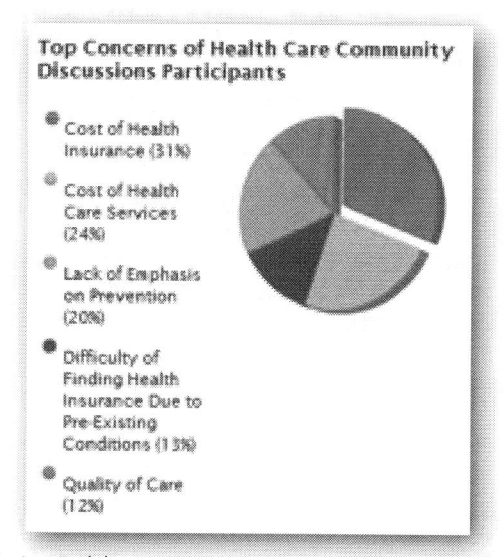

Top Concerns of Health Care Community Discussions Participants
- Cost of Health Insurance (31%)
- Cost of Health Care Services (24%)
- Lack of Emphasis on Prevention (20%)
- Difficulty of Finding Health Insurance Due to Pre-Existing Conditions (13%)
- Quality of Care (12%)

Graph 1 – Public Concerns about Healthcare in the US

In his address to 150 stakeholders from diverse sectors of the healthcare provider community during the White House Forum on Health Reform held in Washington, DC on March 6, 2009,[10] President Obama vowed to sign into law a major reform bill that would create a more equitable and cost-effective health system in America before the end of 2009. President Obama stated to the assembly:

A clear consensus that the need for health care reform is here and now…If there is a way of getting this done [healthcare reform], where we're driving down costs and people are getting health insurance at an affordable rate and have choice of doctor, have flexibility in terms of their plans, and we could do that entirely through the market, I'd be happy to do it that way. If there was a way of doing it that involved more government regulation

---

[10] For a list of invited participants, see http://www.whitehouse.gov/the_press_office/White-House-Forum-on-Health-Reform-Attendees, Office of the White House Press Secretary, March 5, 2009.

and involvement, I'm happy to do it that way as well. I just want to figure out what works. But that requires US to actually look at the evidence and try to figure out, based on the experience that now has been accumulated for a lot of years, you know, how we can improve the system...There is a moral imperative to health care. I get 40,000 letters, I guess, every day here in the White House...I can tell you that on average, out of the ten (the President's staff selects for him to read) at least three every single day relate to somebody who's having a health care crisis.[11]

The President went on to clarify the principles of his belief on why it was essential for Congress to balance *moral obligation* with fiscal responsibility.

[*Also see graphs contained in* Centers for Medicare & Medicaid Services (CMS); and the Kaiser Foundation; and the Health Research and Educational Trust.][12]

Today's prevalent rhetoric about healthcare reform is focused primarily on controlling costs of health services and its economic impact on national stability. A distant secondary concern pertains to the fundamental human inequities of access to health services by socially and economically disadvantaged population groups. Finally, there is a genuine concern over quality of care and outcomes, but this area is extremely complex given the difficulty in measuring results of widespread initiatives. The real foundational elements as to *why* the United States healthcare system *should* treat the healthcare system as a limited human right for all citizens has received little or no attention in Congress. We will elaborate on the crucial issues dealing with healthcare fairness and distributive justice more fully in Part 3 of this book.

Starting with the basic premise that healthcare is an essential element for creating a healthier and more productive society, it should be possible to redesign the US healthcare system in such a fashion that it provides a minimum *threshold* level of care regardless of socio-economic status, within fiscal constraints of our nation's capabilities. In other words, economic concerns should *not* necessarily be the driving force behind healthcare reform; it should be governed by an improved delivery system that offers a reasonable array of basic health services that facilitate health maintenance as well as an appropriate measure of sick care for those who suffer from congenital, acute and chronic illnesses. Perhaps the crux of present-day healthcare reform discussions should answer these three questions: (1) what are the foundational issues that policymakers should be concerned with and, whom should the reformed healthcare system benefit? (2) which delivery forms and payment systems are best designed to insure equitable and affordable distribution of health resources? and (3) how will government officials and leaders of

---

11 The full transcript of the closing remarks by President Obama at the White House Forum on Health Reform is available on the Web; see http://www.whitehouse.gov/the_press_office/Closing-Remarks-by-the-President-at-White-House-Forum-on-Health-Reform, Office of the White House Press Secretary, March 5, 2009.
12 Laura Mecker, *The Wall Street Journal,* March 6, 2009, page A4; and Richard Wolf, *USA Today,* Friday, March 6, 2009, page 4A.

the private sector effectively implement reform plans and initiatives in a cost-sensitive manner? From this perspective, financial viability should be the by-product of a well-engineered healthcare reform process.

Two

Current State of Healthcare System

2.1 -- Market-Based Healthcare

A few important national health statistics derived from reliable governmental and private sources[13] help substantiate the staggering impact that the healthcare system has had on the United States:

1. The estimated healthcare tab for 2008 totaled $2.3 trillion.
2. Healthcare expenditures per person topped $7,800 in 2008.
3. In 2008, the United States had nearly 46 million uninsured and another estimated 30 million underinsured citizens (these figures exclude hundreds of thousands of illegal immigrants who seek care in the United States every year).
4. Healthcare spending has increased an average of 6.8% annually since 2000, while inflation was half that figure.
5. There were 969,000 hospital beds at 5,708 hospitals in the US in 2008.
6. There were 673,596 hospital discharges in 2006 for patients with heart failure-related diagnosis (DRG 127) alone in the US
7. Invasive cardiologists had an average income of $456,901, while primary care family physicians averaged $175,918 per year (38% of the invasive cardiologist rate) in 2007.
8. Financial investment in preventive services was minimal in relation to the substantial dollars supporting the sick-care system – approximately 3% of the total national expenditures.
9. Healthcare presently consumes approximately 18% of the GDP.

---

13 US Department of Health and Human Services; Espicom Business Intelligence, Medical Markets Fact Book 2007; US Census Bureau; US Department of Commerce and Department of Labor; Thomson Reuters; Medical Group Management Association (MGMA); American Hospital Association.

The unfortunate reality is that Americans paid way more for healthcare than any other industrialized nation on earth, yet they enjoyed *fair* overall health status (as measured by life expectancy, infant mortality and morbidity rates) compared with Japan, France and Canada, each with a per capita health spending close to ¼ of the rate in the US

With the impending influx of Baby Boomers turning 65 years of age during the next 15 years, the number of seniors will double in the US, driving up healthcare utilization to an unprecedented level. Seniors consume an average of three times more health resources than the under-65 populations – the projected healthcare utilization in the next 20 years is simply *not* sustainable from an economic standpoint. Graph 3 compares the US spending rate on healthcare with 5 other developed nations on the basis of purchasing power parity and GDP. The United States is way off the charts.

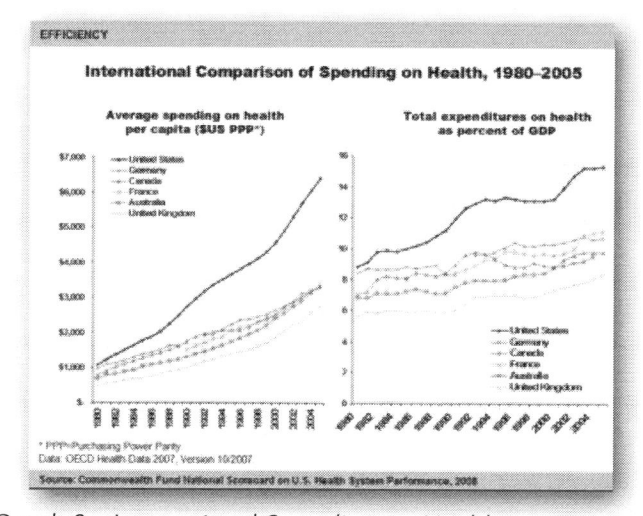

Graph 2 – International Spending on Healthcare Services

To overcome strong resistance to healthcare reform by powerful special interest provider groups, it will be necessary for policymakers to hold steadfast to a new paradigm for our financially driven sick-care system in the United States. In the words of former Senate Majority Leader Tom Daschle:

We shouldn't shy away from making the moral argument for change. It is simply unconscionable that in a nation as wealthy and powerful as ours, citizens are forced to go without medical care that could relieve their suffering and extend their lives. (Daschle, 2008, p. 197)

A national policy defining healthcare as a limited human right could reshape the delivery system into a more humane, accessible, and cost-effective resource for all Americans. This approach should also transform the US healthcare system into a national resource instead of a market-driven commodity.

2.2 -- Competition, Duplication of Services, and Spiraling Costs

The US healthcare system evolved into one of the largest business enterprises in this country over the past 60 years. The hallmark of entrepreneurial success for the healthcare industry has been aggressive competition among providers seeking to garner a larger share of the patient care market. In many instances, it has been a matter of *do or die*. Providers have had to offer comprehensive and state-of-the-art services that represent the most advanced care in the world. Our magnificent medical centers are both the most sophisticated and most expensive among developed nations. The downside of the US healthcare "arms race" is that it has created vast duplication of services and wasted resources. The McKinsey Global Institute estimated that excessive spending in the US has resulted in the following notable statistics (reported in *Medical Economics*, January 23, 2009):

- $650 billion → the amount overspent by the United States on healthcare in 2006 compared to other industrialized nations.
- $436 billion → wasted costs on outpatient care in the US
- $98 billion → wasted costs on drugs in the US
- $91 billion → wasted costs on health administration and insurance in the US

Compared to other countries, the United States out-spends others by at least a factor of 3 to 1 on the basis of per capita healthcare costs, according to figures released by the US Office on Economic Development. The largest share of increased cost has been attributed to health insurance administrative overhead rather than actual delivery of health services, as shown in Graphs 4 and 5.

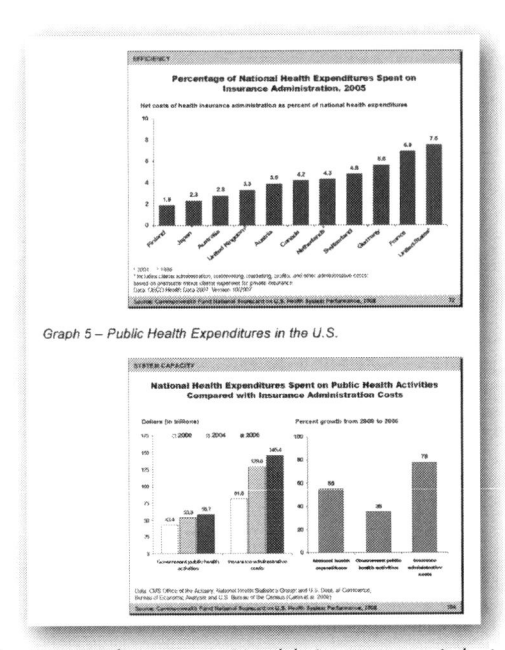

Graph 5 – Public Health Expenditures in the U.S.

Graph 3 – Expenditures on Health Insurance Administration

How has this dramatic increase in healthcare spending in the United States since 1990 contributed to overall improvement (or lack thereof) in the quality of care, cost-effectiveness, and health status of Americans? The US health system's performance in a variety of important areas was analyzed in 2008 by *The Commonwealth Fund*, and selected summary charts from their report are presented below accompanied by brief commentary.

1. *The Commonwealth Fund* used a customized scoring methodology to determine what major considerations constituted a high performance health system in America. With few exceptions, several key indicators of health status declined during the period from 2006 to 2008, with an overall score reduction of 2 points.
2. During the two-year period in the late 1990s and early 2000s, all industrialized countries showed major improvement in the crude death rate for persons under age 75 years (age-standardized death rate per 100,000 population). The United States experienced the smallest gain compared to the other nations: from 115 in 1997 to 1998 to 110 in 2002 to 2003.
3. One of the main indicators of health status of a population is the infant mortality rate (infant deaths per 1,000 live births). Although the US infant death rate dropped gradually between 1998 to 2004, our nation's infant mortality average rate (6.8 / 1,000 live births) was nearly 2.5 times greater than Japan's (2.8 / 1,000 live births), and 1.5 / 1,000 worse than Canada's (5.3 / 1,000 live births). The range between the 10 bottom and top states in the US had a rate spread from 10.1 and 4.7, respectively.
4. Concerning preventive health services, the national percentage of adults who received adequate care remained virtually unchanged between 2004 and 2005, at an average of only half the population. The fact that uninsured and underinsured Americans were worse off than the population as a whole was not a surprise to researchers.
5. Closely related to key indicators of preventive health services was the percentage of adults (19 to 64 years old) that accessed primary care providers between 2002 and 2005 – approximately two-thirds of the US population. The disparity was largest among Hispanic minorities and Whites as well as uninsured and underinsured individuals.
6. Disadvantaged children also were least likely to have a "medical home" providing coordinated primary and preventive care in a *culturally sensitive environment*. The American Pediatric Association has strongly advocated the creation of the "medical home" concept to enhance the overall quality of care for children in the United States.[14] While the average number of children with a medical home was 46% in 2003, the rate for uninsured dropped to a low of only 23%. Hispanic children were also less likely to have a medical home – 30% compared to 53% of White children.

---

14 See details at http://www.medicalhomeinfo.org/

Why The United States Healthcare System Should Be A Limited Human Right For All

7. While the US has the most expensive health system in the world, access to physicians as determined by the ability of sicker patients to schedule appointments the same or the next day, was not appreciably better than our Canadian neighbors (with an established national health system). The average percentage of Americans in 2007 that were able to see a physician within 48 hours was 47%, compared to over 60% in New Zealand, the Netherlands, and Germany.

    Another serious problem affecting coordination of care among treating physicians is the lack of electronic medical records systems. Limited access to patient records and historical information tends to contribute to duplication of tests and procedures, inappropriate prescription of medications, contradictory treatment plans, delayed or harmful care, and billing errors – all these factors drive up healthcare costs to consumers and payers, as depicted in Graphs 12 A below. American physicians have been slow to adopt electronic medical records systems that could improve patient management appreciably.

8. *The Commonwealth Fund Biennial Health Insurance Survey* in 2003 and 2007 indicated that the number of adults ages 19 to 64 who were uninsured or underinsured climbed from 35% to 42%; in 2007, the ratio of uninsured to underinsured persons amounted to 28% and 14%, respectively. Underinsured persons were covered by health insurance plans during the year; however, they experienced medical expenses totaling more than 10% or out-of-pocket healthcare costs of five percent or more of their annual income.

    The main reason given for not accessing healthcare services was the result of high costs, as shown in Graphs 13 A, B, and C below, which is far more common than the other developed nations compared with the US, according to results of *The Commonwealth Fund's International Health Policy Survey* (2003 and 2007).

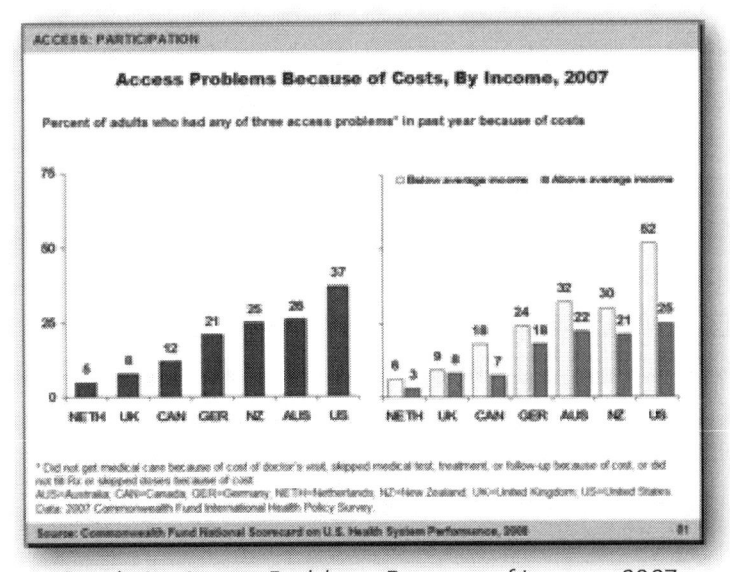

Graph 4 – Access Problems Because of Income: 2007

9. The unintended consequence of inadequate insurance coverage for many citizens in the United States has resulted in terribly congested emergency departments (ED) in hospitals throughout this country. Using the ED instead of the primary care provider's office is very inefficient and costly – ED utilization for non-emergent care in the United States is nearly three times the rate in Germany, the Netherlands, and New Zealand.

Three

The Perfect Healthcare Storm

3.1 -- Political Climate and Rhetoric

Mounting discontent among politicians over healthcare in the US is being blamed on two issues: (1) the runaway cost of Medicare and Medicaid expenditures, and (2) increasing numbers of uninsured and underinsured Americans. According to the CMS projections prepared by Chief Actuary Richard Foster, Medicare's hospital insurance trust fund expenditures are expected to exceed its income from taxes starting in 2011 (DoBias, 2007). The gap between income and spending is widening rapidly because fewer workers are contributing to the government's health security system (Medicare), as compared to the number of seniors who are consuming more health resources as their life expectancy is being extended and the Baby Boom generation reaches age 65, starting in 2015.

Concurrently, the number of uninsured and underinsured Americans under age 65 reached close to 70 million in 2006. The *Kaiser Commission on Medicaid and the Uninsured* found that most of the uninsured were part of working families with the following profile:

- One full-time-worker → 55.7%
- At least two full-time workers → 13.6%
- At least one part-time worker → 12.1%
- No workers → 18.6%

The American Hospital Association (AHA) recently unveiled its recommendations for healthcare reform, which includes five goals: (1) a focus on wellness, (2) efficient and affordable care, (3) highest-quality care, (4) information-based patient management, and (5) health coverage for all, paid by all (AHA, 2007). The AHA advocates equal access for all Americans to quality healthcare services – a *social right* rather than privilege for those that can afford to purchase health insurance.

A Web-poll conducted by *Medical Economics* tested the waters with its physician members regarding acceptance of a *single-payer* health insurance program, controlled by the Federal government, and found the following sentiments:

Question -- Would the US be better off with a single-payer, government-run healthcare insurer? (*Medical Economics*, 2007)

- 20% indicated yes, that they would be paid more consistently.
- 35% said yes, insurance companies are making too much profit.
- 18% said no, it would create too much of a monopoly.
- 27% indicated they were opposed, because it would decrease the quality of service.

This physician poll found that the majority of practitioners (55%) supported a government-sponsored, single-payer insurance system -- a radical change from survey findings gleamed from a prior years' survey. The Web Poll included voluntary respondents and might not necessarily comprise a statistically measurable sampling. Nevertheless, these results represent a surprising and significant shift in physician opinions.

The issue of healthcare reform became a central platform during the 2008 presidential election campaign. "Health care is second only to the war in Iraq among voters concerns, so everyone with an eye on the White House wants a winning answer," wrote *The Economist* (2007). Judge Richard Posner expressed his doubts that any of the candidates' proposals would actually deal effectively with the healthcare crisis facing the nation. He argued that the only way to control escalating healthcare costs is to ration services or force down the price of individual units of care. Judge Posner cautioned that "we should be wary of proposals that, if adopted, would not reduce aggregate costs, but instead would shift the costs to another class of payees, such as taxpayers" (Posner, 2007).

Engstrom and Robison (2006, p. 267) concluded in their book, *Health Care Reform: Ethics and Politics*, that meaningful healthcare reform ought to entail a keen "understanding of the current system's moral failures and, moreover, an understanding of how consistent moral grounding, seen in the context of specific institutional circumstances, can help to overcome those failures". They stressed the importance of *grass roots* involvement in the redesign process and that healthcare must be elevated to the status of a "public resource serving the entire populace." There is mounting evidence that healthcare should be treated as a foundational (moral and ethical) issue as opposed to simply accepting healthcare as being a commodity – "no society can long sustain itself if the health of its citizens diminishes beyond some tip point where citizens cannot be productive, but become a burden to the system" (p. 271). For instance, the Canadian universal health system is based on the presumption that healthy citizens produce a healthy economy.

3.2 -- Obama-Biden Health Reform Recipe

President Barack Obama outlined his proposal for major healthcare reform in the United States during the 2008 election campaign:

> The Obama-Biden [health] plan provides affordable, accessible health care for all Americans, builds on the existing health care system, and uses existing providers, doctors, and plans. Under the Obama-Biden plan, patients will be able to make health care decisions with their doctors, instead of being blocked by insurance company bureaucrats.
>
> Under the plan, if you like your current health insurance, nothing changes, except your costs will go down by as much as $2,500 per year. If you don't have health insurance, you will have a choice of new, affordable health insurance options.

Make Health Insurance Work for People and Businesses -- Not Just Insurance and Drug Companies:

- Require insurance companies to cover pre-existing conditions so all Americans, regardless of their health status or history can get comprehensive benefits at fair and stable premiums.
- Create a new Small Business Health Tax Credit to help small businesses provide affordable health insurance to their employees.
- Lower costs for businesses by covering a portion of the catastrophic health costs they pay in return for lower premiums for employees.
- Prevent insurers from overcharging doctors for their malpractice insurance and invest in proven strategies to reduce preventable medical errors.
- Make employer contributions fairer by requiring large employers that do not offer coverage or make a meaningful contribution to the cost of quality health coverage for their employees to contribute a percentage of payrolls toward the costs of their employees' health care.
- Establish a National Health Insurance Exchange with a range of private insurance options as well as a new public plan based on benefits available to members of Congress that will allow individuals and small businesses to buy affordable health coverage.
- Ensure everyone who needs it will receive a tax credit for their premiums.

Reduce Costs and Save a Typical American Family up to $2,500 as Reforms Phase in:

- Lower drug costs by allowing the importation of safe medicines from other developed countries, increasing the use of generic drugs in public programs, and taking on drug companies that block cheaper generic medicines from the market.

- Require hospitals to collect and report health care cost[s] and quality data.
- Reduce the costs of catastrophic illnesses for employers and their employees.
- Reform the insurance market to increase competition by taking on anticompetitive activity that drives up prices without improving quality of care.

The Obama-Biden Plan will Promote Public Health: It will require coverage of preventive services, including cancer screenings, and increase state and local preparedness for terrorist attacks and natural disasters.

A Commitment to Fiscal Responsibility: Barack Obama will pay for his $50 - $65 billion health care reform effort by rolling back the Bush tax cuts for Americans earning over $250,000 per year and retaining the estate tax at its 2009 level (see web site http://change.gov/agenda/health_care_agenda).

The Commonwealth Fund teamed up with *Modern Healthcare* in December 2008 and conducted an extensive survey of healthcare leaders concerning their priorities and degree of support for Federal healthcare reform legislation. The results of this survey were published in the January 19, 2009 issue of *Modern Healthcare* – they found that the majority (92%) of the respondents favored the creation of a national health insurance exchange to provide coverage for the estimated 70 million uninsured and underinsured Americans caught in the health insurance cost squeeze. Other top priorities noted by the healthcare leadership group are shown below:

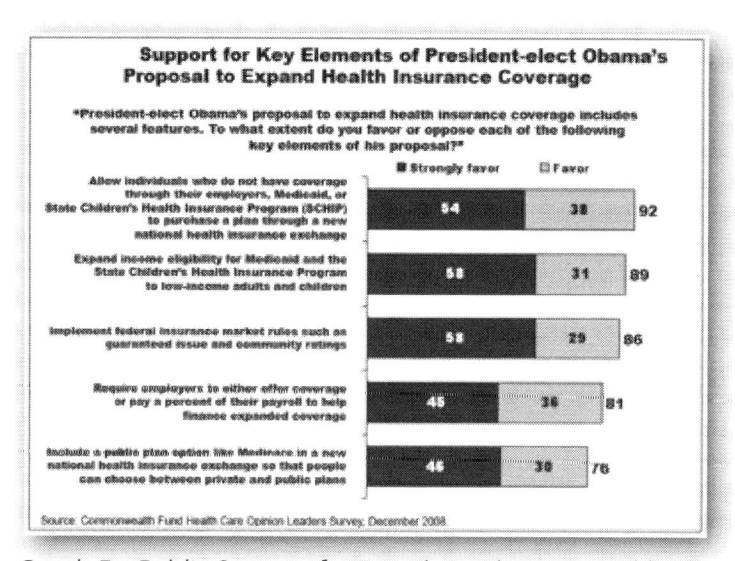

Graph 5 – Public Support for President Obama's Health Plan

The positive spin on the present-day Congressional debate is the recognition that something drastic must be done soon, or the day of reckoning for America's healthcare system will arrive sometime around 2018. The consensus among healthcare experts is that the future healthcare delivery system (i.e., over the next 25 years) in the United States will not look anything similar to today's situation because of the impending *perfect storm* that is closing in on Americans who are confronted with worsening access problems, escalating healthcare costs, poor outcomes, and the *Age Wave* (Dychtwald & Flower, 1989). A new approach – a paradigm shift -- for the US healthcare delivery system must emerge from the present deliberations of politicians and policymakers in Washington, D.C.

Part 2
Problem Statement

Four

Major Issues and Concerns

As President Obama and his critics prepare for the climactic battle over health care, they face a seeming paradox: Millions of Americans say the system is broken and needs fixing. Yet most Americans also say they're pretty satisfied with their health care. The explanation for the apparent contradiction – and a big reason health care has turned into such an incendiary fight – is it's not one crisis, it's a bundle of crises.

1. *The 'cost curve'*
2. *Employers want out*
3. *Growing ranks of uninsured*
4. *Medical bill bankruptcy*
5. *Medicare's exploding cost*

By James Oliphant and Kim Geiger, Chicago Tribune, reprinted in the Tulsa World, September 7, 2009, A16

According to the AHA, the impetus for heightened concern in 2009 over healthcare reform in the United States by the American public, political representatives, government officials, and healthcare providers is fueled by four major trends that are forming the perfect healthcare tempest:

- The impending arrival of the Baby Boom generation which will double the number of seniors (65+) and dramatically increase healthcare utilization (Graph 17 below).
- The escalating number of the uninsured and underinsured population that is closing in on 70 million Americans.

- The unsustainable increase in overall cost of healthcare projected to top 20% of the GDP in the United States by 2018, unless drastic cost containment measures are implemented in the very near future.
- Lack of serious commitment to preventive and public health initiatives that have proven they can mitigate acute care and chronic health services utilization as well as improve disease management measures and overall quality life for millions of Americans.

While the timing for significant healthcare reform in this country appears to be favorable (ten years after the Clinton health reform was defeated), the daunting questions on everyone's mind are what should be done, how should the plan be carried out, how much change is necessary, and when will it have a visible impact on health status? The foundational change that must occur before progress can be realized is how Americans perceive the healthcare system – is it a commodity or human right -- and should it be considered a shared responsibility of all citizens? The challenge for legislators is figure out how to manage the tremendous cost of healthcare in this country while providing sufficient services to achieve improved health status for majority of Americans. And to accomplish this feat without bankrupting future generations!

Our unending appetite for demanding the latest and greatest technological wonders of modern medicine have exacerbated the economic concerns because they are so costly. Yet patient outcomes data and health status indicators suggest that we may not be much better off than earlier times with the traditional hands-on diagnostic and treatment protocols. No doubt that many new diagnostic tests and equipment can pinpoint maladies at much earlier stages when interventions can prevent serious complications. Oftentimes, expensive technology like magnetic resonance imaging (MRI) can replace higher-risk invasive procedures and avoid unnecessary exploratory surgery – early intervention is the most effective treatment for cancer and numerous other ailments. Perhaps this is the justification for the healthcare technological arms-race and why Americans believe so strongly that the best medicine has to be high-tech and expensive.

Hospitals must continuously upgrade their technology in order to remain competitive. For instance, a new MRI with new accommodations and installation can easily amount to a $3 million investment. Most hospitals in larger communities have their own MRI, even though the combined utilization capacity of all these machines far exceeds the demand for services. In short, the equipment is largely underutilized because of competition and duplication of services. This causes higher cost per test than if each machine were working at 80 or 90 percent of its designed capacity. By comparison, consider the fact that Houston, Texas, with approximately 5 million inhabitants, has more MRI machines than the entire country of the Netherlands in Europe, which has an estimated population of 16.5 million. The combination of a fascination for high tech equipment and excess acute care bed capacity (i.e., more hospital beds than the area requires for normal utilization, leading to high vacancy rates) have contributed to a steep "cost curve" in the United States.

When the US economy slumped into a deep recession in 2008, it triggered the largest deficit this country had experienced since the Great Depression. By mid-2009, the government's red ink totaled nearly $2 trillion. Understandably, Congress has been cautious about taking on additional healthcare debt projected at $1 trillion over a ten year period to pay for major healthcare reform and extending health insurance coverage to most Americans.[15] However, many policymakers believe that healthcare reform is the only hope for slowing down and possibly reversing the rising cost of healthcare in the United States. The financial quandary is that we are damned if we don't, and damned if we do.

A group of experts assembled by the Engelberg Center for Health Care Reform at the Brookings Institute and the Robert Wood Johnson Foundation decided that legislation proposed by the Senate Finance Committee -- a principle player in the Congressional reform effort -- could offer opportunities for slowing long term growth if we were to

1. Create an independent entity (a patient centered outcomes research institute) to allocate comparative effectiveness research funding.
2. Increase payment levels to primary care physicians.
3. Establish several steps to increase the link between provider reimbursement and quality of care and efficiency, including the establishment of *Accountable Care Organizations* (ACOs).
4. Expand and streamline the Center for Medicare and Medicaid Services by piloting programs and offering special resources to support the testing, evaluation, and expansion or modification of new payment models in the government health sector, such as *patient centered medical homes*.
5. Move Medicare Advantage to a competitive bidding system.
6. Establish a mandatory individual health insurance requirement, insurance exchanges, rating regulations, and sliding scale subsidies to ensure that insurers compete on price and quality, and help consumers make better health plan decisions.
7. Reduce expenditures on high cost health plans by imposing an excise tax on insurers if the value of health coverage exceeds a certain capped amount. (Simmons, 2009, October 12)

---

[15] In both the Senate and the House, the five Congressional proposals for healthcare reform included a price tag of between $860 billion to $1.8 trillion over a ten-year period according to calculations from the independent assessment agency in Washington, D.C. – the Congressional Budget Office (CBO).

What appears to be sorely lacking in this legislative discourse in Washington, D.C. is attention to the moral and ethical aspects of health and healthcare pertaining to the development of reform initiatives. The central focus of the debate is on the economics of healthcare. The structural design of the healthcare system and how it serves the population would be dramatically different than if the main objectives were to enhance the human benefits of an improved healthcare system in America. Part 3 – The Foundational Elements of Healthcare -- will cover this topic at length.

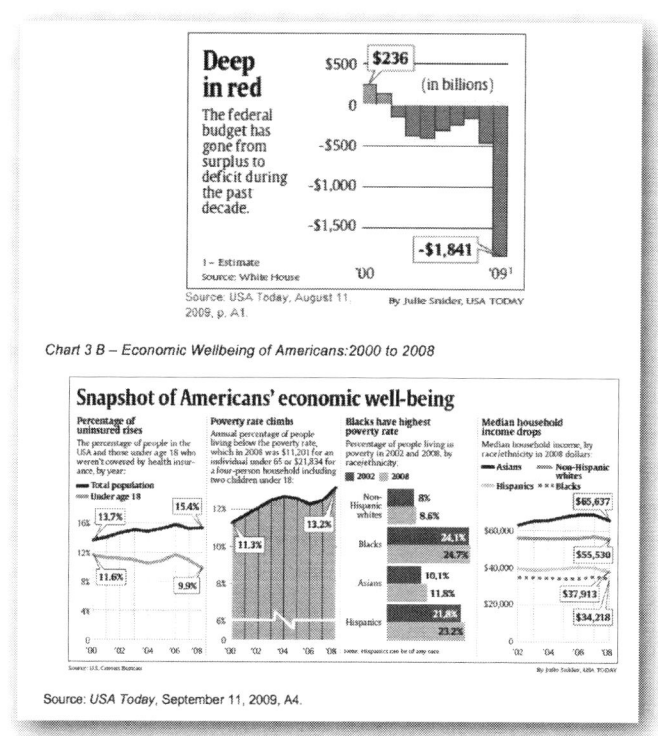

Chart 3 – Federal Budget Surplus and Deficit Trend
Source: *USA Today*, September 11, 2009, A4.

4.1 -- Physician-Hospital Evolution

Although the traditional sick-care system in 2008 consumed about $2.3 trillion overall, only minimal dollars were expended on preventive and public health measures – approximately 3% of national expenditures. Prevention and wellness measures have a proven track record for effectively reducing acute maladies and chronic diseases. With the percentage of seniors reaching over 20% of the US population by the year 2020 (presently it is around 13%), the dramatic growth of chronic illnesses, cardiovascular diseases, and cancer will bring the current health system to its knees due to the overwhelming economic burden, unless significant changes are implemented. A brief tour of key issues relating to the evolution of physician-hospital practices is presented below.

The US healthcare system is ill-equipped to handle a dramatic rise in the number of older Americans (Dychtwald & Flowers, 1989). The senior population will quadruple in 20 years thanks to medical advancements and increasing life expectancy. This Baby Boom generation has been characterized as the arrival of the American healthcare *tidal wave*. A particularly challenging situation is the unprecedented growth in the number of persons over 85 years of age (identified by Dychtwald as the old-old generation) by the year 2050 that will tax the healthcare system with a surge of acute and chronic illnesses far greater than any other age cohort in the history of modern medicine. Generally, the over-60 age group is more sophisticated and knowledgeable than previous generations and will command a controlling block of votes that shape the political process in the near future. This cohort is regarded as the power generation, and they will exercise their consumer preferences as well as demand resources and services to meet their *wants* and *needs* (Dychtwald, 1999).

The United States is not alone in facing the unprecedented growth in the aging population. The direct impact of an aging world is apparent in highly populated countries around the globe: India, China, US, France, United Kingdom, Italy, and Japan. AARP recently sponsored an international conference on aging, *Health Care '08*, that called attention to the growth of older persons internationally -- for AARP, the news in not necessarily bad, since this leading senior-oriented organization has the opportunity to sell its "grey-purchasing power" to an expanding market:

> *We will continue to pursue our vision of a society in which everyone ages with dignity and purpose and in which AARP helps people fulfill their goals and dreams. By going global, we'll be able to make even more of a difference. (AARP, 2008, p. 24)*[16]

Over a span of twenty years, Japan tops the international list with a projected over-60 population growing from 23.2% to 33.7% between 2000 and 2020, or a 10% increase.

The global aging phenomenon is the result of an overall improvement in human health conditions and economic prosperity that is shifting more resources away from younger cohorts and straining the social security and health systems that are dependent on a steady stream of tax contributions from workers to fund these programs.

4.2 -- Lack of Commitment to Prevention and Public Health Initiatives

In order to demonstrate the contrasting approaches to prevention and public health in North America, we will briefly outline the Canadian and US healthcare philosophies. Considerable

---

[16] See also Mary Robinson, William Novelli, Clarence Pearson, and Laurie Norris (eds.), (2007), *Global Health and Global Aging*, New York: Jossey-Bass.

research has been devoted to the merits of preventive health services by the Canadian National Health and Welfare Ministry during the development of the nationalized health care in this country.

Marc LaLonde (1981), who was the Minister of Health and Welfare in the 1970s, championed the national initiative to improve health status of the Canadian population as a way to boost worker productivity and promote "a full, happy, long and illness-free life" (p. 6). The Canadian healthcare system had been heavily influenced by the English and Welsh medical treatment philosophy that focused on illness care by physicians and hospitals. Minimal attention and resources had been committed to preventive care and public health measures during the pre-nationalized medicine era. LaLonde was determined to change the prevailing Canadian perspective on healthcare and emphasized the importance of fostering improvements in the environment (pollutants and other safety hazards), reducing self-imposed risks (lifestyle), and enhancing knowledge of human biology (the biological and organic make-up of individuals) in a public movement that he called the Health Field Concept. As the debate about this "Concept" evolved, LaLonde recognized:

The ultimate philosophical issue raised by the Concept is whether, and to what extent, government can get into the business of modifying human behavior, even if it does so to improve health. (p. 36)

The Canadian debates ultimately led to the implementation of a *multi-disciplinary* (rather than the sole dependence on the medical model) universal healthcare system covering all Canadians, and it was completely funded by the government through across-the-board taxation. This socialized medicine approach to health and wellness was dramatically different from the employer-sponsored, market-driven healthcare system that developed in the United States. The point here is not to hold out the Canadian system as the model for American legislator to emulate -- by no means is the Canadian system a Utopia. We are simply emphasizing the foundational philosophy of their healthcare system. For instance, a serious shortcoming of the Canadian system is that healthcare is heavily rationed and the delivery of care is plagued with long delays and access problems.

Unlike our Canadian neighbors, Americans have resisted major governmental intrusion in their personal health matters. The Institute of Medicine's Report (2001) identifies this natural resistance in the interdisciplinary research focusing on the determinants of healthy behavior and the interplay of biological, behavioral, and societal influences. The IOM Report emphasizes that "individuals and families are embedded within social, political, and economic systems that shape behaviors and constrain access to resources necessary to maintain health" (p. 241). It is not that Americans do not recognize the importance of preventive care and wellness measures for maintaining health; we would rather fix the problems after the fact instead of changing our unhealthy behaviors that have a detrimental effect on health status. It is difficult to change organizational and community culture – the main problem associated with implementing a national strategy to improve health status is that Americans have a strong tendency to act independently when it comes to personal health concerns.

4.3 -- Complementary Medicine and Wellness Approach

Natural Health, Natural Medicine (1995, updated in 2004) was written "to cut through the confusion and provide a basic collection of strategies and methods to maintain optimum health and treat common ailments," states author Andrew Weil, MD in his introductory remarks.[17] Dr. Weil dedicated his practice to preventive health measures that incorporate alternative and integrative practices into the traditional allopathic medicine. As a biologist and physician, Dr. Weil outlines his prescription for better health in four distinct sections of his book: (1) preventive maintenance, (2) specific prevention approaches, (3) basic natural treatments, and (4) home remedies for common illnesses. Dr. Weil notes the importance of vitamins and supplements, and the medicinal effect they can have on the body. Dr. Weil asserts that *Mother Nature* provides an arsenal of natural remedies that offer curative miracles if we know what to look for and where (pp. 257-275). It is undisputed that caring for our bodies and eating healthy foods has a direct impact on health status.

The problem is that unhealthy foods and habits are far more palatable than the alternative health discipline. The American healthcare system offers few economic incentives to maintain a healthy lifestyle as long as insurers pay for the cost of illnesses resulting from poor nutritional habits and lack of physical maintenance. If that is hard to believe, Dr. Weil's book is a valuable review of the benefits of complementary medicine for augmenting the traditional medical care system.

4.4 -- Economic (Dis)Incentives of America's Health System

The majority of America's healthcare is provided through the distribution of approximately one million physicians who care for patients in 4,897 community hospitals[18] throughout the US, according to AHA's 2007 Annual Hospital Survey. The basic classification of these hospitals falls into three broad categories: (1) non-government, not-for-profit hospitals (2,913, or 59.5%); (2) state and local government hospitals (1,111, or 22.7%); and (3) investor-owned, for-profit hos-

---

[17] See also discussion by Ali Mokdad, James Marks, Donna Stroup, and Julie Gerberding, "Actual Causes of Death in the US, 2000," *JAMA*, Vol. 291, No. 10

[18] The American Hospital Association defines "community hospitals" as: All nonfederal, short-term general, and special hospitals whose facilities and services are available to the public. Short-term general and special children's hospitals are also considered to be community hospitals.

pitals (873, or 17.8%). The US has experienced a gradual decline in the total number of community hospitals over the past couple of decades. There were 714 fewer hospitals in operation in 2007 compared to 1987. The most dramatic decline occurred in rural America; a reduction of 602 community hospitals in rural areas versus 112 fewer in urban settings. Presently, 59.2% of all community hospitals are located in urban areas (Tables 1 A and B).

Table 1 A – Number of US Hospitals by Class: 2007

Number of US Hospitals by Class: 2007 Survey

All US Registered Hospitals	5,708	
Community Hospitals	4,897	100.0%
Non-government Not-for-Profit Hospitals	2,913	59.5%
Investor-Owned Hospitals	873	17.8%
State and Local Government Hospitals	1,111	22.7%
Staff Beds for All Community Hospitals	800,892	
Admissions in All Community Hospitals	35,345,986	

Source: American Hospital Association, Annual Hospital Survey: 2007, Fast Facts of US Hospitals, http://www.aha.org/aha/resource-center/statistics-and-studies/fast-facts.html

Table 1 B – Number of Hospitals Trended: 1987-2007

Trend of All Community Hospitals: 1987-2007

Total	Urban	Rural	% Rural
5,611	3,012	2,599	46.3%
5,057	2,852	2,205	43.6%
4,897	2,900	1,997	40.8%
-714	-112	-602	

Source: American Hospital Association, Annual Hospital Survey - TrendWatch Chartbook 2009, Table 2.1

The median (50th percentile) operating margin for community hospitals was strongest among for-profit and rural referral centers, where the overall profit grew close to 19% from

2002 to 2006, i.e. 2.8 to 3.45 percent, respectively. For-profit hospitals outperformed their non-profit counterparts, nearly doubling profit margins at the 50th percentile of the range (see Table 1 C).

Table 1 C – 50th Percentile Total Operating Profit of Hospitals: 2002-2006

50th Percentile Total Operating Profit Margin for US Hospitals: 2002 and 2006

Class	2006	2002	% Change
All Hospitals	3.45	2.8	18.8%
Urban	3.46	2.68	22.5%
Rural	3.44	3.01	12.5%
Teaching	3.74	2.35	37.2%
Rural Referral Centers	5.14	3.74	27.2%
Not-for-Profit	3.35	2.52	24.8%
For-Profit	6.63	6.57	0.9%
Government	3.04	2.3	24.3%
High Profitability	11.32	6.29	44.4%
Low Profitability	-3.61	0.45	-112.5%

Source: Thomson Reuters, The Sourcebook 2008 (All rights reserved)

In addition to the declining number of community hospitals, the US also had 155,637 fewer beds to care for patients during the period from 1987 to 2007. The major reasons for the shrinking number of community hospital beds involved a continuing shift from inpatient to outpatient care facilitated by technological advances, and a shorter average-length-of-stay (ALOS) for nearly all in-patient classifications, according to the AHA.[19] This declining bed availability has had a dramatic impact on the ratio of community hospital beds per 1,000 population nationwide – the ratio has dropped from 3.95 to 2.66 beds per 1,000 population between 1987 and 2006, respectively (Table 2).

---

19 For example, obstetrical deliveries during the early 1980s had an ALOS of over 10 days; today moms spend an average of less than two days in the hospital following delivery of newborns.

Table 2 – US Bed Supply Trend: 1987-2007

US Beds Availability Trend: 1987-2007

Year	# Beds	Beds/1,000 Pop	% Change
1987	956,529	3.95	
1997	853,287	3.19	-19.2%
2007	800,892	2.66	-16.6%
Absolute Change			
87-97	-155,637	-1.29	

Source: American Hospital Association, Annual Hospital Survey - TrendWatch Chartbook 2009, Table 2.2

The distribution of community hospitals and number of inpatient beds do not necessarily correlate with specific healthcare needs of local populations across the country. The mal-distribution of healthcare resources in rural and urban areas has been the subject of intense political debate since the 1950s and has lead to several failed attempts to encourage more practitioners to service rural communities. The impediments for attracting younger physicians to rural areas revolve around (1) social and professional isolation, (2) a limited number of subspecialists to help with complicated patient care issues, and (3) a higher rate of uninsured patients and indigent care that affects income potential. The problems relating to the increasing number of uninsured and underinsured in the country have reached a crisis level – politicians are being pressured to deal with mal-distribution of healthcare resources and the escalating costs of medical care. The last significant Congressional effort to address these issues was in the early 1990s during the Clinton Healthcare Reform administration. The reform initiative failed to move forward because of pressure from special interest groups to preserve the status quo in healthcare.

In *The Future US Healthcare System* (Altman, Reinhardt & Shields, 1998), the editors highlight the challenges Americans face in redirecting the structure of our healthcare system: "an effort to disseminate some of the most recent thinking about the problem and possible solution and to spur renewed efforts aimed at stemming the rising tide of Americans with no health insurance and uncertain access to needed medical attention" must be addressed in order to avert disaster (p.2). They characterize the present state of the United States' healthcare policy as a "crisis in serious need of reform."

According to John Holahan (1998), one of the book's contributors, the US dependence on the Medicaid program as its main safety-net for the poor and lower-income working families is not a sustainable solution over the long term because state officials constantly struggle with budgetary shortfalls and make programmatic cuts to meet multiple social demands. Unfortunately, the rising demand for care and declining per capita subsidization from the federal government to states for public programs has reached its breaking point. Another serious concern is the lack of coordination of health policies and programs, which makes it nearly impossible to render continuity of quality care to the burgeoning, needy, indigent population. For instance, Grady Health System, with its 1,000 beds and status as one of the largest public hospitals in the country located in downtown Atlanta, is on the brink of failure due to the extraordinary load of uninsured and underinsured patients from this metropolitan region. Although the vast healthcare system in Atlanta recognizes the need for a publicly supported hospital and academic medical center to accommodate the less fortunate and provide training for future physicians, few administrators are willing to open their doors to patients who cannot pay for services. Consequently, Grady is on the verge of bankruptcy and is losing millions of dollars each month. The saga of public hospitals is being played out in nearly every major metropolitan city in America, with no real solution in sight.

Another contributor, Alain Enthoven (1998), a distinguished member of the Jackson Hole Group founded in 1992, expounds on the concept of incremental healthcare reform in his article: "There is little to lose and much to gain by cutting today's link between jobs and health insurance" (p. 311). He outlines an eight-step process that builds on the employment-based system and includes government-regulated insurance plans for small employer groups in all states. Enthoven introduces the idea of creating a national Health Insurance Purchasing Cooperative (HIPC) to encourage competition among health insurance monopolies and bringing down the cost of premiums, especially for small employer groups and privately insured policy holders who do not have leverage to negotiate with health insurance companies.

The final essay in *The Future US Healthcare System* by Thomas Rice calls for urgent implementation of a universal health insurance program in the United States. Rice's premise is that access to basic healthcare is a matter of "social justice and fairness" for all Americans (p.389). Normal economic and market conditions do not take into account the concept of social justice and fairness. Rice attributes his perspective in large part to the work done by John Rawls in his book, *A Theory of Justice* (1971). Rice summarizes his call-to-action, favoring universal health insurance coverage in his following statement:

> …the case for universal coverage is very strong. Universal coverage is consistent with prevailing notions of fairness; people should not be penalized for circumstances – such as their socio-demographic background or their current state of health – over which they may have little control…It is thus no surprise that nearly every developed nation is committed to providing healthcare to its population regardless of ability to pay. The United States has much to learn from these societies that have found it worth their while to provide universal health insurance coverage. (p. 401-402)

Healthcare in the United States is regarded as *big business*. Our national policy does not view healthcare as a social right for all individuals. Health insurance is tied to employment and small firms, and individuals are at the mercy of for-profit insurers who prefer to spread their risk over large employer groups. Until the attitude that health insurance and healthcare is a commodity for those who can afford to pay for it fades away, only incremental progress, if any, will be possible. If the number of uninsured and underinsured continues to escalate and reaches the projected 25% of the total population within the next five years, the healthcare crisis will no longer be a topic of discussion for the coffee shops in America; it will demand the full attention from politicians, policymakers, and tax payers to institute a fair and equitable universal healthcare system in the United States, or face the collapse of the entire system. There is still limited time to take preemptive steps to improve the healthcare delivery system in the US

4.5 -- Assuming Personal Responsibility for Health and Wellness

The Institute of Medicine's (IOM) 2001 Committee Report, *Health and Behavior: The Interplay of Biological, Behavioral, and Societal Influences*, is the culmination of three years of collaborative and interdisciplinary research including experts in the fields of public health, clinical and social psychology, medicine, epidemiology, health education, law and ethics, psychiatry, and family therapy. This landmark report is a sequel to the original work published in 1982 – *Health and Behavior: Frontiers of Research in the Biobehavioral Sciences*. According to the 2001 IOM report, health is defined as the state of *positive wellbeing*, as opposed to the common perception of the absence of illness or disease (pp. 3 and 21-25). The authors of the Report discussed several interrelated factors that directly affect individual and communal health, including biobehavioral, psychological, social, environmental, and physiological conditions.

The Committee alludes to the "bi-directional, multilevel relationships" that are intrinsic to health status (pp. 27 and 40), and the significant impact that *stressors* (and differential coping abilities) have on behavioral and physiological responses of individuals to similar ecological conditions (pp. 42-70). The Report discusses how personal and collective healthy conditions are the by-product of the interplay between various circumstances that are both in and outside of our spheres of personal control. For example, tobacco-related mortality amounted to over 400,000 deaths of American adults in 2000 (p. 88) – certainly within the direct influence of individual smokers. Hundreds of thousands of smokers are afflicted by various chronic diseases that impede their quality of life and result in billions of dollars of (avoidable) healthcare costs annually.

Longer life spans attributed to aggressive public health initiatives in developing nations around the world that stem the spread of infectious diseases and mitigate unhealthy lifestyle practices are also contributing to a growth in chronic conditions such as obesity, diabetes, smoking-related cancer, etc. (p. 50). Prior to these public health achievements, most of the population did not survive long enough to be afflicted by debilitating conditions in later years. It seems ironic that "progress" in developing nations is contributing to increased healthcare utilization and cost. It is imperative to shift international health initiatives away from simply treating the spread of infectious diseases in poor and middle-class nations and to enhance comprehensive healthcare management that improves the overall quality-of-life during the entire life cycle. The IOM report notes that chronic illnesses in developing nations are projected to grow at an unprecedented rate through 2015, compared to the more affluent countries (*The Economist*, 2007, p. 50). Since the United States and other wealthy nations are the central source of funding for many of the public health initiatives around the world, we share in the responsibility to influence the type and scope of public health programs to enhance the overall health status of developing countries.

    The healthcare industry is a multi-billion-dollar business that will grow exponentially as the Baby Boom generation marches toward age 65 throughout the next couple decades. In every corner of the world, people are living longer, and consumption of limited healthcare resources is rising. We have incontrovertible evidence that a significant portion of growth in the traditional medical care field is the result of our success in conquering the spread of communicable diseases and treatable illnesses -- the by-product of this success is resulting in more chronic health problems (i.e., lung cancer, hypertension, cardiovascular disease, poor nutrition, accidents, etc.). It makes no sense to ignore the value of prevention and wellness programs and continue to invest minimally in research and public education about how to maximize our wellbeing throughout our increasing life span (Garrett, 2000).

Five

The Hippocratic Oath

*The function of protecting and developing health must rank
even above that of restoring it when it is impaired.*

By Hippocrates of Kos, "The Father of Medicine"

Physicians were expected to abide by the professional standards set forth in the *Hippocratic Oath* which has been the guide for the ethical practice of medicine dating back to the 4th Century B.C. At this point in history, Hippocrates was believed to have laid out his prescription for the medical profession. David Cantor (2002) notes in his collection of accounts by various scholars about Hippocrates that there is little concrete evidence about the actual works that have been attributed to this noted Greek philosopher and prominent figure of medicine. Cantor discusses one of the most popular documents from the Hippocratic era – the *Hippocratic Corpus*[20] – which may have actually been a series of contemporary stories about the practice of medicine by numerous authors rather than Hippocrates himself. Whether or not Hippocrates was the *mythical* father of modern medicine, he undoubtedly was regarded by physicians around the world as the ancestral *authority* that helped shape today's medical profession.

Hippocrates insisted that there is a very special and unique relationship between healer and patient handed down through the generations since the inception of medicine. Unlike other professions, physicians (healers) are first and foremost committed to care for their patients and hold their interests above all other matters. It is believed that the Hippocratic Oath (Figure 4) ascended to the forefront of American medical practice during the 1930s when the document was showcased in the original Broadway production created by Sidney Kingsley. It was this classical *Oath* that came to represent the highest standard of ethics for the practice of medicine

---

20 The *Hippocratic Corpus* – see http://www.ucl.ac.uk/~ucgajpd/medicina%20antiqua/Medant/hippint.htm

and stipulated the *moral conditions* and *codes of behavior* for all practitioners. In essence, the *Hippocratic Oath* symbolizes a commitment to medical excellence and progressive thinking that should be the hallmark of the noble profession of medicine.

Figure 3 – Hippocratic Oath for Physicians

I swear by Apollo the Physician, and Asklepios and Hygieia, and all the Gods and Goddesses that, according to my ability and judgment, I will keep this oath and this syngraphe ('contract'):

to consider him who taught me this Art as dear to me as my parent, to share my substance with him, and to relieve his necessities if required; to look upon his offspring as equivalent to my own brothers, and to teach them this Art, if they wish to learn it, without fee or stipulation;

and that by precept, lecture, and every other form of instruction, I will impart a knowledge of the Art to my own sons, and those of my teachers, and to disciples bound by a stipulation and oath according to the law of medicine, but to none others.

I will follow that system of regimen which, according to my ability and judgment, I consider for the benefit of my patients and abstain from whatever is harmful and mischievous.

I will give no deadly medicine to anyone if asked, nor suggest any such advice; likewise, I will not give a pessary to a woman to induce abortion.

I will live my life and practice my art with purity and holiness.

I will not cut persons suffering from 'the stone', but will leave this to be done by men who are practitioners of this skill. Whatever houses I enter, I will enter for the benefit of the sick, and will abstain from every voluntary act of mischief and corruption, and especially from the seduction of females or males, of free persons or slaves.

Whatever I see or hear in connection with my professional practice or not in the life of men, which should not be made public, I will not divulge, considering that all such knowledge should remain secret.

As long as I continue to keep this Oath inviolate, may it be granted to me to enjoy life and the practice of the Art, respected by all men, at all times. But if I should trespass and violate this Oath, may the opposite be my lot.

Source: George Sarton, A History of Science I (Cambridge: Harvard 1952) 376; Ludwig Edelstein, *The Hippocratic Oath: Text, translation, and interpretation* (Baltimore: Johns Hopkins 1943).

An updated version of the Hippocratic Oath was created by Dr. Louis Lasagna in 1964 while serving as the Dean of the Sackler School of graduate Biomedical Sciences at Tuffs University Medical School, Boston. The modern-day "Physician's Oath" urges practitioners:

- Never to deliberately harm anyone for anyone else's interest
- To avoid violating the morals of the community
- To maintain the good of the patient as the highest priority

Both versions of the Physician's Oath incorporate a blend of science and philosophy into the practical application of medicine and ethics. It also describes the ideal expectation for the exchange between the healer or medical practitioner and patient – the relationship must be special, personal, trusting, emotional, and private (even though it is considered sometimes too *paternalistic*). In *Medicine & Philosophy: A Twenty-Century Introduction*, authors Ingvar Johansson and Niels Lynoe (2008) discuss the distinction between the scientific and philosophical concerns involving the patient-physician relationship: (1) medicine is based on natural scientific facts. and (2) moral philosophy is the normative science of meaning and purpose of human behavior or ethos:[21] "where a moral system is accepted, it regulates the life of human beings" (p. 267). They characterize the interrelationship of medicine and ethics (practice and theory) as synonymous with *knowing how* and *knowing that* (borrowed from Donald Schon, in *The Reflective Practitioner*):

> *In the varied topography of professional practice, there is a high, hard ground where practitioners can make effective use of research-based-theory and technique, and there is a swampy lowland where situations are confusing 'messes' incapable of technical solutions. (p. 269).*

Johansson and Lynoe elaborate: "we regard this [continuum between the high, hard ground and swampy lowland] as being as true of medical ethics as of medical practice." This intrinsic connection between medicine and ethics is what is so unique about the medical profession.

James Marcum (2008) argues that there should be a *philosophy of medicine* that serves to *humanize modern medicine*. Marcum believes in the philosophical approach to modern medicine because "the quality-of-care crisis is really a crisis over the nature of medicine" (pp. 49-61). The philosophy of medicine, Marcum writes, helps define the true purpose of medicine. The goal of the physician should be to take care of the whole person (patient), not only the mechanical body (medical impairment or disease). Marcum defines the physician's highest priority as the fulfillment of the Hippocratic Oath – to protect the best interests of his patients above all else. Marcum clarifies that instead of being rationally concerned for his patient in an emotionally detached manner (in keeping with advocates of the biomedical model), it is more important to assume a humanistic or humane stance, showing that the practitioner cares both emotionally and rationally for the health of his patient *qua* person (p. 276).

---

21 *Ethos* = n : the distinguishing character, sentiment, moral nature, or guiding beliefs of a person, group or institution; *Merriam-Webster's Dictionary and Thesaurus*, 2006.

US federal and state regulatory licensing requirements for physicians have reinforced their authority to direct the care of patients to consist of *admitting* patients to healthcare facilities; *ordering,* not simply requesting or suggesting that specific care plans be carried out; and conducting tests and treatments administered by technical staff and caregivers. Unlike other professionals that normally take direction from their employer or systems' manager, physicians exercise a unique external control over the allocation and consumption of healthcare resources. This exclusive circumstance gives physicians a special role for driving the economic engine of the health system. In most cases, physicians have enjoyed higher social status and wealth than the average professional because of their unique expertise, authority, and inherent control over the medical marketplace (pp. 18-29).

5.1 -- Patient-Physician Relationship

To better understand the uniqueness of the patient-physician relationship, it is necessary to reflect upon the *nature* of the relationship itself. Marcum (2008) poses the question: "What is medicine? Is it an *art* or a *science* – or a combination thereof?" The answer to this question has been the subject of intense debate around the world since the time of Hippocrates. Marcum postulates that there are two basic schools of thought regarding the definition of medicine (pp. 301-303):

> *Evidence-based* → biomedical model envisions medicine as a science; 'medical knowledge and practice is viewed as rational, observational and inductive, mainly in physio-chemical or vitalistic terms.'
> *Patient-centered* → humanistic model perceives medicine as an art; 'the art of medicine concerns itself not only with the sick individual but with the totality of his environment – his family, his occupation, his social and pecuniary status, indeed with everything that can favor or retard his recovery from illness' (derived from Reisman, 1931).

He claims that the quality-of-care crisis stemmed from an over-emphasis on the natural sciences starting in the 20th Century. According to Marcum, medicine should have a different connotation for physicians and patients.

> 'Medicine,' from the physician's perspective, 'is very much what he cares to make it' (derived from Black, 1968). In other words, medicine is a profession in which the physician can specialize. Medicine, from the patient's perspective, however, 'should mean simply help in sickness – help which comes promptly, is given willingly, which is manifestly efficient, and does not cripple him financially' (derived from Black, 1968).

Medicine is based on a *healing relationship* between patient and physician, Marcum decides.

For medicine to be most effective, the physician must approach the relationship with his patient from both a personal and organic perspective. He should incorporate a humanistic dimension in the treatment process. In other words, the medical practitioner is not simply a skilled technician working on body parts to restore normal functioning of the subject. According to Marcum "for contemporary medicine to resolve its quality-of-care crisis, it must connect with its *pathos*[22] in terms of both the patients' suffering from illness and the physician's suffering to heal that illness" (p. 325). The pathos Marcum refers to is the transformation of the biomedical scientist into a "wise and loving healer." Physicians must work diligently on the quality of the patient-physician relationship; not just treating the physical body of the patient but instead treating the *persona* (pp. 49-61). Marcum urges contemporary practitioners to resume the role of caring for patients and not merely curing diseases (derived from E. Cassel, 1991).

The subject of medical ethics is part and parcel of the physician's duty to attend to the overall needs of patients according to the best of his or her abilities. Patricia and Arthur Parsons (1995) published a how-to book for patients so they could better appreciate a patient's rights and responsibilities, as well as to encourage an open, meaningful, and frank dialogue with their practitioner in order to achieve the most beneficial results from the interaction. In *Hippocrates Now! Is Your Doctor Ethical?* the Parsons advise patients to take an active role in the decision-making process. It is not sufficient for the patient to assume the role of passive subject and not question the reasoning behind certain procedures and treatment protocols that the doctor orders for the patient.

Full disclosure is critical to building a bi-directional trusting relationship between the patient and physician. Conflicts-of-interest arise when the physician's primary motivation for ordering tests or conducting diagnostic procedures is to make a profit. On the other hand, the patient who ignores his physician's care-plan is also wasting precious healthcare resources and the caregiver's time. It is incumbent on both the patient and healthcare professional to do everything possible to maximize positive outcomes for the sake of the relationship and economic wellbeing of society.

The unique nature of the patient-physician relationship is protected in most instances by the ethical standards for medical professionalism. Christine Cassel, president of the American Board of Internal Medicine, and Jeffery Harris, president of the American College of Physicians, comment that the charter (Physician Charter on Medical Professionalism), which is "endorsed by more than 100 medical societies worldwide, embraces three principles of professional responsibility that our healthcare system must also support: (1) promoting patient welfare, (2) respecting patient autonomy, and (3) achieving social justice" (*Modern Healthcare*, 2009, p. 21). There is real danger of developing a conflict-of-interest when physicians try to adhere to the stringent standards of integrity outlined in the Charter, while at the same time attending to the financial pressures of the *business of medicine* in their practice. This potential conflict was evident in the results of a recent survey of physicians published in the *Annals of Internal Medicine*:

---

22 *Pathos* = n. an element inexperience or artistic representation evoking pity or compassion; *Merriam-Webster's Dictionary and Thesaurus*, 2006.

While physicians support the idea of medical professionalism, some have trouble living up to those ideals. For instance, while 96% believe that patient needs trump financial interests, 24% of physicians say that they would refer a patient to an imaging facility they own – without informing that patient of the potential conflict. (p. 21)

In the context of today's healthcare reform debate, medical professionalism and the special role of the patient-physician relations must remain a dominant theme rather than focusing on controlling the spiraling costs of (sick) care. Cassel and Harris' commentary stresses that "reform provides an opportunity to engage patients and physicians in shaping a system that serves patients well and fosters trust and medical professionalism" (p. 21).

The reality for most physicians is that insurance companies and healthcare organizations are exercising greater control over the patient management and referral process. These institutions are driving a wedge between patient-physician relationships because of financial considerations. Changing referral patterns, controlling choice of patient treatment protocols, determining admission and discharge criteria, and dictating medication formularies, etc. all have the effect of detracting from the special relationship physicians are charged with regarding the care of their patients. To add to the complexities of the patient-physician relationship, employers are seeking to contain their healthcare benefits cost by renegotiating health insurance terms and even switching insurers; employees are often forced to change providers because of penalties imposed on patients that go outside of insurance-designated health networks. These constraints combine to deeply impact the nature of the traditional patient-physician bond.

Physician satisfaction with the medical profession is at an all time low. This is especially true for primary care providers. The top complaints from practitioners are (1) not enough time to spend with patients to do the job right; (2) too many hassles associated with dealing with insurance carriers to gain permission to treat patients; (3) the rising cost of providing quality care is outpacing reimbursement increases, which results in declining income; (4) excessive paperwork required by government regulations; (5) outrageous malpractice insurance premiums and frivolous litigation; (6) inadequate payment for primary and preventive services (compensation for specialty care is significantly higher than primary care); (7) not enough time for family and lifestyle opportunities; and (8) excessive educational debt. Personal *time* is perhaps one of the most precious assets a physician has to share with patients (Cassell, 2004). These issues are depriving physicians from devoting the necessary time and passion to care for patients the way they believe is appropriate.

Eric Cassell, MD (2004), who is a practicing physician at The New York-Presbyterian Hospital and professor of public health at Weill Medical College of Cornell University, claims that the primary goal of medicine should be to mitigate human pain and suffering. Cassell states that pain and suffering are related, but vastly different manifestations or afflictions:

Suffering is an affliction of the person, not the body. For example, a forty-seven-year-old single woman, in whom the sudden appearance of widespread metastatic breast cancer caused her to be hospitalized and near death, suffers. But it is not primarily the weakness, profound anorexia, and generalized swelling, as distressing as they are, that are the source of her suffering, but the loss of control and inability to prevent the evaporation of her career, whose brilliant promise had finally been realized a few months earlier. (pp. xii-xv)

Contemporary practitioners are not well trained to treat *suffering*, which deals with the whole person; instead, physicians are typically focused on the technical aspects of disease management. The objective nature of the body and its diseases has existed in Western medicine since its beginnings in ancient Greece (450 B.C.). There is a tendency toward objectivity and hard facts rather than a more subjective approach to patient care. This creates an impersonal relationship between the patient and physician. The emphasis in this type of impersonal exchange is centered on the disease process instead of the person, focusing on the source of pain instead of suffering (the entire realm affecting the wellbeing of the patient), notes Cassell.

Cassell vigorously criticizes the bioethical movement in medical training programs because it produces physicians who revere the scientific aspects of medicine instead of promoting "healers and professionals" that are concerned with the human dimensions of the patient-physician relationship. The changing facets of *standardized* (as compared to *personalized*) medicine has created serious challenges for physicians according to Cassell:

1. It emphasizes the scientific method based on the belief that it is "value free;" it deemphasizes the qualitative nature of the relationship and the importance of the individual in the exchange process.
2. It places excessive reliance on technology, encouraging the practitioner to seek the "ultimate truth" about the cause of the disease or illness – referred to as "evidence-based medicine;" people are infinitely complex, and uncertainty cannot be explained without due consideration of the whole environmental circumstance of the patient – this can only be accomplished through personalized interaction between the parties.
3. The most influential groups of physicians in the United States have transformed themselves from traditional clinicians into full-time medical researchers; this transformation has served to distance the physician from his patients through an artificial reliance on concrete external technological factors as opposed to intuitive knowledge that characterizes the "art" of medical care prevalent in the past.
4. Mass communication and the explosion of scientific knowledge available to patients has demystified the paternalistic (a belief that "doctor knows best") role of the physician in medical treatment; patients now-a-days want more autonomy and are insisting on actively participating role in the care plan. (pp. 16-28)

These key factors, notes Cassell, are profoundly changing modern medicine. He cautions: "Medicine is fundamentally a moral enterprise because it is devoted to the welfare of the persons it treats…Science and morality are not opposed – they are joined in medicine. Science cannot be the dominant force in medicine because it is in the service of something larger than itself" (p. 27). Prolonging life at any cost when death is inevitable may simply cause needless suffering for the patient and loved ones (Cassell discusses at length the natural process of "the illness called dying"). Fear also causes suffering; therefore, understanding fear can contribute to improved patient wellbeing, even if a cure may not be a likely alternative. The physician and patient should share in the decision-making process that can lead to death, Cassell asserts (pp. 243-259).

The theoretical framework for strengthening the nature of the medical profession presented by Cassell offers a unique perspective regarding the preservation of patient-physician relationship. He ends his essay with these insightful words:

The doctor-patient relationship is the vehicle through which the relief of suffering is achieved. One cannot avoid 'becoming involved' with the patient and at the same time effectively deal with suffering…As one problem is resolved, others appear. It is inevitable, therefore, that in the face of emergent dilemmas current medical technologies will be inadequate and the skills and concepts of physicians will fall short…It is the responsibility of physicians to care for the sick even with imperfect means in a sea of uncertainty. This is the source of their grace. Thus it has always been and thus it is now – the relief of suffering is the fundamental goal of medicine. (p. 259)

Cassell is encouraging physicians to return to the practice of personalized medicine and rely more on *intuitive* medical knowledge in order to assist patients to attain healthier lifestyles and personal wellbeing. A graphic representation of Cassell's postulate concerning key physician attributes is presented below:

Table 3 – Physician-Patient Alignment

Alignment of Physician Attributes: Importance to Patients

	Present	Future
Ability Training, Skills, and Medical Expertise	#1	#3
Accessibility Location, Willingness to Accept Patients and Payers	#2	#2
Affability Closeness to Patients, Openness, and Genuine Concern	#3	#1

Source: Mark Tozzio, 2009.

The relative importance of a physician's *affability* (humanistic traits) relating to patient care should continue to shift to the top of the chart. Technical *ability* (scientific capabilities) is taken for granted or assumed to be a reasonable degree of competence as a result of regulatory oversight by professional and state organizations. *Accessibility* (availability of physician resources) should remain the second-most important priority on the chart and will become a more serious concern as the demand for healthcare services increases and the ratio of physicians to the population continues to decline.

5.2 -- Corporatization of Healthcare and the Oath

During the 1970s, the economics of modern medicine and rapid diffusion of expensive technology began shifting the balance of traditional healthcare power from physicians into the hands of business managers of corporate health delivery systems and large, privately-managed-care insurance organizations who had access to vast amounts of capital resources (Starr, 1982). Eventually, politicians and public policymakers became more comfortable with the concept of the "right of equal access to medical care," which also "meant that cost control had to be built into the medical system" (p. 393). The reimbursement system in the United States gradually moved away from the fee-for-service to a *prospective payment* methodology (global prospective payment based on diagnosis related groups or DRGs) in order to get a better handle on the run-away cost of healthcare. The growth of corporate medicine and the concept of universal health insurance seemed inevitable to Starr (pp. 420-430).

Arnold Relman, MD, professor emeritus of social medicine at Harvard Medical School, Boston, Massachusetts, and well-respected former editor of the *New England Journal of Medicine* (from 1977 to1991), authored several books on the topic of healthcare reform in the US He was particularly critical of the transformation of healthcare from a social and beneficent institution to a profit-making business. In his recent (Relman, 2008) critique of Ezekiel Emanuel's book published in *The New York Review of Books* (2009), Relman recounts the turning point of the American healthcare system: "The behavior of US physicians has been changed by the commercialization of medical care, and this too has increased costs."[23] He further notes that prior to 1975, the AMA upheld the professional standard claiming that the medical practice was a *pure profession*, rather than a market-based business enterprise. The AMA's ethical guidelines advised physicians to limit their income to reasonable earnings from the care of patients, and to refrain from advertising and from entering into financial arrangements with drug and device manufacturers.

---

[23] Interestingly, Ezekeil Emanuel is the older brother of President Obama's chief of staff, Rahm Emanuel, who is also the chair of the Department of Bioethics at the National Institutes of Health and is medical advisor to Peter Orszag, director of the cabinet-level Office of Management and Budget (OMB).

Why The United States Healthcare System Should Be A Limited Human Right For All

The AMA reversed its original stance after the US Supreme Court's landmark decision in 1975 that ruled that professionals, such as attorneys and physicians, were actually engaged in interstate commerce and had to follow antitrust legislation. By 1980, the AMA considered the practice of medicine to be "both a business and a profession," as long as their behavior did not harm patients. Relman argued over the years that the present employer-sponsored market-driven (for-profit) insurance system must be replaced by a single-payer, not-for-profit payment system similar to the Medicare program for older Americans. His vision was to provide universal care with cost controls through "a public agency but managed entirely on a not-for-profit basis by privately organized doctors and hospitals… [with] multispecialty groups of salaried physicians and other professionals [like the Mayo Clinic and other successful integrated healthcare delivery systems], which would include adequate numbers of primary care doctors." No doubt, implementation of such a system would entail a dramatic paradigm shift in the modern American healthcare delivery system.

Over the past 50 years, the solo-primary care physician has gradually been replaced by higher-earning *specialists* and *proceduralists* (oriented to expensive surgical procedures, complex technology, and specialized facilities) who are typically part of an integrated healthcare network or system that contracts for patient care with health insurance companies (*USA Today*, 2009). Nevertheless, Relman believed that the simple, humanistic patient-physician relationship should remain the essential focus of a reformed healthcare system in the United States. Another ongoing struggle for physicians has been the growing burden of malpractice insurance and expensive litigation resulting in *defensive medicine* that unnecessarily drives up the cost of care and limits the precious time that providers can spend with patients.

These and other physician concerns have lead to a decline in the number of seniors graduating from medical training programs and an increase in those opting out of Family Practice residencies. There has been a drop by 54 percent since 1997 in the enrollment in Family Practice, according to the American Academy of Family Practice.

The AMA found that more physicians are discouraging their children from entering into the healing profession. They say that personal satisfaction and return-on-investment is just not there any longer. This situation is creating a growing shortage of healthcare professionals in primary care and some sub-specialty fields. The dissatisfaction problem is a serious concern that must be addressed soon in order to maintain a sufficient number of health providers in the training pipeline to care for our growing and aging society. Obviously, the availability of dedicated and well-trained primary care physicians seriously impacts the accessibility of patients to quality medical care; this issue is particularly troublesome because of the growing number of senior citizens in the US who will require more medical services as they age.

Six

Ethics and Modern Medicine

6.1 -- Ethics, Fairness, Justice, and Healthcare in the United States

> *There must be a national health care policy, the system must be reformed, patients must receive care that they need and from which they can benefit, and there must be a single level of access and delivery of health care. The more than $700 billion of current health care costs must be reallocated in a rational way without arbitrary rationing. And there must be neither slaves nor slave doctors.*
>
> By Stephen M. Ayres, "Rationality, Not Rationing, in Health Care," in Rationing American's Medical Care: The Oregon Plan and Beyond, 1992

Advocacy groups across America have fought for "affordable and readily accessible healthcare for all those in need" since the early 1960s.[24] President Franklin D. Roosevelt pushed for national health insurance coverage during The Great Depression as part of the *New Deal* policies, to no avail. Finally, in 1966, the compulsory federal Medicare program covering all persons over 65 years of age, along with the Medicaid program for the poor, were implemented in President Lyndon B. Johnson's term during the *Great Society* era. Healthcare reform was also a controversial political campaign theme during the 2008 Presidential runoff between Republican contender John McCain and his Democratic rival Barack Obama.

---

[24] The idea of national health insurance came about around 1915 when the group American Association for Labor Legislation attempted to introduce a medical insurance bill to some state legislatures; see John Dennis Chasse, (1991), The American Association for Labor Legislation: An episode in Institutionalist policy, *Journal of Economic Issues*, Vol. 25, Retrieved April 26, 2009, from http://.

Inequality of access, cost, and quality of health services has been a persistent challenge throughout the past 100 years of US history. Researchers have repeatedly found that the lower a family's economic status is, the more healthcare inequities exist. Not only do economically disadvantaged families have more limited access to healthcare services, they also tend to receive a lower standard of care because of barriers to access that exist for preventive care. Another important obstacle that poor families face is that they have fewer choices for inpatient and outpatient services because many providers do not accept government health insurance, or indigent patients. This is particularly true for specialized care providers.

In his essay *Why a Two-Tier System of Health Care Delivery is Morally Unavoidable* (1992),[25] Tristram Engelhardt, Jr. (1992) stresses that policymakers seeking to establish a more equitable healthcare system in the US face significant challenges for three reasons:

> *First, there is the desire on the part of most people to postpone death indefinitely; to lower the risk of suffering, disease and disability; to ameliorate their suffering due to disease and disability; and not to spend so much on satisfying the first three desires as not to have enough resources left over to enjoy their lives. Second, there are only limited resources available to achieve the many projects that appeal to humans. Last and most important, there is no generally justifiable secular moral vision concerning justice, fairness, or the final significance and meaning of human life that will enable secular societies to discover how they should rank the first four desires. (p. 204)*

In order to overcome these issues, he believed that it is necessary to involve the community-at-large in a fair prioritization and distribution process to allocate finite health resources. In this manner, policies would more accurately reflect the community authority and the diversity of moral sentiments concerning access to healthcare.

Economists claim that the shortcomings of the American healthcare system are rooted in the economic and cultural (moral and ethical beliefs) fabric of our nation. Amiel and Cowell (1999) present a cross-section of economists' perspectives dealing with inequality in their book, *Thinking About Inequality*. Their interesting compilation of essays is particularly relevant and applicable to this analysis since it focuses on ethical considerations involving modern medicine. The authors contend that "in passing from the topic of inequality to the topic of social welfare much more is involved than just replacing a negative with a positive" (p. 66). Inequality and social welfare are inextricably intertwined in social and political systems and are usually related to popular definitions of poverty based on some sort of financial ranking criteria of income distribution in a society (pp. 89-113). The actual measurements of inequality within a society,

---

[25] The definition of a two-tiered healthcare system according to Tristram Engelhardt, Jr. is a system that includes both private and governmental segments.

according to Amiel and Cowell, are heavily influenced by a *cross-cultural perspective* (p.114). The editors clarify:

Nevertheless, it is evident that 'culture' – interpreted very broadly as the universe in which a person acquires his values – may have an impact upon distributional judgments at a fundamental level. For example, it might be argued that whether a person comes from a society with an 'individualistic culture' (such as the United States) or a culture that accepts as part of the order of things a benevolent interventionist state (Sweden?) may affect not only the value that the person places on inequality relative to other social issues but also on the meaning to be given to inequality rankings when comparing income distributions. (p. 115)

I have correlated Amiel and Cowell's interpretation of the economic cross-cultural perspective of inequality (and its relationship to poverty) with the persistent resistance of US policymakers to move *away* from the employer-based market-driven healthcare system toward a universal healthcare model that offers a basic healthcare benefits package to all citizens, regardless of economic status. In other words, it seems that the American healthcare philosophy is heavily vested in the system whereby employers offer health insurance benefits to employees as an enticement to work for the company, and workers share in a portion of the cost of healthcare insurance premiums. The larger the company and the more employees that participate in the health insurance plan, the greater the bargaining power to control costs (at least in theory). Under the employer-sponsored health insurance system, the unemployed, underemployed, self-employed, and economically disadvantaged who cannot afford to pay health insurance premiums are left to the whims of providers outside of the mainstream healthcare system. The disenfranchised from the employer-sponsored coverage program total some 70 million Americans (uninsured and underinsured individuals).

Volumes of research and scholarly articles have described the inherent inequities of the current employer-sponsored, market-driven healthcare structure in the United States. The common thread among all these studies is the reality that the sick care (the traditional healthcare system continuum) as well as preventive health services are regarded as a *privilege* for approximately three-quarters of the population, rather than a limited human right for all citizens. That leaves about 50 to 70 million Americans who are uninsured or underinsured, according to the estimated count in 2008, to fend for themselves and to access healthcare mostly through hospital emergency departments throughout the nation. To rectify the present sad reality, meaningful healthcare reform in the US will have to bring about a drastic paradigm shift.

6.2 -- Medicine for Profit

It is important to stress at the onset of this section that in spite of all the problems with the US healthcare system, the majority of healthcare professionals working in hospitals and health-related businesses in this country are dedicated, honest, and hardworking individuals who subscribe to the highest standards of care and ethical conduct in their roles as caregivers and support personnel. There is nothing immoral about making a reasonable return on investments in the business of healthcare. In fact, without a sufficient profit margin, there cannot be a healing mission. This section concentrates on some aberrations within our healthcare system that tend to give the healing profession a "black eye" – these situations must be rectified in order to restore the respect to the profession that is so deserved.

The emphasis on market-based competition and profit-making within the corporate practice of medicine has generated immense pressure on decision-makers who must deal with difficult ethical considerations in rural and urban communities throughout this country. Few contemporary healthcare providers, politicians, regulators, consumers, and the public-at-large would dispute the claim that the American healthcare system is perceived as a lucrative *business enterprise* that relies on growing the volume of procedures and treating more sick patients in order to fuel its economic engine. As the saying goes, a greater number of sicker paying patients generally equates to greater income potential and higher profitability for healthcare operators. The economic incentives (with a myriad of reimbursement schemes) of the US healthcare system do not encourage providers to foster a healthier community – this would put them out of business in the long run. The traditional employer-sponsored, market-driven health insurance system and government reimbursement programs encourage (over)utilization of healthcare resources. Only a miniscule amount of the national funding for healthcare is devoted to public health initiatives and preventive health and wellness services – about three percent of the total $2.3 trillion healthcare dollars spent in 2008.

Typically, healthcare providers are motivated to aggressively market to privately insured patients, as opposed to government-funded beneficiaries in the Medicare and Medicaid programs, to strengthen reimbursement and profitability. Few, if any, providers are proactively seeking indigent patients. This is especially true for proprietary for-profit providers. Although 82.2% of general acute care community hospitals in this country are classified as *non-profit*, tax-exempt organizations serving a charitable purpose, nearly all non-governmental insurance companies are classified as *for-profit* entities. Non-profit hospitals and health services organizations, by law, cannot distribute their *excess revenue (profit)* to private entities or investors (this is considered a violation of the inurnment law). However, they can accumulate reserves for future use and invest "profits" in growth strategies that garner a larger share of patients in their defined service areas -- and consequently more paying patients results in additional marginal income. This has resulted in continuous expansion of facilities and programs among non-profit hospitals and health systems.

Table 4 – Number of US Hospitals by Class: 2007

Number of US Hospitals By Class: 2007 Survey

All US Registered Hospitals	5,708	
Community Hospitals	4,897	100.0%
Non-government Not-for-Profit Hospitals	2,913	59.5%
Investor-Owned Hospitals	873	17.8%
State and Local Government Hospitals	1,111	22.7%
Staff Beds for All Community Hospitals	800,892	
Admissions in All Community Hospitals	35,345,986	

Source: American Hospital Association, Annual Hospital Survey: 2007, Fast Facts of US Hospitals, http://www.aha.org/aha/resource-center/statistics-and-studies/fast-facts.html

During the golden era of healthcare spanning from the 1960s to early 1980s, consumers experienced unprecedented and uncontrolled cost increases from healthcare providers and insurance companies. The federal and state governments did little to directly regulate profits of health insurance companies, pharmaceutical firms, medical equipment vendors, or healthcare providers. There were virtually no efforts to tie community needs to the availability of healthcare resources (duplication of services). Healthcare utilization climbed exponentially, inflation escalated, and the cost of health insurance premiums provided by for-profit private companies skyrocketed. During the 1970s, the government instituted a national health planning and development program including quasi-regulatory entities throughout the nation to grant approval to health providers -- Certificate of Need (CON) -- to build new facilities and acquire major medical equipment. The CON was intended to prevent unnecessary expenditures and costly duplication of services; instead, the program created a costly legal bureaucracy that had minimal effect on healthcare enhancement and cost containment. The CON program was eventually phased out by the end of the 1980s. The annual bill for healthcare services grew from seven percent of the GDP in 1970 to over 14% by 1995 (Fisk, 2000).

The lucrative healthcare industry climate of the 1980s and 1990s attracted ambitious entrepreneurs who developed mega for-profit hospital corporations that were able to (1) access massive sums of capital from Wall Street investors to acquire independent non-profit hospitals, (2) leverage economies of scale within their chains of hospitals to better control operating expenses and administrative overhead, (3) employ physicians to work for the corporations and redirect patients to their facilities, and (4) maximize profitability for stockholders and private investor groups. The 1970s and 1980s ushered in the corporate practice of medicine, which contributed to "the decline of compassion and solidarity" in the healthcare system, according to Fisk.[26] This was also an era when hospital corporations' top leaders lost sight of their mission and reaped vast sums of money from the medical industry. This abuse of power caused national embarrassment, shame, and punitive fines for healthcare leaders primarily in the for-profit hospital industry.

The philosophy of US policymakers has been to foster market-based competition in the healthcare arena based on the belief that economic forces would be self-regulating and self-limiting and that healthcare *players* would promote affordable and accessible health services to the communities they served. By 2008, healthcare consumed 18% of the United States' GDP and topped $2.3 trillion. So much for managing the rising healthcare costs.

Case Study #1

Maggie Mahar's (2006) book on *Money-Driven Medicine* reads like a Mafioso novel as she recounts the rise and fall of huge for-profit hospital chains in the US: *Hospital Corporation of America* (HCA), founded in 1968 by Thomas Fearn Harrison Frist Sr. (father of Dr. William Harrison "Bill" Frist, presently a US Republican Senator from Tennessee and former Senate Majority Leader), Dr. Thomas Frist Jr., and Jack Massey (HCA merged with *Columbia Healthcare*, founded by financer Rick Scott in 1994); *National Medical Enterprise* (NME), founded in 1969 by lawyer and certified account Richard K. Eamer; *Tenet*, created in 1994 from the merger of the fallen NME, *American Medical Holdings* (formerly American Medical International – AMI), and *OrNda HealthCorp*, lead by Jeffrey Barbakow, a Wall Street dealmaker and banker; and *HealthSouth*, founded in 1994 by Richard M. Scrushy. Each of these individuals earned millions of dollars during their tenures at the helm of these multi-billion-dollar hospital corporations. Each of the companies listed above was investigated by federal and state agencies for suspected fraudulent and unethical business practices – collectively they paid fines for criminal, civil, and punitive damages totaling nearly $4 billion.

These examples were not restricted to the for-profit hospital industry. There were similar stories about abusive leaders in not-for-profit corporations, pharmaceutical companies, insurance organizations, device makers, etc. The astonishing fact is that these situations persisted over 50 years without radical healthcare system payment reform and only piecemeal regulatory changes. The solution to the corporate practice of medicine misfortunes, according to Mahar, is

---

26 Milton Fisk, (2000), *Toward a Healthy Society: The Morality and Politics of American Health Care*, Lawrence, Kansas: University Press of Kansas, pp. 21-64.

to return the practice of medicine to a *trusting* relationship between the patient and physician. She summarizes her proposition as such:

> *If the patient assumes that health care is an industry like any other, then the consumer advocates are right – the patient cannot expect the marketplace to put his interests first. Corporate retailers like Wal-Mart and McDonald's are expected to be honest, but they are not expected to be selfless – they are not expected to put their customers' interests ahead of their stockholders'. But physicians are not retailers, and health care is not a retail industry or even a service industry in the ordinary sense of the term…It's not enough to prevent the abuses or cure the excesses of money-driven medicine, but at least it changes the terms of the discussion, making it clear that the doctor is not marketing a commodity, he is practicing his profession – and as a member of the healing profession, his responsibility is to give his patient not what he thinks the patient [or the corporate manager] wants, but what he has reason to believe will yield the best results [for the patient]. (pp. 343-344)*

Mahar's book is an eye-opener for those who have not worked close to the corporate practice of medicine world. It also serves as a startling reminder of the importance of ethical and moral responsibilities that are expected of healthcare leaders as they carry out their fiduciary roles within the medical system.

Case Study #2

In June 2009, McAllen, Texas became the *showcase* for the risks of modern-day for-profit greed in America medicine. Prominent Harvard Medical School surgeon Atul Gawande, MD published an article in the June 1, 2009 edition of *The New Yorker* that brought national attention to McAllen. He noted that this community had the second-highest Medicare cost-per-enrollee in the entire United States without necessarily demonstrating significant health status problems to justify this unfortunate claim to fame.[27]

Comparing McAllen to El Paso, Texas, which are demographically similar communities some 800 miles apart from each other (both are located on the west-Texas border with Mexico), Gawande uncovered evidence that Medicare was paying nearly $7,500 more per enrollee in McAllen (average payment of $14,946) than in El Paso, where the average payment was $7,504 for similar medical care. His analysis of the higher healthcare utilization and costs disparities for residents in McAllen compared to El Paso was based on data from reliable government

---

[27] Dr. Gawande is a general and endocrine surgeon and is Associate Professor at the Harvard School of Public Health and the Harvard Medical School in Boston, Massachusetts. He served as advisor to the US Department of Health and Human Services during the Clinton Administration and is also Director of the world Health Organization's Global Patient Safety Challenge program.

sources including the US Department of Health and Human Services – Centers for Medicare and Medicaid (CMS), Dartmouth's Institute for Health Policy and Clinical Practice, D2Hawkeye, Ingenix (UnitedHealth's data-analysis company), and others.

Gawande's information clearly indicates that the higher cost of healthcare in McAllen was *not* the result of superior medical care (which could explain a higher cost differential), nor unusually poor health status or higher morbidity in the population in this border community. He reasons that the higher cost of healthcare was correlated with (1) overutilization of health services prescribed by attending physicians, (2) excessive entrepreneurial practices by local physicians (lots of privately owned healthcare facilities and diagnostic services), and (3) a general lack of accountability throughout the healthcare system to ensure a balance between quality and cost-effectiveness of service delivery.

Gawande's article about healthcare practices in McAllen also highlights a couple of important ethical considerations that he gleaned from interviews with local healthcare professionals who were actually disillusioned about the strong for-profit mentality in this Texas border community:

1. About fifteen years ago, it seems, something began to change in McAllen. A few leaders of local institutions took profit growth to be a legitimate ethic in the practice of medicine. Not all the doctors accepted this. But they failed to discourage those who did. So here, along the banks of the Rio Grande, in the Square Dance Capital of the World, a medical community came to treat patients the way subprime-mortgage lenders treated home buyers - as profit centers.
2. When you look across the spectrum from Grand Junction to McAllen – and the almost threefold difference in the cost of care – you come to realize that we are witnessing a battle for the soul of American medicine. Somewhere in the United States at this moment, a patient with chest pain, or tumor, or a cough is seeing a doctor. And the damning question we have to ask is whether the doctor is set up to meet the needs of the patient, first and foremost, or to maximize revenue. (pp. 8 and 10).

These are profound observations about healthcare services and medical professionals in these two demographically similar Texas communities.

President Barack Obama referenced Dr. Gawande's article about the excessive cost of healthcare in McAllen, Texas at one point his town-hall forum at Northern Virginia Community College in Annandale during his broadcast to the nation. He was responding to a comment made by a Texas physician who took issue about the role of medical malpractice insurance in the rising cost of healthcare. The physician's contention was that defensive medicine (overutilization of services) was being practiced to protect physicians from outrageous malpractice judgments – this was the main culprit for rising healthcare costs in America. Citing the case of McAllen, Texas, President Obama retorted that the real culprit behind excessive healthcare costs was directly attributed to the variation in physician practice patterns, and was not caused by the threat of malpractice suits. President Obama went on to emphasize that his administration was committed to bring about comprehensive healthcare reform that would incentivize providers and insurers to focus more attention on health improvement and prevention for all Americans, as well as drive down the overall cost of healthcare. President Obama stated that healthcare reform was "a moral imperative." President Obama urged Americans to pressure their Congressional representatives to pass healthcare reform legislation during the 2009-2010 Congressional session. Two significant statements stood out in President Obama's July 1st town-hall address -- first, what did President Obama actually mean by his reference to healthcare reform being "a moral imperative;" and second, did he truly believe that an appeal to the American people urging them to contact their Congressional legislators to approve a comprehensive reform bill would actually result in the approval of basic universal coverage for all Americans – or was this simply political rhetoric?

In a follow-up article on June 23, 2009, Gawande reiterated that "the cause that I found locally [in McAllen, Texas] was a system of care that was highly fragmented for patients and often driven to maximize revenues over patient needs" (p. x). Responding to critics of his June 1st account in *The New Yorker*, Gawande presented additional information about McAllen and El Paso that showed that "by any measure, McAllen's poverty and poor health fails to account for its differences from El Paso," and that healthcare expenditures were virtually the same in both places during the early 1990s. Things have not changed much population-wise since that period, except for overutilization of health resources, reiterated Gawande.

Case Study #3

On another important healthcare front, most healthcare advocacy groups are classified by the Internal Revenue Service (IRS) as not-for-profit organizations that are supported by membership dues paid by providers – hospitals, insurance companies, surgery centers, home health agencies, various physician specialty groups, information technology firms, etc. Advocacy organizations do not offer direct healthcare services or treat patients. Their mission is to serve the needs of their members and primarily monitor and influence national and local legislation in an effort to preserve the status quo (most advocacy groups also provide policy support and practice guidelines services to their members). The leadership teams of these non-profit advocacy groups and associations can command hefty compensation packages, which recently raised the eyebrows of the public and government officials; *Modern Healthcare* summarized the compensation packages paid to executives of major healthcare advocacy organizations in 2006 and 2007 (Carlson, 2009). These figures were obtained from the healthcare associations' published annual reports furnished to the IRS's on Form 990.[28] *Modern Healthcare* wrote:

---

[28] The Form 990 is required of not-for-profits describing operations, revenue and expenses filed with the Internal Revenue Service every tax year.

Of the $1.5 trillion in revenue collected by all not-for-profits in 2007, about 60% of that went to healthcare organizations, which includes hospitals and health systems as well as associations and societies that support them…By comparison, the second-most-lucrative category of tax-exempt organizations is education, which accounted for only 17% of the total revenue. (pp. 24-29)

Concerning specific association executives' compensations, *Modern Healthcare* noted that the "high executive salaries reported by some of the healthcare associations probably reflect the high visibility of the industry they serve, particularly in light of the ongoing reform efforts (these comments were attributed to Linda Lampkin, research director at the Economic Research Institute in Washington, DC). Table 5 displays the executive compensation packages for the top ten income earners at healthcare advocacy organizations in 2007 totaling $15.5 million. The entire group of association executives "received an average salary of $640,162, a 23% increase over the previous year." The report did not include the compensation for the rest of the not-for-profit associations' senior-management team, which would add substantially to the overall total.

Table 5 – Health Association's Executive Compensation: 2007

2007 Health Association Executive Compensation Survey and Percent Change from 2006

Executive / Organization 2007 Compensation /	% Change from 2006
Scott Serota, CEO, Blue Cross and Blue Shield Association, Chicago	$2,611,116 / 7.8%
C. Duane Dauner, CEO, California Hospital Association, Sacramento	$2,403,669 / 236.0%
Kenneth Raske, CEO, Greater New York Hospital Association, New York	$1,746,000 / 4.9%
Karen Ignagni, CEO, America's Health Insurance Plans, Washington	$1,619,377 / 16.4%
James Castle, CEO, Ohio Hospital Association, Columbus	$1,451,557 / 128.4%
Richard Umbdenstock, CEO, American Hospital Association, Chicago	$1,342,173 / NA
Dennis O'Leary, CEO, Joint Commission on Accreditation on Healthcare Organizations, Oakbrook Terrace, Il	$1,174,446 / 37.8%
Spencer Johnson, CEO, Michigan Health & Hospital Association, Lansing	$1,133,867 / 2.5%
Chip Kahn, CEO, Federation of American Hospitals, Washington	$1,068,449 / 6.9%
Carolyn Scanlan, CEO, Hospital and Health System Association of Pennsylvania, Harrisburg	$955,300 / 9.2%

Source: Modern Healthcare, Special Report, April 27, 2009, p. 25.

Discussion

These three anecdotes were presented for the purpose of highlighting the moral shortcomings of our present healthcare system that poorly defines the purpose and primary goal for healthcare organizations in the US What should the corporate objective for healthcare providers be in America – should it be structured to generate as much profit as possible for its "stakeholders," or is the main goal to offer the most comprehensive, effective, and highest-quality care to needy patients? These examples of corporate abuse and profiteering within the healthcare industry justify the need to enforce reasonable parameters for personal gain derived from businesses that are largely supported by public funds. Few rational people would disagree with the statement that these three case studies represent extreme abuses in our healthcare system. Unfortunately, they also represent a tendency in the healthcare industry to pressure executives to generate as much profit or excess revenue as possible without regard to the overall impact on health status improvement of the populations these organizations were established to serve.

If healthcare is to be considered a limited human right, and healthcare providers are expected to enhance the overall population's wellbeing, then the ground rules of the game must be changed from the traditional market-driven commodity and/or profit-making business approach. It seems evident that the healthcare industry has had few incentives to police itself. The types of problems described in these three case studies are the manifestation of a much larger set of issues and problems, according to Milton Fisk (2000). Fisk attributes these situations to a lack of *political morality*. Until there is a much clearer definition of the social and moral goals associated with health and healthcare in the US, these types of problems (selfishness, excessive profiteering, and corporate abuses of the system) will continue to proliferate. Fisk discusses the root cause of these healthcare challenges from a political morality aspect:

> *Social goals give a direction to appeals for action coming from a political morality; concern for others is needed to have a motive for advancing social goals, which here are adopted for changing the way a people live together. Such goals can be realized only by a type of cooperation that involves concern for others. This might seem like a very strong condition to put on social goals and political morality because under it social goals would become irrelevant for purely self-interested agents, as would political morality…My argument will support the view that the [healthcare] system must be a public good (p. 14 and 88).*

The concerns alluded to in this section about abuses of power in the healthcare system relate to appropriateness of channeling huge sums of public tax dollars and monetary subsidies to individuals and stockholders instead of directing the money for essential patient care. After all, American taxpayers presently fund nearly 60% of the nation's healthcare tab through Medicare, Medicaid, and other federally subsidized programs (Mahar, 2006). Is there a *moral* issue to be addressed here?

Why The United States Healthcare System Should Be A Limited Human Right For All

There are several bona fide, profit-oriented business systems operating throughout the United States and the world. Most serve a beneficial human purpose. Yet other business enterprises can be viewed as immoral and detrimental to society (pp. 3-20). The purpose of the discussion in this section is to highlight the foundational difference for society between healthcare in the US and other market-driven ventures. If we choose to classify healthcare:

- As a market-driven commodity – *it remains a profit making business.*
- As a foundational element of US society – *it is transformed into a public good.*

Economists Cowan and Rizzo (1995) present an objective essay about the pros and cons of "whether [business] profits and profit-making are moral or immoral" (p. 2). They underscore in their introductory remarks that successful businesses in a capitalistic society thrive on profits, and "that the moral status of profits is a complex issue, understanding of which demands examination both of profits and of aspects of morality" (p. 17). Their book presents two specific chapters dealing with the subject of *normal* business profits:[29] (1) the nature of profits by Israel Kirzner, (pp. 22-47), and (2) the cultural justification of unearned income, or distributive justice, by Robert Cooter and James Gordley (pp. 150-175). We will briefly consider how these two concepts fit with a profit-making mentality in the US healthcare industry.

Kirzner reviewed various theories advanced by scholars that described how justly-earned profits emerge in a normal business environment. There are two widely accepted economic axioms addressing ethical profit making in business, according to Kirzner. First, there is the notion of *sweat equity*, which entitles an individual to profit from the benefits of her labor – a just wage or salary for one's individual efforts. Second, there is the commonly accepted notion of the *symbolic* fruit-of-a-tree that is owned by an individual and should rightly yield a profit to its owner. In both these instances, profit-making is ethically appropriate. There is another instance described by Kirzner that applies to the nature of "pure economic profit" derived not necessarily from one's sweat or either from the fruit-of-a-tree, but instead it is generated from the entrepreneurial circumstance itself. In this situation "understanding the economic nature of pure entrepreneurial profit may well open up fresh insights concerning the ethical acceptability of business profits as broadly understood in everyday discourse" (p. 22). In the latter instance, one cannot attribute the nature of pure entrepreneurial profit to either of the aforementioned ethically acceptable profit-making conditions; there is *no* implicit connection between the entrepreneurial profit generation and the justification for such an entitlement (i.e., in the case of windfall profits). Of course, scarcity of resources, degree of risk, luck, future insight, leadership

---

[29] Cowan and Rizzo defined: "Normal profits are the return to the owner of a firm that operates in a perfectly competitive market, in long-run equilibrium…when a firm maximizes profits, each factor of production will receive a per unit payment exactly equal to what it produces at the margin." See p. 3.

qualities, state of disequilibrium conditions (untapped opportunities awaiting discovery), relative supply and demand, and market conditions are a few other key variables that influence the general level and sustainability of entrepreneurial profit-making (pp. 27-41). Kirzner defends the position that there is a role within distributive justice theory for accepting pure entrepreneurial profit as an acceptable ethical condition in society:

> *It is our position, indeed, that in confining attention to the issue of how given output, or given resources, are to be justly distributed, theorists of economic justice have illegitimately blocked from consideration a most important series of possibilities. These possibilities arise out of the circumstance that, in the real world or open-ended uncertainty, an enormous contribution to the total size of output is made by those whose alertness has brought to society's attention the availability of resources, the availability of techniques, and the desirability to consumers of specific kinds of output. Appropriate rewards (and incentives) for this kind of contribution requires that we step outside the framework of a given available set of goodies that must be shared out...The theory of pure profit outlined in this chapter finds its place in such a broader-gauged approach to economic justice. (p. 47)*

How does economic theory apply to profit-making (or excess margin) in the US healthcare industry? Overall, Kirzner's broader-gauged approach to economic justice generally does relate to the healthcare industry from a theoretical standpoint. However, profit-making in healthcare should not supersede the notion that it is wrong for providers and insurers to deliberately exclude any particular population group requiring basic health services; those people should not be excluded due to an economic hardship or the excessive cost of health insurance protection, as is the case for millions of uninsured and underinsured consumers.

> *For [Frank H.] Knight luck is a decisive factor generating profit; for [Ludwig von] Mises superior vision is the decisive factor in the grasping of pure profit...We wish to insist that a third possible source of economic gain, a source entailing ethical implications of an entirely different character, must be recognized. This source is deliberate human discovery, not to be attributed to unaided luck but (at least in part) to the alert attitude on the part of the discoverer. It is the alertness of human beings that enables them to notice and profit from what they find."*
>
> BY ISRAEL M. KIRZNER, IN PROFITS AND MORALITY, 1995

My contention is that if healthcare were considered a public service entity, then the entire healthcare industry and the taxpayers would have an ethical and moral responsibility to *reinvest* a substantial portion of the profits or excess margins generated from caring for the sick in order to improve the wellbeing of the community. Applying the "fruit-of-a-tree" concept to healthcare would encourage the development of initiatives that actually enhance the community's health status in the same manner that our nation regards basic education as a right for all American children for the benefit of future generations.

The healthcare industry's vested interest in *growing* the business of sick care for the sake of pure profit-making seems contradictory to the philosophical goal of fostering a healthier and more productive nation. When individual corporate leaders[30] and stockholders siphon off excessive profits outside of the healthcare system, it prevents society from improving the health status of the nation. This concept is especially valid if the corporate strategy also supports policies that deliberately exclude caring for government-funded and indigent patients. Unless healthcare's economic incentives for providers are radically changed (the paradigm shift alluded to above), the consequence of fostering a mentality of profiting from sick care will ultimately push the US in the direction of declining social and economic conditions; our healthcare system does not seem to fit the normal entrepreneurial models outlined by Kirzner.

Turning to the article by Cooter and Gordley (1995) in *Profits and Morality*, their contention is that (1) socio-cultural activities and (2) business ventures do not have the same utility and moral purposes for society. Referring to the original Aristotelian grouping of mankind's activities, the authors discuss the intrinsic nature of *liberal* and *illiberal* activities in society (p. 151). In the case of liberal activities, they exist "for their own sake, independent of any further end to be achieved" (i.e. poetry, philosophy, and athletics). On the flip side, illiberal activities are engaged in only for the sake of their effects (e.g., medicine, masonry, agriculture, etc.), and without these fundamental activities, human life would extinguish altogether. This was Aristotle's basis for believing that "disparities in the value of actions ultimately justifies disparities in wealth and power [social inequalities]", noted Cooter and Gordley (p. 152). In keeping with these Aristotelian principles, limited resources allocation (or redistribution and rationing) in a democratic society is subject to the degree of *equality* and *liberty* of its members (p. 166). Practically, these principles are rebalanced due to (1) the tension that emerges between freedom in the economic sphere and equality; (2) preservation of incentives for savings, investments, and risk-taking all require unequal wealth; and (3) the intrinsic value perceived by society of certain non-economic activities like liberal education and the arts. The evolution of major political and economic theories since the

---

30 According to the Securities and Exchange Commission filings for 2007 and 2008, certain for-profit healthcare leaders earned the following total compensation packages (annual salaries, deferred comp, bonus (exercised stock options): Wayne Smith, CEO, Community Health Systems, $9.8 million – 2007 and $13,943,867 – 2008, respectively; Alan Miller, CEO, Universal Health Services, 8.5 million and $7,00,312; Trevor Fetter, CEO Tenet Healthcare Corp., $7.5 million and $8,657,735; Ronald Williams, CEO Aetna Insurance, $43 million and $10,762,798; H. Edward Hanway, CEO Cigna Corp. (Insurance), $31 million and $10,216,798; Michael McCallister, CEO Human (Insurance), $24.5 million and $2,387,670; Steven Shulman, CEO Magellan Health Services, $32.2 million and $3,517,875; Kent Thiry, CEO DaVita (Dialysis), $22.9 million and 10,579,827; and John Byrnes, CEO Lincare Holdings, $16.7 million and $11,709,723.

time of Aristotle have followed both distinctive and intertwined paths, described Cooter and Gordley:

According to the utilitarian tradition, the value of something is the total pleasure that individuals obtain from it…according to the market tradition, the value of something is the total amount that individuals are willing to pay for it." (p. 157).

Utilitarian advocates argue that income redistribution and equal access to basic necessities of life (through income taxation for social services, the arts, and socialized medicine for instance) are justified because the "value of wealth is the pleasure it affords to people." *Market-based* advocates, on the other hand, claim there is no way to adequately measure the actual value of wealth among different groups from an economic viewpoint and, therefore, it is best for the government to stay clear of the redistribution of income dilemma and "give the individual the greatest liberty and wealth to satisfy his private preferences." Market economists evidently prevailed during the mid-20th Century when the American industrial revolution took hold, and the private and public sectors solidified their respective roles in society. The authors assert:

The modern case for economic equality rests upon the belief that equal is fair. Opposed to it is the belief that exchange should be free and free exchange is efficient. Thus the modern debate about redistribution turns upon the ideals of equality, liberty, and efficiency. The ancient debate, however, focused more on cultural values. The best should have more, according to the ancient argument, for the sake of cultural excellence. We have tried to rethink the cultural argument for unearned income in order to situate it in a Democratic society. (p. 172)

Freedom of choice and the acquisition of wealth (capitalism) have been the driving forces of American democracy and represent common measures of personal success in a market-driven economy.

The literature reviewed during the preparation of this book did not justify *extraordinary* entrepreneurial profiteering and personal acquisition of wealth as a result of denying necessary healthcare services to the needy. Healthcare is perceived as a vital service that improves the health status of society. It stands to reason that promoting an unhealthy population is a recipe for disaster for any nation. We can also deduce from the literature that universal healthcare is a logical strategy for the nation because it enhances the overall wellbeing of all citizens – to their maximum potentiality. Then why is it so difficult to adopt a policy in the United States that guarantees basic healthcare for all citizens? After all, healthier citizens are definitely more productive members of society than sickly ones. Healthier individuals ultimately consume fewer medical resources, which also saves public and private dollars (Fisk, 2000). There are many economic advantages to offer everyone reasonable access the basic healthcare services in the long run.

If one accepts the premise that healthcare in the United States *should* be a limited human right for all, it is also necessary to realize that the implementation of such a paradigm shift must be grounded in the moral principles of democracy, fairness, distributive justice, and shared responsibility for funding such a system. The overarching challenge for policymakers is to address the dichotomy of the US healthcare system being a *commodity* versus a *public good*. The next priority is to determine what truly constitutes *basic* healthcare services. Perhaps the most politically and morally charged issue is how (methodologies, criteria, policies, regulations, etc.) policymakers should *limit* or *ration* healthcare services, since national funding for foundational services are finite. Finally, it will be critical to ascertain who should administer and oversee the healthcare distribution process and regulate unreasonable profiteering from the sick care system.

Seven

TWO CONTRASTING APPROACHES FOR PROVIDING UNIVERSAL HEALTH COVERAGE

Let us take a look at a couple of examples of applied universal healthcare administered by public bodies and their attempts to address the moral and ethical challenges of health improvement and maintenance – The Netherlands and Oregon, US

7.1 -- The Dutch Health System Experience

In this first example, we review with work of Hank A.M.J. ten Have (1993)[31], who discusses the process of resource allocation of health services in The Netherlands starting in the 1970s. The Dutch government has been grappling with the development and implementation of the basic principles by which a state-run universal health system's insurance program would be "conducted in a social context in which two [ethical] values – *solidarity* and *equity* – are generally accepted as fundamental" (p. 43). The Dutch health system covers all its citizens on a cost basis, proportional to an individual's income level, although a parallel private insurance system is also available for those who want and can afford it. *Equity* refers to the philosophical belief that everyone in the community is entitled to basic health services. *Solidarity* places the responsibility of paying for universal healthcare and social securing on the people through the government by means of a relatively high taxation rate (36% of wages). During the past 25 years, the publicly-funded healthcare system in The Netherlands has faced increasing pressure to balance the breadth of services with growing utilization (associated with the aging of the population and increasing demand for health services due to chronic and degenerative illnesses among seniors) and the rapidly rising cost to tax payers to support their system. The Dutch government has also

---
[31] Henk A.M.J. ten Have is Professor with the Department of Ethics, Philosophy and History of Medicine, Catholic University of Nijmegen, The Netherlands.

faced the ethical dilemma of rationing certain healthcare services using the subsequent criteria for making *fair* choices:

> *The starting-point for the Committee's [Committee for Choices in Health Care appointed by the Dutch State Secretary for Welfare, Health and Cultural Affairs, in August 1990] argument is the proposition that everyone who needs health care must be able to obtain it. However, equal access to health care should not be determined by demands but needs. In order to have just distribution of services, it is not important that all services are equally accessible, what is crucial is what services are accessible. Not every health care service is equally relevant for maintaining or restoring health. It is important to identify 'basic care', 'essential services' or 'core health services' focused on basic health care needs in contradistinction to individual preferences, demands or wants. (p. 45)*

This approach for determining what constitutes *basic* and *necessary* health services relates to works of philosopher Norman Daniels (1985), who classifies *appropriate* healthcare as that which "enables persons to maintain a normal range of opportunities to realize their life plans in a given society." The appropriateness of healthcare distribution was evaluated by the Committee using three distinctive yet interrelated approaches:

- *The individual approach* – mainly self-determined.
- *The medical professional approach* – defined by the medical profession as being free from disease.
- *The community-oriented approach* – determined in the context of specific (and changing) normative and socio-economic values and expectations espoused by the Dutch society.

Ten Have explains that the Dutch *normative framework* dictated how the healthcare system would be divided into three descending levels of providers: (1) facilities dedicated to the frail and disabled (custodial care), (2) facilities designed in the implementation to maximize wellness and restorative care (acute and emergent care), and (3) facilities for disease management and triage (p. 46). In this system, solidarity implied that the autonomous individual learned to recognize that his own interests are best served by promoting the common good, and placing needs before wants as it related to rationing basic health services in The Netherlands.

In another article on the Dutch health system, Hub Zwart (1993)[32] talks about the ethical dilemmas associated with healthcare *rationing* in The Netherlands. The debate over basic health care and rationing pivoted on two opposing ethical beliefs: i.e., *liberalism* and *communitarianism*, according to Zwart. In the case of liberalism, advocates "consider the individuals as a moral

---

32 Hub Zwart is Professor of Philosophy with the Centre for Ethics, Catholic University of Nijmegen, The Netherlands.

agent who should define his own moral goals and design his personal life plan." The *communitarianism faction* held that "the moral community provides the individual with a moral 'space' in which he inevitably finds himself located, and from which he derives the resources by means of which moral problem-situations can be evaluated" (pp. 53-54). The Committee followed a quasi-communitarianism (although there are also vestiges of liberal perspectives in the implementation of rationing) philosophy when they adopted the foundational elements of the Dutch health care system, called the community-oriented approach (p. 54). Zwart points out that the citizens, either explicitly or tacitly, consented to the community-oriented approach in order for the government to be able to implement the rationing system. Referring to comments about maximizing the *good life*, Zwart explains that "traditional views on human existence often contain some notion of a natural life span [intrinsic limits to human life]… at old age, death should no longer be considered a tragedy that is to be postponed at all costs… [rather, it] should be the final chapter of a full and meaningful file" (p. 55). This did not signify that the Dutch system sanctioned withholding medical care to older persons because their benefit to society was less meaningful than for younger persons. Zwart elaborates:

> *The Committee, however, rejects this view [of withholding medical services to the elderly], claiming that it 'would conflict with the universal right to self-determination.' Every individual patient is to decide for himself at what moment his life can be considered complete. On this issue, the Committee clings to a liberal perspective on health care. (p. 56)*

Although rationing seems to be an inevitable part of any universal health system because of the need for governmental cost-containment and exponential demand for finite resources, the process for implementing any definitive selection criteria is always problematic. In the first place, there is the challenge of dealing with individual rights of self-determination, which can often conflict with the *greater good* concept. Secondly, it seems arbitrary and capricious to draw a line in the sand and establish categorical and impersonal criteria for determining who should live or die based on chronological age or some other nominal standard. Nonetheless, it is a fact of life that most health resources that an individual will consume in a lifetime occur in the final two to three years of life. It seems wasteful from a societal viewpoint to expend extraordinary measures in order to extend an individual's life beyond a "reasonable" point (whom is qualified to determine what is reasonable?). According to Zwart, "in the life history of an elderly patient a point may emerge where the inclination to intervene should give way to the readiness to accept."

Despite the lively political debate about fair criteria and the necessity for rationing healthcare in The Netherlands, the Committee has yet to devise a *morally acceptable* formula for dispensing services that are considered relevant for maintaining or restoring health (Have, 1993). The Committee's failure to implement a basic healthcare plan for universal coverage in The Netherlands, including a balanced allocation of resources and fiscal controls, will undoubtedly result in mandatory rationing for the entire population. Ten Have states that the per capita health costs have steadily climbed during the past 25 years by an annual factor of 0.6%. He stands by his earlier contention that "in The Netherlands the main issue has not been the question of how to distribute scarce resources, but how to find a [new] balance between individual interests and the general welfare [state]." (p. 43)[33]

Although policymakers in The Netherlands have deemed healthcare a social and moral right for its citizens, so far they have not established a functional and rational methodology for implementing an equitable policy that offers both *basic health services* and *financial constraints* relative to the nation's healthcare providers and consumers.

Table 6 – By the Numbers- How the US Compares with Other Developed Nations

BY THE NUMBERS / How the U.S. compares

How the U.S. health care system stacks medical indicators:

	USA	Germany	Sweden	Canada	Italy
Percentage of health expenses as a share of gross domestic product, 2007	16%	10.4%	9.1%	10.1%	8.7%
Percentage of health expenses paid with public funds, 2007	45.4%	76.9%	81.7%	70%	76.5%
Life expectancy at birth, 2009[1] (in years)	78.1	79.3	80.9	81.2	80.2
Infant mortality rate per 1,000 live births, 2009[1]	6.3	4	2.8	5	5.5
Uninsured population, 2007	15.1%[5]	0.2%	0%	0%	0%[3]
Percentage of people who want to completely change the health care system, 2008	33%	17%	NA	12%[2]	20%
Inpatient surgical procedures per 1,000 population, 2004	90	79	62	45	53
Hospital bed occupancy, 2005	67%	76%	NA	90%	76%

1–estimate; 2–2007; 3–2006; 4–2002; 5–2008   Sources: McKinsey; The Commonwealth Fund; Organization for Economic Cooperation and Development

	Spain	Australia	Netherlands	United Kingdom	France
Percentage of health expenses as a share of gross domestic product, 2007	8.5%	8.7%[3]	9.8%[3]	8.4%	11%[1]
Percentage of health expenses paid with public funds, 2007	71.8%	67.7%[5]	62.5%[4]	81.7%	79%
Life expectancy at birth, 2009[1] (in years)	80.1	81.6	79.4	79	81
Infant mortality rate per 1,000 live births, 2009[1]	4.2	4.8	4.7	4.9	3.3
Uninsured population, 2007	1.7%[3]	0%[5]	1.4%	0%	0.1%
Percentage of people who want to completely change the health care system, 2008	12%	18%[2]	9%[2]	15%	15%
Inpatient surgical procedures per 1,000 population, 2004	51	51	40	63	NA
Hospital bed occupancy, 2005	71.6%	71%	64%	84%	75%

1–estimate; 2–2007; 3–2006; 4–2002; 5–2008   ent; Central Intelligence Agency; The Harris Poll; Spanish Ministry of Health and Consumer Affairs; U.S. Census

Source: *USA Today*, September 23, 2009, 7E; McKinsey; The Commonwealth Fund; Organization for Economic Cooperation and Development; US Central Intelligence Agency; The Harris Poll; Spanish Ministry of Health and Consumer Affairs; and US Census Bureau.

---

[33] This conclusion was part of his early work published in 1988 (pp. 23-39), Ethics and economics in health care: A medical philosopher's view; in *Medical ethics and economics in healthcare*, ed. By G. Mooney and A. McGuire, Oxford: Oxford University Press.

Compared to the US, The Netherlands spends 6.2% less of their GDP on healthcare, enjoys slightly higher life expectancy at birth (2009), has a significantly lower infant mortality, and has only 1.4% uninsured population. The Dutch circumstance is very similar to other European nations as well as Canada, according to an analysis published by *USA Today* on September 23, 2009 (Table 6) in a special issue on healthcare compiled from various reliable government and institutional think tanks. It is noteworthy that 9% of the population remains unsatisfied with the healthcare system in The Netherlands.

7.2 -- The Oregon Health Program Experience

> *Is it better to let hundreds of thousands of impoverished Oregonians go without health care or to insure more people but limit their benefits? Oregon chose the latter course, using the world's first Prioritized List of Health Services that remains the only one in the US today. It limits services to those that are most effective and draws a "line" to keep services within available budget dollars.*
>
> BY OREGON DIVISION OF MEDICAL ASSISTANCE PROGRAMS, DRAFT NEWS RELEASE, NOVEMBER 6, 2008

While the overall healthcare system in the United States is based on a free-market competitive philosophy, several individual states have devised sub-systems in an effort to deal with unique economic constraints fueled by swelling numbers of uninsured and underinsured residents. The states' governmental burden and runaway costs for maintaining the Medicaid program covering lower-income families (mothers and children) limits other key social services that are considered critical to the wellbeing of the community-at-large (i.e., education, public safety, sanitation, transportation, etc.).

Oregon was the first state (and remains the only state) in the nation to publically tackle the moral and economic challenges of allocating basic healthcare services to the poor on a formal and prioritized list over the past twenty years. The controversial Medicaid *rationing* program was part of the enactment of the *Oregon Basic Health Services Act of 1989*. After approximately five years of public and political debate, the State of Oregon implemented the *Prioritized List of Health Services* for its Medicaid population. The program is administered by the Oregon Health Services Commission (OHSC).[34]

The methodology employed by the OHSC in 1991 was originally based on Kaplan's *Quality of Well-Being Scale* (QWB) "because it appeared to encompass considerations of total health

---

[34] Personal discussions in April 2009 with Darren Coffman, Executive Director of the Oregon Health Services Commission, Office for Oregon Health Policy and Research, (503) 373-1616.

which was data and values driven" (Brannigan, 1993). The program has effectively enabled policymakers and regulators to introduce a measured "control" mechanism on the rising cost of Medicaid services in Oregon, yet extend coverage to about 120,000 additional beneficiaries compared to the guidelines of the traditional federal-state program, emphasized Darren Coffman, a twenty-year veteran and senior staff for the 11-member Health Services Commission. Coffman recently clarified that "the introduction of the list caused about a five-percent shift of the cost curve downward after it was introduced, then other cost drivers kept the curve moving up at the same rate it would have taken without the list in place from that point on."[35]

The problems associated with rationing certain health care services continued to intensify because of treatment of a wider range of catastrophic medical circumstances than was anticipated early on, since current ethical and medical standards demanded saving lives at any cost. For instance, organ transplantation services, trauma and burn centers, care for premature newborns, all run into the hundreds of thousands of dollars' range, according to the American Hospital Association. This example highlights a complex moral dilemma: who is adequately qualified to make these inevitably complex healthcare rationing decisions -- the individual; healthcare professionals; ethicists; politicians; or society, through government regulatory institutions?

Brannigan (1993) evaluated *Oregon's Experiment* during its inception. His analysis is "primarily a descriptive [report] aiming to provide a clear synopsis of the Oregon project's history, complex methodology, and strengths and weaknesses" (p. 15). A brief recapitulation of Brannigan's findings should be helpful to better understand the underlying technical, moral, and ethical concerns that Oregon policymakers wrestled with during the formative stages of Oregon's healthcare rationing program implemented in 1994.

The concept of rationing health services to Medicaid enrollees emerged from the proceedings of the *1982 Governor's Conference on Health Care for the Medically Poor*. The task of developing a fair process and rational criteria for apportioning healthcare resources within the Oregon Medicaid program was assigned to a voluntary group called the Oregon Health Decisions, Inc. (OHD). The OHD involved approximately 5,000 participants in over 300 public forums throughout the state. Their report, *Society Must Decide*, concluded that "health care rationing, cost containment, and health resources allocation were seen, first and foremost, as community matters" (p. 15). This *grass-roots* initiative guided the entire evolution of Oregon's universal access and distribution of finite health services to the state's Medicaid population after the adoption of three legislative bills mandating the provision of basic health care services to nearly all of the uninsured (p. 17).[36] These three interrelated bills constituted the *Oregon Basic Health Services Act* (OBHSA), which was approved by the state legislature and became law in July 1989.

---

[35] Personal correspondence from Darren Coffman on May 26, 2009.
[36] The three bill included SB 27, the Basic Health Benefits Act, SB 534, the State Health Risk Pool, and SB 935, the Health Insurance Partnership Act.

Since this unprecedented state legislation also affected Oregon's participation in the federal Medicaid program, which funded a large portion of the program, it required a *waiver* of certain guidelines stipulated by the US Department of Health and Human Services (DHHS). The OBHSA did not become operational until January 1, 1994.[37] The OBHSA established an eleven-member Health Services Commission to oversee the operation of the Oregon Health Plan. Brannigan clarifies:

The fundamental axiom underlying the OBHSA is that all persons have a right to basic health care, that 'floor beneath which no person should fall'...Its prioritized listing is a formative step requiring constant monitoring and reassessment. The Health Services Commission's 1991 report, Prioritization of Health Services, describes the list as a 'prototype for ensuing development and refinement of the prioritization process.' (pp. 15-32)

The initial methodology proposed for creating the prioritized list of services covered by the Oregon Medicaid Program was based on three guiding principles: (1) use of empirical data of medical effectiveness of treatment, (2) degree of effect on the quality of life of the individual, and (3) compliance with healthcare values from the community's perspective. According to Coffman, the following guidelines were used to develop the *blueprint* for healthcare delivery to Medicaid participants in Oregon:

- All citizens should have universal access to basic level of care.
- Society is responsible for financing care for poor people.
- There must be a process to define a "basic" level of care.
- The process must be based on criteria that are publicly debated, reflect a consensus of social values, and consider the good of society as a whole.
- The healthcare delivery system must encourage use of services and procedures which are effective and appropriate, and discourage over-treatment.
- Healthcare is one important factor affecting health; funding for healthcare must be balanced with other programs which also affect health.
- Funding must be explicit and economically sustainable.
- There must be clear accountability for allocating resources and for the human consequences of funding decisions (personal communication).

As noted above, one of the original assessment tools for determining the overall impact of health services on the wellbeing of Oregonians was the adoption of Kaplan's QWB methodology. The

---

[37] The Oregon Plan was approved by Donna Shalala, Secretary of the US Health and Human Services, on March 19, 1993.

QWB approach was used because it combined both a data and a values-measurement system. Without getting into the intricacies of the prioritization methodology, disease and treatment groupings were categorized into three broad ranges:

Categories 1 to 9 (highest priority) – essential health services
Categories 10 to 13 -- very important health services
Categories 14 to 17 – health services important to certain individuals

Preventable or readily treatable conditions automatically were given higher priority on the list. In May 1991, the OHSC released its first prioritization list, containing 709 items. The Oregon legislature reviewed the list and was able to fund items one through 587 based on available resources – referred to as the *cut-off line*. "Net benefits and medical effectiveness were arrived at by considering, in order of descending priority, the treatment's ability to (1) maintain life, (2) restore one to an asymptomatic state, (3) be cost effective, and (4) be consistent with community values," notes Brannigan (p. 25).

However, Coffman clarified in recent correspondence that this methodology was never actually implemented and is not significant from a historical perspective. He further stated that the methodology that was finally approved resulted in the prioritized list implemented in February 1994, providing this services prioritization: (1) the treatment's ability to prevent death and (2) treatment cost. Subsequently, the Health Services Commission moved 75% of the lines based on one or more *subjective criteria* crafted primarily from the public values comments [gathered during the hearings].[38]

Bob DiPrete and Darren Coffman (2007) recount the historical progression of Oregon's health services prioritization on the OHSC web site: "The strategy was to move away from 'rationing' by excluding people from health coverage or reducing access through underpayment [for Medicaid eligible persons]" (p. 2.). The methodology evolved into 17 ranked categories in 1993, and eventually was pared down to nine ranked categories in 2006, with greater emphasis on preventive services and chronic disease management in order to reduce costly crisis intervention for morbidity and mortality (Oregon is the only state that allows physician assisted-suicide, legalized in 1997). DiPrete and Coffman note that "over 1.2 million Oregonians have been covered under the prioritized list" since the program was implemented in 1993 (p. 5). Although the OHSC claimed to move away from rationing health services, this novel approach is certainly intended to *rationalize* the distribution of limited health resources according to the "relative importance of a condition-treatment pair" that excludes payment for conditions ranking above the cutoff on the prioritized list (i.e., their numerical ranking is higher than the cutoff threshold); this is certainly an allocation methodology, regardless of what it has been labeled.

---

38 Personal correspondence from Darren Coffman, on May 26, 2009.

The Oregon Health Plan has elicited both praise and criticism from consumers, policymakers, healthcare providers, community leaders, and ethicists. Although the OHP admittedly has its flaws, Brannigan (1993) points out that policymakers were to be commended for going beyond an arbitrary and capricious methodology for doling out healthcare to the poor; typically, Medicaid eligibility is determined using random percentages of the federal poverty level guidelines in order to fit local available tax dollars to a distribution system at various points in time (pp. 27-28). Brannigan's assessment of Oregon's allocation approach concluded:

Oregon's strategy tackles a monumental challenge: how is it possible to expand access to quality health care and still manage to control health care spending? Yet, it struggles within the same political and economic environment from which features of the American health care crisis emanate. It ranks treatment[s] according to their overall medical effectiveness, and draws a cut-off line essentially determined by fiscal realities within a market-oriented health system. A pernicious consequence of a market-driven health care system is that it turns out to be ultimately profit-conscious with services evaluated primarily in terms of their investment return, rather than on health care needs. And problems spiral since we tend to confuse 'health care needs' with 'health-related desires.' Rationing cannot replace the circumstances which give rise to the need for rationing. (pp. 31-32)

Congressman Ron Wyden, Senior Senator from Oregon (and one of the architects of the Oregon Health Plan), shared his sentiments about the evolution of the OHP with the assembly at the Annual Public Policy Conference and Business Exposition of the Federation of American Hospitals (FAH)[39] held on March 2, 2004 (transcript by Kaisernetwork.org, Kaiser Family Foundation):[40]

Now, suffice it to say I can understand why anybody in this room or outside it would be skeptical about this or anything else that is labeled a health care reform. But I will tell you I have seen in my home state that it works to involve the public like this! How many of you have heard of the Oregon Health Plan? I can see you out there. Who's heard of the Oregon Health Plan? [Applause] We've got some Oregonians clapping. Oregon, my home state, is the first place on the planet to say that health care is a social and ethical good.

You'll never have enough money to do everything and you've got to have a debate about the kind of tough choices that I've described. That's how we built the Oregon Health Plan. It has expanded coverage significantly. It's meant a lot of people who used to have nothing now have access to a decent package of benefits and it's often described

---

[39] The Federation of American Hospitals (FAH), founded in 1966, is the national representative of investor-owned or managed community hospitals and health systems throughout the United States and one of Washington, DC's most respected and influential health policy and advocacy organizations.
[40] See http://www.kaisernetwork.org/health_cast/uploaded_files/030204_fah_transcript.pdf.

as the first health care rationing plan in America. It's not rationing because you can't ration care from people who get none. We have people who used to get nothing and after we made these tough choices, now they get access to a decent package of benefits, perhaps not everything, but a decent package of benefits.

And so what I have done, I haven't taken the whole plan—the rating of everything, 1–800 and much of what you've read about it—but the basic concept of saying that we've got to make tough choices that health care is an ecosystem and what you do in one corner will affect everything everywhere else and we've now enacted it into law with the support of the Federation. The Federation was an integral supporter of this effort early on. I'm very grateful that Chip and the Federation has been willing to think outside the box about how to pass real health care reform. (pp. 11-12)

The OHP remains in effect to this date, and the list has continued to undergo further refinements. Presently, the Plan funds 503 of the 680 conditions and treatment pairs on the prioritized list and provides basic health coverage for a significant portion of the state's indigent population that would otherwise remain uninsured because of state and federal funding shortfalls.[41] According to Coffman, "the savings to Oregon of $17.81 PMPM [per member, per month] translates to an estimated annual savings in federal funds of $48.5 million." Coffman also reveals that the *2005 Report to the National Governor's Association* demonstrates how the adoption of the OHP approach could generate savings of around $4.8 billion in healthcare savings annually for the US (pp. 4-5).

Table 7 – Current Examples of Conditions-Treatment Pairs on the OHP Prioritized List

Current Examples of Condition-Treatment Pairs on the OHP List Funded
- *Gallbladder surgery is covered for gallstones and cholecystitis, but not for asymptomatic gallstones w/o cholecystitis*
- *Any preventive service with a recommendation level of A or B from the*
- *US Preventive Services Task Force*
- *Vision exams and eyeglasses, but not contact lenses or Lasik surgery*
- *Treatment for hip fractures*
- *Treatment of HIV/AIDS*
- *Tobacco cessation services*

---

41 Personal correspondence from Darren Coffman on May 26, 2009 – "After having reached a high of nearly 120,000 expansion eligible participants, we dropped to under 18,000 about two years ago, and we are now inching our way back up (I can't find any current numbers on the web, but I think we've added about 10,000 back and the legislature is now considering a proposal to add back another 60,000+). This is in comparison to about 600,000 uninsured, so clearly a way to go. The OHP overall does cover around 450,000 though, but most would qualify under the old Medicaid rules."

Unfunded
- *Treatment of inflammatory bowel syndrome*
- *Treatment for low back pain that does not have nerve involvement (i.e., muscular)*
- *Liver transplant for cancer of the liver*
- *Bariatric surgery for morbid obesity, but is covered if in conjunction with Type II Diabetes*
- *Correction of deformities of feet that do not significantly impact ability to walk*
- *Treatment for uncomplicated hernias, unless in children*

Source: Personal correspondence from Darren Coffman on May 26, 2009.

Stephen Ayres' essay published in the *Brookings Institute's* text *Rationing America's Medical Care – The Oregon Plan and Beyond* (Strosberg, et al., 1992) echoes other physicians' reluctance to embrace the radical approach to healthcare management in Oregon. He stresses in *Rationality, Not Rationing, in Health Care* that the problems related to America's healthcare system were not directly the result of scarcity; they were the result of mal-distribution of resources. Society's insatiable quest for longevity and perfect health were the real culprits for driving up the cost of healthcare beyond reasonableness. Ayres calls for politicians to face the fact "that the United States is the only country in the developed world that does not provide health care for all its citizens" (p. 134). The government is not capable of providing *rational* rationing, Ayres contends, and notes that the personal physician must remain in control (the primary care gatekeeper concept) of the distribution of our nation's wealth of health services. Ayres wrote:

> *There must be a national health care policy, the system must be reformed, patients must receive care that they need and from which they can benefit, and there must be a single level of access and delivery of health care. The more than $700 billion of current health care costs must be reallocated in a rational way without arbitrary rationing [what would Ayres say about the $2.3 trillion healthcare bill in 2008?]. And there must be neither slaves nor slave doctors. (p. 142)*

The foundational premise for the Oregon legislature establishing the OHP was that rationing certain health services on the basis of effectiveness and benefit to Medicaid recipients was necessary in order to allow the state to place greater emphasis on preventive care and proven medical interventions. At the same time, they were also convinced that limiting payment for treatment (of certain types of sick care) that ranked lower on the *prioritization scale* as far as medical efficacy and community values would provide *more* resources to overall program participants in the long term. It seems that Oregon's policymakers are on their way to achieving the basic goals laid out for the state's healthcare reform plan – *to improve health outcomes through financing clinically effective treatments within public budgetary constraints.*

In yet another pioneering move toward universal healthcare reform, the Oregon legislature passed HB 2009 on June 11, 2009, recommending the creation of the *Oregon Health Fund Board.* Governor Ted Kulongoski praised the establishment of the Oregon Health Authority (OHA) to "transform the state's system to make quality health care accessible and affordable for *every* Oregonian…by 2015." According to Governor Kulongoski, ultimately all current state healthcare functions will fall under the auspices of the OHA. One of the main responsibilities of the newly formed OHA is to develop a *health benefit package* that will serve as a minimal guideline for the Oregon Health Insurance Exchange to be implemented by December 31, 2010. Bruce Goldberg, MD, Director of the Oregon Department of Human Services, referred to the creation of the OHA as "a historic accomplishment in health care," and exclaimed that "health care coverage is both a *moral and an economic imperative*…that will make things better in Oregon now and in the future" (2009, June 12).

On June 20, 2009, the Oregon Health Fund Board published its initial recommendations regarding the implementation of the *Essential Benefit Package* (EBP) aimed at broadening health insurance coverage to all government employees in the state. The Committee explained that the EBP "is an affordable, sustainable package of benefits which emphasizes evidence-based care provided in the integrated health home…This package would provide the foundation that defines what is considered essential coverage" (Oregon Health Fund Board, p. 1). The EBP design is predicated on a similar concept as the basic healthcare coverage advocated in this book – national healthcare reform should include a basic set of foundational or basic benefits, emphasizing preventive and wellness services, that are available universally at minimal or no cost to participants.

Eight

Sick Care vs. Preventive Health Measures

8.1 -- Health Care Equals Sick Care

Industrial nations are progressing toward a greater and greater sense of health care as a communal property.

By Melvin Konner, MD, Medicine at the Crossroads, 1993.

The World Health Organization (WHO) is the international public health agency founded by the United Nations in 1948 with headquarters in Geneva, Switzerland. WHO defines *health* as the goal of the practice of medicine. Health relates the presence or absence of somatic disease to larger concerns such as the relationship of individuals to the environment and society. Jerry Avorn (1983) argues that health is primarily regarded as *somatic* (physiological and anatomical aspects of the human body) in nature (pp. 183-197). However, Avorn comments that there are significant distinctions between what individuals actually *need* in the way of healthcare, versus their *wants*, *demands*, and *interests*.

The difficulty for healthcare practitioners is to apply scientific knowledge to the healing process and at the same time convince patients that they must use the directions to better health – through lifestyle modification, proper administration of medication, mental health initiatives, physical exercise, improved eating habits, rest and relaxation, disease prevention measures, responsible driving habits, etc. The predominant attitude of patients is that doctors can fix any problems. This is a fallacy because the patient has control over her wellbeing, not the physician. Our approach to healthcare in America is to seek medical attention *after* the fact. The "health" system is geared to care for sick people and has little, if any, incentive to maintain the health and wellbeing of the community. After all, *heads in beds* is what pays bills and generates profits. CMS reported that in 2007, national healthcare expenditures amounted to $2,241,200,000, and that government funding for public health prevention activities totaled $64 billion, or only 3 percent of the US healthcare bill (see Figure 7). This strategy is the most expensive method for promoting community health status improvement.

Of course, there is a need for an efficient and effective acute care system to treat illness and mitigate suffering and pain. There is a definite role for a first-class healthcare system that is designed to restore health to individuals (sick care). The point I am making here is that the majority of attention and funding in America has been devoted to the treatment of patients *after* the onset of disease, illness, or accidental injury. Without earlier intervention into the illness-disease cycle and preventive care, the need for more healthcare services will continue to grow exponentially.

Human beings have been preoccupied with living a healthy and productive life for as long as possible. Modern medicine has certainly contributed to improving the quality and longevity of human life around the world. In the United States, life expectancy[42] for women born in 1996 was estimated to reach an average 79 years of age; their male counterparts averaged 73 years. By comparison, the average life span in America during the mid-1800s was estimated to be 40 for women and 38 for men. The longest average life span in the developed world is found in Japan, where women born in 1993 will average 82.5 years, and men are expected to average 76 years. The 2009 worldwide average life expectancy is estimated at 65 years of age. It is recognized that the single most important factor impacting the huge jump in life expectancy is attributed to the implementation of aggressive public health measures during the 1850s through the 1950s – e.g., water purification, sanitation improvement, immunization, pasteurization, nutritional education, etc. (Garrett, 2000).

Melvin Konner, MD highlights the fact that average life expectancy is only part of the human longevity equation. In *Medicine at the Crossroads*, Konner (1993) discusses the upper limits of *long-lived people,* which is believed to be around 110 years, depending upon positive health habits and good medical care (p. 175). This being the case, there is room for improvement in the average life expectancy for Americans if they choose to foster better lifestyles and administer the best and most appropriate preventive care and medical services to all citizens. Konner questions whether people die of diseases or chronic illnesses, or if the body breaks down because of old age? Konner's quandary is an important medical concern, since future heroic measures might be able to reduce death from the top killer diseases (i.e., cardiovascular, cancer, and neurological) and ameliorate suffering from chronic illnesses through modern remedies and

---

42 The US Census Bureau tracks statistics about Americans including life expectancy – the number of years of life remaining at a given age adjusted for race, gender, socioeconomic status, geographic location, and other group characteristics (life expectancy index). Actuarial tables are generated for men and women separately.

treatment techniques (joint replacements, pain blockers, hearing / visual aids, and diabetes control). However, there is nothing medical science can do to avert death from old age (at least at this juncture of scientific knowledge). This poses a significant problem for the US healthcare system, as we are able to stretch the average life expectancy toward 100 years old because medical utilization increases exponentially as the overall population ages. The age cohort over 65 consumes nearly four times the amount of health resources than the under-65 age cohort, and most of this care is rendered in the last couple of years of life.

Chart 4 – Differential Inpatient Utilization Rates

Differential Inpatient Utilization Rates

Age Groups	Utilization Rate / 1,000 Pop
18-64	<129.0
65+	>358.8

Source: CDC, 2004

Konner warns:

> Daniel Callahan, director of the Hastings Center in New York, a think tank for biomedical ethics, has spoken out frequently on this problem…By the year 2040, it has been projected that the elderly will represent 21 percent of the population [in the United States] and consume 45 percent of all health-care expenditures. How can costs of that magnitude be borne? (p. 177)

In his epilogue, Konner offers a physician's perspective and a new way of thinking about the direction medicine Americans should strive for in the 21st century:

1. We must try to restore trust between doctor and patient.
2. A massive shift in emphasis, through both training and reimbursement, must restore a healthier balance between primary care and specialization.
3. We must overcome the tendency to see drugs as miracle cures.
4. The promise of mastery over human biology presented by the new science of genes must be pursued with exceptional caution.
5. The role of surgery and related interventions in the body must be reevaluated.
6. Our treatment of serious mental illness is both inhumane and wasteful.

7. The aging of our population is certain to supply an unending source of new and greater medical expenditures unless we begin to face some hard choices; but these choices are only more frequent for the elderly, not limited to them. (pp. 227-231)

The US Census Bureau indicated that the number of residents over the age of 100 grew dramatically from approximately 15,000 in the 1980 census to over 77,000 in 2000, a five-fold increase. It is estimated that the worldwide number of centenarians alive today exceeds the total number of persons that ever lived to be 100 during the entire history of humankind! The very-old cohort (85+ years) is the fastest growing population segment in the US The safety-net infrastructure in this country was not designed to support the needs of this special group in terms of Social Security benefits, Medicare services, assisted living, and nursing home care, in-home support systems, and so forth. In the final analysis, the term *healthcare* system is a misnomer; the US has a sophisticated and advanced *sick care* system which does a great job (at a very high cost to taxpayers) of treating patients after the onset of illness and injury.

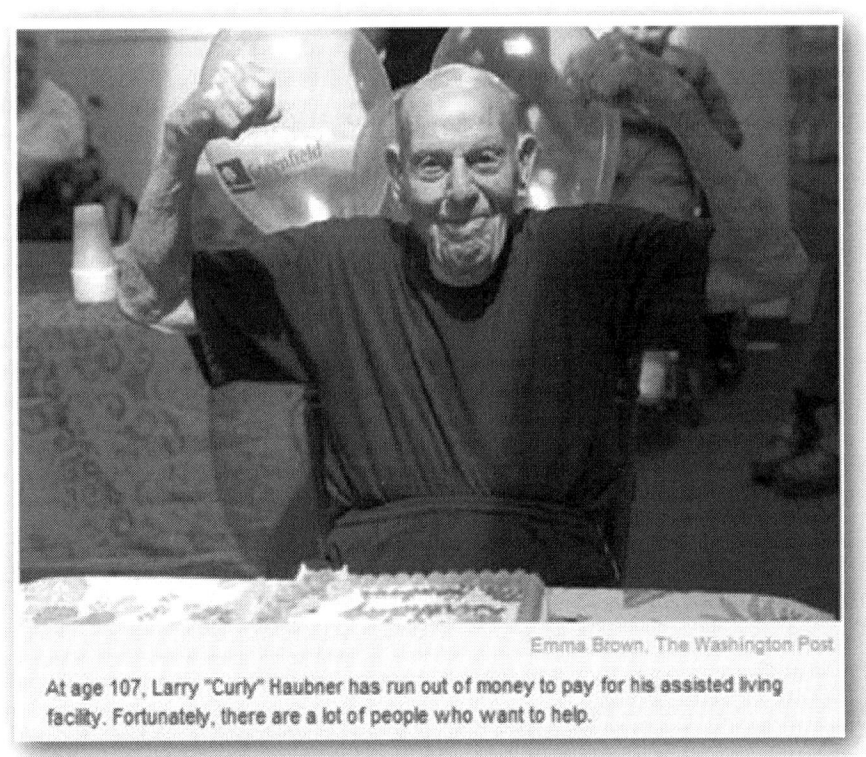

Figure 4 – Larry "Curly" Haubner at Age 107

Source: Emma Brown, *The Washington Post*. Caption – "At age 107, Larry 'Curly' Haubner has run out of money to pay for his assisted living facility. Fortunately, there are a lot of people who want to help."

8.2 -- Preventive Health Measures and ROI

America's future well-being is inextricably tied to our health.

By Trust for America's Health, July 2008 Issue Report.

Mokdad, et al. (2004) researched the principal causes of death in the United States and proved that the leading causes of mortality in 2000 were directly related to preventable health problems – i.e., tobacco smoking, poor diet and physical inactivity, and excessive drug and alcohol consumption. They argued that the findings of their study persuasively showed the need to establish a stronger preventive care orientation within health care and the public health systems in the United States. This was the exact same conclusion that Hippocrates reached way back in 400 B.C. – and that healthcare was not necessarily the state's sole responsibility. Each individual must exercise her moral obligation to maximize health status to the extent possible, within the constraints presented by our respective environmental circumstances and lifestyle habitats.

An authoritative report published in July 2009 by the *Trust for America's Health*, a non-profit advocacy organization, and the *Robert Wood Johnson Foundation*, shows how America has failed miserably regarding its epidemic of overweight and obese children and adults. The findings of this alarming report – *F as in Fat 2009: How Obesity Policies are Failing America* – found that the states in the deep-south fared much worse than other regions of the country, and also noted that Mississippi ranked among the top 3 worst states in America, with a rate of 32.5% of adults classified as obese for the fifth year in a row. Children did not fare any better than the adults; 44.4% of children ages 10 to 17 were classified as overweight or obese in Mississippi. Overall, 23 states in the US increased their adult *fat* rating, while no state showed a decline from the prior year: "in addition, the percentage of obese and overweight children is at or above 30% in 30 states," the TFAH report noted. Furthermore, researchers discovered that the Baby Boom generation turning 65 within this decade has a higher obesity rate than previous generations, which will result in serious health implications and costing Medicare dearly.

To combat this American obesity epidemic, the TFAH report recommends that the following health policy measures be implemented immediately:

- Ensure that every adult and child has access to coverage for preventive medical services, including nutrition and obesity counseling and screening for obesity-related diseases, such as type-2 diabetes.
- Increase the number of programs available in communities, schools, and childcare settings that help make nutritious foods more affordable and accessible and provide safe and healthy places for people to engage in physical activity.

- Reduce Medicare expenditures by promoting proven programs that improve nutrition and increase physical activity among adults 55 to 64.

As far as governmental institutions are concerned, there must be a better balance between (1) improving access to a wide range of healthcare services, and (2) health promotion, communicable and chronic-disease management, health education, and personal and environmental safety. The current public and private funding for healthcare disproportionately favors certain types of sick care rather than public health initiatives and prevention services. The data suggest that public health measures and preventive services deliver a big return-on-investment (ROI)! The efficacy of public health interventions was extensively evaluated by the TFAH, which published their results in a detailed report in 2008 – *Prevention for a Healthier America: Investments in Disease Prevention Yield Significant Savings and Stronger Communities* (Levi, Segal & Juliano, 2008). The TFAH's project was supported by multi-agency grants from The Robert Wood Johnson Foundation, Kaiser Foundation, The Urban Institute, US Department of Health and Human Services, CDC, and US Environmental Protection Agency. The report summarizes over 300 scientific studies focusing on health status impact and ROI pertaining to a wide range of disease prevention and health initiatives piloted across the nation. According to TFAH:

> *This study shows that the country could save substantial amounts on health care costs if we invest strategically in community-based disease prevention programs. We could see significant returns for as little as a $10 investment per person into evidence-based programs that improve physical activity and nutrition and lower smoking rates in communities. Not only could we save money, many more Americans would have the opportunity to live healthier lives...There is a wide range of other disease prevention efforts that target these and other health problems and have a beneficial impact on the health of Americans. Until the country starts making a sustained investment into disease prevention programs, we will not realize the potential savings. (p. 55)*

The US public health initiatives totaled an estimated $64.1 billion, including CDC's expenditures on public health programs at the state level. Unfortunately, this represents only about *three percent* (around $213 per person) of the $2.1 trillion (around $7,400 per person) national healthcare bill in 2007 that was committed to prevention and wellness (CMS, Office of Actuary, 2009).

An annual increase investment of as little as $10 (approximately $3 billion) per capita in proven community-based prevention programs and services throughout the US could result in an average twenty-year return of 6.2:1 -- nearly $18.5 billion annual savings annually in relative 2004 healthcare dollars. The report states: "this return on investment represents medical cost savings only and does not include significant gains that could be achieved in worker productivity, reduced absenteeism at work and school, and enhanced quality of life." (p. 3). Net savings to Medicare and Medicaid programs could yield $8 billion annually. The group classified the recommended public health initiatives into three broad areas:

Primary prevention – measures before problems arise (clean air, water and sewage systems, food and nutrition improvements, immunizations, etc.)
Secondary prevention – measures for early detection and intervention (tracking and containment)
Tertiary prevention – reduction of further complications of existing disease problems (treatment and rehabilitation)

The TFAH report cites three central factors that could have the largest impact on individual health: (1) improved physical activity, (3) better nutrition for children and adults, and (3) reduction in tobacco smoking initiatives. A state-by-state analysis of the estimated ROI based on a $10 per person public health investment shows the following results for selected US states:

Table 8 – ROI Impact of Preventive Health Initiatives

Impact of Preventive Initiatives Comparative ROI – Selected States

State	Annual Investment	10-20 Year Savings Per Annum	10-20 Year ROI
Arizona	$57. 4 million	$329.1 million	4.73:1
California	$358.4 million	$2.3 billion	5.41:1
Wash,, DC	$5.8 million	$69.1 million	10.93:1
Kansas	$27.4 million	$200.8 million	6.34:1
Oklahoma	$35.2 million	$240.4 million	5.83:1
Texas	$225.2 million	$1.5 billion	5.22:1
Utah	$24.2 million	$124.7 million	4.15:1
United States	$3 billion	$18.5 billion	6.2:1

Source: Issues Report, Trust for America's Health (2008).

Every state in the country had a substantial positive ROI projection, with the lowest being 4.15:1 in Utah and the highest being 10.93:1 in Washington, DC. TFAH's *Blueprint* for healthcare reform is as follows:

- Setting new, realistic short and long-term health goals for the country;
- Investing in disease prevention as a cornerstone of health care reform;
- Ensuring a stable and reliable funding stream for core public health functions and preventive services, such as immunizations and screening, public health emergency preparedness, and promoting physical activity, good nutrition, and smoking prevention.
- Creating an independent, science-driven National Public Health Board;
- Implementing a National Health and Prevention Strategy focused on lowering disease rates, including a strategy to combat obesity;
- Increasing accountability by tying tax-payer investments to improving the health of Americans and improving federal, state, and local coordination;
- Addressing the public health workforce crisis with stepped-up recruitment efforts;
- Clearly defining public health emergency preparedness and response roles and responsibilities;
- Establishing an emergency health benefit for use by uninsured and underinsured Americans during major disasters and disease outbreaks; and
- Fixing the food safety system.

In spite of the compelling evidence that preventive health services and public health initiatives could pay dramatic dividends, the United States healthcare system remains focused on the profit-making business of sick care (Figure 7). To reiterate the obvious, there are very few economic incentives in the present reimbursement scheme for providers (hospitals, private insurers, physicians, rehab centers, nursing facilities, etc.) to encourage them to work collaboratively to achieve a healthier society. Increasing competition for patients in strategic markets where health status could show improvement would mean lower profits and excess margins across the board for a cadre of healthcare providers vested in sick care. This is the big conundrum for healthcare reform in the United States!

Obesity Costs US $147 Billion Annually

The United States is spending as much as $147 billion each year for obesity-related healthcare – representing nearly 10% of all annual medical costs ... "obesity will continue to impose a significant burden on the healthcare system as long as the prevalence of obesity remains high" Overall, the study reports that obese people spent $1,429 (42%) more for medical care in 2006 than did normal weight people...In addition to the study, CDC has issued its first comprehensive set of evidence-based recommendations to help communities tackle the problem of obesity through programs and policies that promote healthy eating and physical activity (Published by HealthLeaders Media).

Study by Eric Finkelstein, Director of the Prevention and Research Triangle Institute in collaboration with the Centers for Disease Control (CDC), July 27, 2009.

A random poll conducted by Greenberg Quinian Rosner Research between May 7 and 12, 2009, also sponsored by the Robert Wood Johnson Foundation and Trust for America's Health, including 1,014 respondents, found that "an overwhelming number of Americans of all political stripes supported increased funding for preventive health services" (*Modern Healthcare*, June 15, 2009, p. 9). The findings show that support for additional spending for preventive health services was strongest among respondents claiming an affiliation with the Democratic Party, or 86%, followed by Republicans and Independents, 71% and 70%, respectively (3.1. percentage margin of error). Unfortunately, this same political solidarity has yet to translate into legislative action in the halls of the US Congress.

How should the private and governmental health insurers in America be restructured in such a way that healthier behavior and a wellness and prevention orientation are rewarded throughout the country? The monumental challenge that politicians and policymakers at all levels are facing is not to succumb to the overwhelming pressure from special interest groups and advocacy associations determined to maintain the status quo of the healthcare system. It does not seem prudent to attempt to expand healthcare coverage for another 70 million uninsured and underinsured Americans until we seriously address the merits of major investments in prevention and wellness programs throughout the United States – this approach could definitely help offset the rising cost of sick care. Compared to the projected doubling of the traditional sick care budget by 2018 to close to $4 trillion, even if meaningful healthcare reform plans being discussed today were enacted by 2010, a serious commitment to prevention and wellness seems like a "no brainer."[43]

Newly appointed US Health and Human Services (DHHS) Secretary Kathleen Sebelius (former Governor of Kansas) called attention to "a recent national health care *status quo* report" released in June 2009, which indicates that there were serious health problems in every state in America. Health insurance premiums have steadily climbed across the board in the United States since 2000. Most states have experienced insurance premium increases in excess of 100% over the eight-year study horizon. The report highlights the dangerous prevalence of obesity among children -- one of the fastest growing epidemics in this country -- with major healthcare repercussions down the road as these individuals suffer from medical complications from diabetes and associated debilities, further driving up the healthcare tab (Table 10 presents a sampling of the report's results for selected states).

---

[43] The National Coalition on Health Care projects that the figure could reach $4 trillion by 2015, or 20 percent of the nation's GDP.

Table 9 – Sampling of Healthcare Status Quo of US States

Sampling of Healthcare Status Quo of States

State	Average Family Health Ins. Premium Increase Since 2000	Overall Quality of Care Rating in State	%Obese Children in State
Arizona	97%	Average	18%
California	114%	Average	15%
Washington, DC	103%	Weak	20%
Kansas	105%	Average	16%
Oklahoma	77%	Weak	16%
Texas	104%	Weak	20%
Utah	101%	Average	11%

Source: Health Reports, Health Care Status Quo of States, HealthReform.gov (June 26, 2009).

Secretary Sebelius oversees the operation of the largest US government agency charged with the task of identifying disease prevention and health promotion initiatives – the US Office of Disease Prevention and Health Promotion (ODPHP). The ODPDP is located in Rockville, Maryland. *Healthy People 2010* is one of ODPDP's key publications, which sets forth health and prevention priorities and implementation objectives for the nation. According to *Healthy People 2010*, the two main priorities for America are (1) increasing quality and years of healthy life, and (2) eliminating health disparities. These are laudable priorities, but they will require substantial financial resources to be realized. During the past 50 years, there has been a total disconnect between the stated public health goals and the amount of money the federal government has actually committed to these priorities. The reader is invited to study how the US healthcare spending has been apportioned by industry sector in Figure 6 below, and learn where the *real* priorities have been.

It was encouraging hear that the Senate Finance Committee passed their healthcare reform proposal in October 2009 by a tally of 18 yea and 4 nay votes. The Senate Finance Committee proposal included a provision recognizing the value of monetary rewards for employers

Figure 5 – National Healthcare Spending by Industry Sector: 2006-2007

participating in company-sponsored wellness programs. This was an unprecedented step forward for Congressional representatives to support prevention and wellness initiatives. The sponsors of the "wellness" amendment, Republican Senator John Ensign (NV) and Democratic Senator Thomas Carper (DE), cited evidence that "the key to achieving savings is to provide rewards to people who engage in healthy behaviors... [the focus] is on healthy behaviors and not genetics... we don't penalize people for any genetic problems they might have" (Simmons, 2009, October 1). The inclusion of preventive care language in the preliminary healthcare reform legislation (whether it is finally approved by the entire Congressional body or not) is encouraging and signals an important shift in the public's attitude moving closer to a wellness-oriented model in America.

8.3 -- Can Rationing Be Rationalized?

The appropriate allocation and consumption of finite resources is a necessary component for sustaining a functional system over time. That is a basic law of ecology (Hawley, 1950). This presumption also applies to our healthcare system as well. It is not logical to advocate *unlimited* sick care resources for all citizens; the unabated demand (and perhaps actual need) for healthcare resources will ultimately outstrip the ability of any government to provide such services. This is the principle reason why the US healthcare system cannot be regarded an *unlimited* human right for all. On the other hand, society and community leaders cannot abdicate their moral and ethical responsibilities for insuring that citizens are treated fairly concerning the distribution of basic healthcare resources available within each community. As in the case of other basic human needs (food, shelter, clothing, education, safety, etc.), basic healthcare (prevention, public health services and education, and primary care) should be allocated without regard to an individual's race, ethnicity, religious preference, or economic class. The operative word here is *basic* healthcare rights.

Allocating basic health services fairly means that they should be distributed in such a manner that society has reasonable access to a *threshold level of care* that promotes a general state of wellbeing capable of producing healthier individuals that are productive members in their communities. Rationing is a means for *prioritizing* the distribution of scarce resources, so they can provide the *most good*, for *the most people*, *most of the time*. To avoid discrimination and inequities, consumers should be actively involved in a public process for determining prioritization of healthcare services that conform to community values. Policymakers, governmental regulators, and economic planners should foster diverse alternatives for obtaining broad societal involvement in any rational prioritization process. Once a consensus is reached regarding the *best* allocation methodology, then policymakers can develop criteria for insuring that healthcare resources reach every individual, according to the highest needs and most appropriate utilization in accordance with prescribed goals and moral standards.

As discussed in Section 7.2, the *Oregon Health Plan* implemented in 1994 was designed around the foundational belief that limiting health benefits to needy and justifiable patients is a superior allocation strategy than simply leaving "thousands of impoverished Oregonians without health care" over the long term. The prioritized list for delivering health services to Oregonians is an example of a rationing system that maximizes the common good. In *Rationing America's Medical Care: The Oregon Plan and Beyond*, researchers at the Brookings Institution's (1992) analyze several ethical decisions that should be addressed by leaders contemplating the development of rational approaches for allocating limited health resources:

> The Oregon Plan provides in its most general outline a heuristic procedure [according to the Encarta Dictionary: a helpful procedure for arriving at a solution, but not necessarily a proven solution] for health care policy debates. It is an attempt to address real-life moral

concerns regarding health care in the face of finite moral and philosophical resources… Oregon represents the first substantial attempt to democratize discussions regarding health care allocations. Despite the shortcomings that may beset the plan, Oregon has done better than any other state, or the federal government, in involving citizens as colleagues in the communal project of deciding how much to give to health care and what health care to purchase. (Englehardt, 1992, p. 204)

With continuous oversight from the Health Services Commission and bi-annual recommendations regarding necessary adjustments to the prioritized list submitted to Oregon's legislature, state officials have been able to rationally (as opposed to arbitrarily) match changing community needs and values to budgetary constraints.

An important cautionary note about the OHP is offered by Brookings Institution's work group: "If allocation or explicit rationing of health services is ever to be considered ethical, it must include everyone, rich and poor alike" (Garland, 1992, p. 50). The Health Services Commission only regulates Medicaid services, which is a fraction of the healthcare consumption in Oregon. Critics of the Oregon Health Plan have attacked it because they claim it is based on limited empirical scientific evidence and includes conflicting multi-cultural community opinions about fairness and healthcare needs (pp. 51-57). No doubt these arguments are worthy of our careful deliberation. However, flawed the OHP may be according to its critics, they also failed to offer a viable alternative to the obvious inequities built into the existing employer-sponsored, market-driven, health insurance system – it excludes access to the working poor and underinsured population that cannot buy adequate health insurance coverage.

Brannigan and Boss (2001) pose the following philosophical question: "What constitutes a just healthcare system"? Several (arbitrary) criteria could be employed to answer this question:

- Distribution according to market and / or ability to pay.
- Distribution according to social merit.
- Distribution according to medical need.
- Distribution according to age.
- Distribution according to queuing – first come, first served.
- Distribution according to random selection.

Each of these criteria could be used to prioritize the distribution of limited health resources, but are they just? Scholars have contended that "healthcare needs encompass more than medical considerations." Brannigan and Boss note: "they [the criteria listed above] imply all sorts of values besides purely medical ones," and state that any distribution methodology must realize that healthcare needs are *foundational* – many other external needs (security, education, housing, etc.) depend on the health status of communities. They claim that "one thing is sure – the notion of healthcare is not a fixed entity" (p. 625-626).

Rationing of limited health resources is an integral step for achieving universal healthcare, which is defined herein as a basic health benefits package for all citizens. Universal healthcare should be a transparent process, free of tricky formulas, complex funding methodologies, or eligibility criteria that detract from the intent of the system. Without a rational methodology for allocating limited health resources in America, we are forced to employ *arbitrary criteria* to distribute healthcare to members of our society. Ultimately, our healthcare distribution choices will boil down to (1) Less for more, or (2) more for less.

> *Access to high-ticket items should not be in the hands of one patient and one physician. There should be a higher level of control, no matter who is paying the bill. This is especially true for futile care. Many billions of dollars are spent on terminal care that simply does not help the patient.*
>
> *What I'm talking about is the rationing of "rescue" care. We may not like the idea, but there is no way to have a sensible and truly helpful system for delivering care to patients without rationing. We already have rationing, but in an irrational form. What we need is a rational system for rationing care.*
>
> By George D. Lundberg, MD, in Severed Trust, 2002.

A creative, yet controversial, health allocation tool for determining the relative disease burden and monetary value of performing various medical interventions was popularized by Milton Weinstein and W.B. Steason in 1977 -- *quality-adjusted life-year* (QALY) indicator.[44] This scheme might be considered the equivalent of a *human treatment* ROI methodology or HTROI, to coin a new acronym. Essentially, the QALY weights the cost-effectiveness and impact on resource utilization against the potential of enhanced health attainment.

Definition of QALY

> *QALY: Quality-adjusted life-year, a year of life adjusted for its quality or its value. A year in perfect health is considered equal to 1.0 QALY. The value of a year in ill health would be discounted. For example, a year bedridden might have a value equal to 0.5 QALY.*

---

[44] *Journal of Health Policy and Planning*, Cary, NC: Oxford University Press. For additional information, see http://heapol.oxfordjournals.org /cgi/content/abstract/21/5/402; http://www.ispor.org/meetings/Invitational/QALY/Paper1.pdf; and http://www.cmaj.ca/cgi/content/full/168/4/433

The chief complaint about the QALY approach is that it does not adequately balance the benefits of treating younger and older patients in terms of remaining years of life; older patients will nearly always have a shorter average life span than younger cohorts. By the same token, the QALY does not account for the special needs of the most disadvantaged or disabled individuals in our society. They too will always be disadvantaged by the QALY methodology in comparison with non-disabled persons (an approach has been devised to mathematically adjust for these special factors -- the disability-adjusted life-years or DALY). Another serious limitation of this tool is that everyone' perceived value of life and life span is different, regardless of socioeconomic circumstances. Therefore, how can QALY or DALY objectively measure the intrinsic value of saving one life versus another without being able to accurately determine the person's perception of the future value of living? Hayry reasons, "many attempts besides the QALY model have been made to define 'scientifically' what individuals want, or what makes their lives good...[however,] how can we define objectively something that is, essentially, also subjective" (Hayry, 2002, p. 60).

In his article published in *The New York Times* on August 25, 2009, Reed Abelson notes that the "R" word is the public's most dreaded fear when it comes to deciding who is entitled to healthcare benefits. Abelson explains that many people believe that greater involvement of government in the healthcare delivery system will eventually lead to a national rationing program based solely on the determination of medical treatment effectiveness and "return-on-investment" formulas. He underscores the fact that health insurance companies already decide which procedures and treatments they will pay for based primarily on cost-effectiveness. The real danger to our healthcare system and its long-term survival may actually hinge on the *failure* of legislators to address universal care and cost controls (an allocation process) through healthcare reform legislation. According to Peter Lee, who oversees health policy for the Pacific Business Group on Health in California, an alliance of large employers: "if nothing is done, health care is going to break the bank of not only the federal government but of every household in America" (Abelson, 2009). Failure to act *rationally* about rationing *is* the double-edged sword that policy-makers and taxpayers are faced with at this critical juncture in American history.

The difficulty with most allocation schemes is that there is no single reliable methodology to efficiently and fairly distribute healthcare services that are truly necessary or desirable by the total population. Workable allocation schemes require *rationality* in order to accommodate diverse healthcare situations. From a purely *Utilitarian* philosophy, healthcare policies pertaining to distribution of health resources should be based on the notion of promoting the greatest wellbeing (or happiness) for humankind (Hayry, 2002).

Nine

Employer-Sponsored Health Insurance

9.1 -- Will the Real Number of Uninsured Persons in the United States Please Come Forward

Ask the average "well-informed" healthcare executive, politician, health researcher or journalist how many uninsured Americans there were in 2008, and they will tell you the number is around 46 million. Where did this figure come from? Most analysts rely on the US Census Bureau for consistent demographic information, so I will do the same and explore how the number of uninsured is determined.

The Census Bureau is the official government agency charged with the responsibility of conducting decennial and periodic census surveys, and it publishes reports on a myriad of facts about people living in the United States. They also collect considerable information about healthcare insurance coverage (or the lack thereof) in the United States. The common database produced by the Census Bureau provides analysts and researchers with the raw demographic information, and typically they apply their own methodologies to interpret the data and make assumptions and projections about future scenarios. A case in point is the report published by the Urban Institute (2009) entitled *Health Reform – The Cost of Failure*. John Holahan, Ph.D. was the project director for the Institute's report that projected the number of uninsured in the United States would grow steadily over the next decade as a result of the shift away from employer-sponsored health insurance and continued deterioration of the US economy:

> *In the worst case scenario, the number of uninsured Americans would increase [from 47 million in 2008] to 57.7 million in 2014 and to 65.7 million in 2019. In the best case, the number grows to 53.1 million in 2014 and 57 million in 2019. All of these estimates assume that states would continue to maintain current eligibility levels for public coverage [Medicaid]. Without this, the number of uninsured would be even higher. (Holahan, et al., 2009, p. 2)*

In a phone conversation with Dr. Holahan,[45] he explained that they used the latest Current Population Survey (CPS) from the *Census Bureau* as the basis of their projections. Then they applied the Institute's sophisticated methodology – *Health Insurance Policy Simulation Model* (HIPSM) – to develop their own future scenarios under various socio-economic conditions. If, as the HIPSM model predicted, 60 million Americans are projected to be without any health insurance over the next ten years, that figure would amount to close to 20% of the US population – a staggering figure to say the least! Assuming that the underlying figures provided by the Census Bureau are correct, the advice to policymakers is that timely health reform is critical to the country's social and economic wellbeing. The Urban Institute's report warns: "While enacting health reform will be difficult and expensive, the cost of failure is substantial" (p. 3).

How reliable are the Census Bureau's baseline health insurance estimates to begin with? Charles T. Nelson, Assistant Division Chief for Income, Poverty, and Health Statistics, Housing, and Economic Household Statistics Division for the Census Bureau, shared the report with me that was actually used by the Urban Institute – *Current Population Reports, P60-235*.[46] In discussing the contents of the *P60-235 Census Report*, Nelson commented that "because people can be covered by more than one type of coverage, you cannot add together the various types of coverage to come up with a total coverage figure."[47]

Studying the *P60-235* Census Report (see Table 11 below), it is apparent that by adding the private health insurance and government health insurance figures together, there is an estimated total of 45.6 million uninsured lives added to the 298 million covered lives – this amounts to 342 million covered and uninsured individuals in the US in 2007. The problem with this information is that the Census Bureau reported that the nation had approximately 300 million citizens at the start of 2008. The discrepancy in these figures is too great to ignore!

Nelson suggested that I review the latest health insurance participation report prepared by the *Centers for Disease Control and Prevention* (CDC) for further details on the most recent statistics concerning the number of uninsured in the US: *Health Insurance Coverage: Early Release of Estimates from the National Health Interview Survey, January to March, 2008* (CDC, 2008). The CDC is part of the US Department of Health and Human Services, National Center for Health Statistics, and is responsible for monitoring the nation's ongoing state of health. The CDC's Health Insurance Coverage report offered the subsequent data relating to the growth of uninsured individuals in the United States through 2008:

---

45 John Holahan, phone conversation May 28, 2009.
46 Reference provided by Charles Nelson, US Census Bureau; Retrieved May 28, 2009, from http://www.census.gov/prod/2008pubs/p60-235.pdf .
47 Charles Nelson, phone conversation May 29, 2009.

- From January to March 2008, the percentage of persons uninsured at the time of the interview [sampling of about 19,000 persons in the Family Core] was 14.3% (42.6 million) for persons of all ages, 16.2% (42.4 million) for persons under the age of 65 years, 19.3% (36.1 million) for persons aged 18-64 years, and 8.5% (6.3 million) for children under the age of 18...There was no significant change in the percentage of people under age 65 who were uninsured at the time of the interview between 2007 and the first 3 months of 2008.
- Based on data from January – March NHIS, a total of 55.3 million (18.5%) persons of all ages were uninsured for at least part of the year prior to the interview...Working-age adults were almost twice as likely to experience this lack of coverage (24.1%) as children under the age of 18 (13.0%).
- From January – March 2008, 19.4% of persons under 65 were covered by public health plans at the time of the interview, and 65.5% were covered by private health insurance plans...More than two-thirds (68.7%) of adults 18-64 years of age were covered by a private plan, compared with 57.5% of children under 18 years...More than one-third of children (35.3%) were covered by a public plan, compared with 13.2% of adults aged 18-64 years.
- There was no significant change in the percentage of children or working age adults covered by private or public plans from 2007 to the first 3 months of 2008.
- Among adults aged 18-64 years, the percentage uninsured for more than a year fluctuated between 11.9% and 14.3% between 1997 and the first 3 months of 2008...By contrast, the percentage of children uninsured for more than a year decreased from 8.4% in 1997 to 5.6% in 2002...Since 2002, the percentage of children uninsured for more than a year has remained steady and has ranged 5.0% and 5.8%.
- Private health coverage rates among both children and working-adults are now significantly lower than in 1997 [Table 3 – Percent Persons Under 65 With *Public Health Plan* Coverage in US 1997 = 13.6%, 2008 = 19.4%; Percent Persons Under 65 With *Private Health Insurance* Coverage in US 1997 = 70.8%, 2008 = 65.6%; and Percent Persons Under 65 *Uninsured* at the Time of Interview in US 1997 = 17.4%, 2008 = 16.2%].

Based on the Census Bureau's figures, there appears to be a total of between 42 and 46 million uninsured persons in this country presently. The CDC's report indicated that the number of uninsured fluctuates during the calendar year, and that approximately 42.6 million residents were without health coverage at the time of the survey (first quarter of 2008). The estimated distribution of uninsured residents by county is presented in Figure 7.

The Commonwealth Fund also published its own projections for the future level of uninsured in the United States. According to their proposal for healthcare reform legislation, they suggested that the number of uninsured could be reduced from 48 million in 2009 to 4 million in 2012 *if* Congress acted swiftly to enact comprehensive healthcare reform (universal coverage).

The Commonwealth Fund's historical estimate of the trend of uninsured by age cohorts is presented in Figures 8 A and B, below:

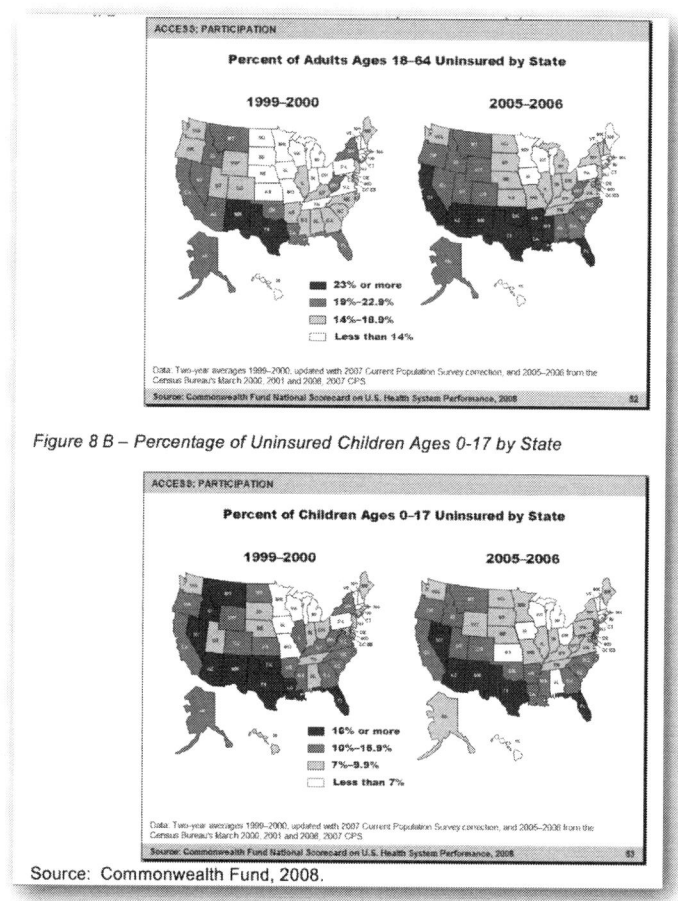

Figure 6 – Percentage of Uninsured Adults 18-64 and Children 0-17 by State
Source: Commonwealth Fund, 2008.

Quantifying the *real* extent of the uninsured and underinsured conundrum is not simple. If one constructs a bottom-up profile of covered lives in America using official records from health insurance companies, it is impossible to reconcile the estimated number of insured and uninsured persons from all these reputable in early 2008, which was close to 300 million. I examined each of the *Annual Reports* for publicly traded for-profit health insurance companies available for the year ending December 31, 2008, and consulted with the *HealthLeaders Interstudy Group*, which monitors health insurance performance of all major insurers in America.

The total number of covered lives for these private insurance companies was 123 million in 2008 (non-duplicative lives). Private insurance companies generated $305 billion in premium revenue with a net income of $11.2 billion and a net profit averaging 4%. Public records for the non-profit Blue Cross and Blue Shield plans (39 plans across the United States) indicate that their total covered lives equaled approximately 50 million during the same timeframe, with an insurance premium revenue of about $100 billion. Government sources reported 125.5 million covered lives overall, and an operating budget of $887 billion. Government sources calculated that excessive overhead costs and built-in wasted costs amounted to $680 to $800 billion annually. Table 12 summarizes my findings:[48]

Table 10 – Health Insurance Providers' Performance: 2008

US Health Insurance Providers' Performance: 2008

Insurer	Net Covered Lives(1)	Health Care Revenue(2)	Net Income (after taxes)	% Net Profit
UnitedHealth Group, Inc.	28,228,939	$81.1 Billion	$5.3 Billion / $3.0 Billion	4.0%
Aetna, Inc.	17,102,192	$28.8 Billion	$2.5 Billion / $1.6 Billion	5.5%
Health Care Service Corp	12,431,136	$16.0 billion	$2.7 Billion / $743 Million	4.6%
CIGNA HealthCare	10,392,882	$17.0 Billion	$? / $665.0 Million	4.0%
Kaiser Foundation Plans.	8,617,076	$37.8 Billion	$? / $2.2 Billion	5.8%
Humana, Inc.	5,681,938	$28.0 Billion	$1.0 Billion / $650 Million	2.3%
BC BS of Michigan	4,937,013	$10.7 Billion	-$118 Million / -$145 Million	-1.3%
EmblemHealth, Inc.	3,449,474	$8.6 Billion	-$128 Million / -$117 Million	-1.4%
HealthNet, Inc.	3,080,865	$15.2 Billion	$147 Million / $95 Million	.06%
Major For-Profits	**122,897,686**	**$304.8 Billion**	**$? / $11.2 Billion**	**3.7%**

---

48 A Press Release from Robert Kelley, Vice President of healthcare analytics with Thomson Reuters, Ann Arbor, Michigan, issued October 26, 2009, indicated that the quantifiable wasted healthcare dollars in the US

BC BS Plans - 39 Plans Nationally

Major Not-Profits	**50,000,000**	**$100 Billion**	Estimate based on BC BS of Michigan figures
Medicare / SSI	45,300,000	$468.0 Billion	
Medicaid (federal and state)	58,714,800	$320.0 Billion	
Military (DOD TriCare / VA)	13,500,000	$65.0 Billion	
Government Employees	8,000,000	$34.0 Billion	
Government	**125,514,800**	**$887.0 Billion**	
Deductible / Co-Insurance / Co-Pay	Most Insured	$500.0 Billion	Estimated
Uninsured (est.) subsidy,	**47,000,000**	**$300.3 Billion**	Estimated (Charity care, DSH uncompensated care, and other subsidized programs)
TOTAL	**345,500,000**	**$2.4 Trillion**	

GAO Estimates that 30% of Cost = Administrative Overhead, overutilization, regional differential charge structure, excessive profits, etc. ($630 Billion)

Sources: (1) Private Insurance Covered lives – HealthLeaders Interstudy; (2) FP – latest company annual reports as of May, 2009; Government - HHS; Medicare and Medicaid information – Kaiser Foundation 2009, www.StateHealthFacts.org; Uninsured estimate - Senate Finance Committee Report May 20, 2009, US Census Bureau CPS Reports, Urban Institute; Table prepared by Mark Tozzio.

As mentioned above, this information indicates that 298 million Americans had some type of health insurance coverage, plus the estimated 47 million uninsured lives – this total *exceeds* the Census Bureau estimate of residents living in this country in 2008. So how does one accurately account for the number of Americans that supposedly did not have any health insurance coverage in 2008? It does not seem plausible that there are 47 million uninsured in this country based on these records. Or are the health insurance companies not telling an accurate story?

Perhaps a plausible explanation regarding the discrepancy in the number of uninsured in the United States was presented by George F. Will, Pulitzer Prize-winning syndicated columnist with the *Washington Post*, in his column titled, "Arguments for Public Health Option Don't Hold Water." Will reports:

Why The United States Healthcare System Should Be A Limited Human Right For All

Radical reform of health care is supposedly necessary because there are 45.7 million uninsured. That number is, however, a 'snapshot' of a nation in which more than 20 million working Americans change jobs every year. Most of them are briefly uninsured between jobs. If all of the uninsured were assembled for a group photograph, and six months later the then-uninsured were assembled for another photograph, about half the people in the photos would be different. Will, 2009, p. B10)

Will postulates that nearly half of the 46 million Americans estimated to be uninsured by public sources were actually (1) non-citizens (9.7 million), (2) individuals eligible for existing government programs who elect not to participate (14 million), and (3) another 9.1 million who have incomes of at least $75,000 per year and could easily afford health insurance. The remaining 12.9 million individuals who are *chronically* uninsured could be covered by "tax credits or debit cards" that Will claim would empower them within the existing healthcare system. His key point is that the number of *chronically* uninsured in the United States is far less than the 46 million individuals identified by the political establishment. Will suggests that there are approximately 13 million chronically uninsured people, and that this figure does not justify a drastic revamping of the US health insurance system; there should be simpler ways to deal with the uninsured problem in America.

Although Will did not cite his sources of information for his article, his general assumptions can be validated using a recent sample of the civilian non-institutionalized population complied by the National Center for Health Statistics (NCHS / NHIS) and published in the *Health Insurance Coverage: Early Release of Estimates from the National Health Interview Survey, January to March 2008*. This survey recognizes three broad categories of residents lacking health insurance coverage nationally: (1) *current*, (2) *intermittent*, and (3) *long term*. The NCHS / NHIS document published in September 2008 reports:

From January to March 2008, 42.8 million persons [residing in the United States] of all ages (14.3%) were uninsured at the time of the interview, 55.3 million (18.5%) had been uninsured for at least part of the year prior to the interview, and 31.2 million (10.5%) had been uninsured for more than a year at the time of the interview. (NCHS / NHIS, 2008, p. 38)

The NCHS / NHIS report also categorizes various other types of public and private health insurance groups covering individuals (NCHS / NHIS cautioned that the early release of the report's information may lead to a variance of 0.1 to 0.3 percentage points compared to the estimates published later in the final publication). First, children under 18 years of age who were uninsured for more than one year at the time of the 2008 survey totaled 5.8% of this cohort, down from 8.4% in the 1997 survey. Second, the population over 65 years of age without health insurance at the time of the survey amounted to an estimated 1.5% of this older cohort (Graph 20).

On September 10, 2009, the US Census Bureau released the latest official number of uninsured Americans during 2008. They estimate that the uninsured rate rose 1.3% over the 2007 figures to become 46.3 million. The percentage of people covered by employer-based health insurance programs declined from 59.3% in 2007 to 58.5% in 2008. The rising cost of private health insurance benefits and the economic downturn since 2007 are identified as major reasons for the continuing shift away from employer-sponsored coverage. Government-insured programs including Medicare, Medicaid, and the Veteran's Administration program climbed 1.2% to a total of 29% in 2008. Coverage for children, a central focus of legislative attention over the past four years, improved noticeably. The number of uninsured children under age 18 fell to its lowest rate since 1987 to 7.3 million, compared to 8.1 million the prior year. This information is derived from the *Annual Housing and Household Economic Status* randomized survey of Americans.

A closer examination of the Census Bureau information on health insurance coverage reveals a gender gap showing that women have a significant disadvantage (inequity) concerning employer-sponsored coverage (Graph 21). One of the obvious reasons for this disparity is the fact that most married couples carry health insurance under the husband's job health plan, leaving women at a higher risk of becoming uninsured in the event of the spouse's unemployment, separation or divorce, or death. Women have a greater tendency to secure private (non-employer-sponsored) insurance than men, which is considerably more costly than employer-sponsored coverage. The Census Bureau identifies two additional areas where there are problems with pricing and access to insurance coverage that discriminated against women: (1) coverage for obstetrical services, and (2) coverage for victims of domestic violence. Most states allow health insurance companies to be selective about certain cohorts or higher risk individuals, which results in a greater number of women and their families being uninsured, underinsured, or eligible for government subsidized care under the Medicaid program.

So there we have it, *clear as mud*. Depending on which "reliable" source one uses for calculating the baseline estimate of covered lives in the United States, the projection of the total uninsured and underinsured population could vary by a factor of several million. A reasonable estimate of the number of *chronically* uninsured Americans in 2009 is probably in the range of 20 million. Add to the uninsured figure another 30 million Americans who are underinsured and at serious risk of financial ruin due to the uncontrolled rising cost of health insurance premiums, co-pays, and deductibles, and we have a real health insurance crisis in this country.

> *Only God knows the actual head count of the uninsured, but let there be no doubt that we will still have massive numbers of Americans who either can't*

afford insurance, don't qualify for it, can't access it, or can't access enough of it. Now, what will this nation do about it? That's an even thornier question.

By David May, Assistant Managing Editor, "Doing a Number on the Uninsured," Modern Healthcare, September 28, 2009

9.2 -- Addressing the Health Insurance Conundrum

Health insurance coverage had its origins in the United States between the 1930s and 1950s (Lundberg and Stacey, 2002). Baylor University Hospital in Dallas, Texas is credited for establishing the first pre-paid health insurance program for teachers in the metropolitan area in 1929. "For six dollars per year, the teachers would be insured for up to twenty-one days of inpatient care at Baylor" (p. 24), Baylor claimed. Soon after Baylor's "success" in the health insurance business, the Blue Cross plans came into existence in America. Blue Cross was originally organized as a tax-exempt charitable health services organization. Lundberg and Stacey noted that the first Blue Cross plans "were created to keep hospitals solvent with a steady income," and not necessarily to benefit patients directly. In the late 1930s and early 1940s, entrepreneur Henry J. Kaiser and his trusted advisor Sidney Garfield, MD developed a first-class pre-paid integrated health delivery system to attend to the medical needs of thousands of construction workers and their families engaged in the Grand Coulee Dam project in Washington and other huge projects in southern California. The plan is known today as *Kaiser Permanente* (pp. 77-88).[49]

The humble beginning of the health insurance industry expanded rapidly in 1946 when the US Congress funded the Veterans Administration hospital system (VA) and approved the Hill-Burton legislation. This sudden infusion of federal money stimulated massive construction of new hospitals, especially in rural America. The caveat for obtaining Hill-Burton funds was that hospital sponsors had to commit to provide a minimum amount of "free care" to indigent patients for a period of up to 40 years. This requirement proved to be a substantial challenge for hospitals during the post-war period in the 1960s when unemployment skyrocketed and the economy plummeted. In 1965, Congress enacted Medicare for seniors and Medicaid for the growing indigent population. "Most observers would single out Medicare as the most powerful engine behind the cost escalation in health care [in the United States]," wrote Lundberg and Stacey (p. 31). The provision of healthcare in the United States and traditional fee-for-service payment mechanisms shifted more lives into the present employer-sponsored market-driven health insurance system during the early 1960s. The next thirty years ushered in the "golden

---

[49] Kaiser Permanente is the corporate entity based in Oakland, California that is made up of three health organizations -- The Kaiser Foundation Health Plans; the Kaiser Foundation Hospitals; and the Permanente Medical Groups. It is the largest fully integrated managed care organization (MCO) in the US with approximately 9 million subscriber members in eight states.

era" for medical providers and the health insurance industry, and the price of healthcare in the US soared.

Attempts by the government to control the dramatic rising cost of healthcare led policymakers to experiment with several types of "managed care" programs: Health Maintenance Organizations (HMOs), Preferred Provider Organizations (PPOs), and Independent Practice Associations (IPAs). The government also instituted the national health planning agencies such as Health Systems Agencies (HSAs), Certificate of Need Program (CON), and other cost-containment organizations to regulate expenditures for new and replacement healthcare facilities and equipment. Finally, in 1983, Congress adopted the prospective payment system – *Diagnosis Related Groups* (DRGs) – developed by Yale University under contract by the Health Care Financing Agency (HCFA) in an effort to restrain the cost of Medicare. Essentially, federal insurers would pay a preset amount for each DRG category, so the traditional fee-for-service charges became virtually irrelevant. This complicated, yet predictable DRG program spread to other private insurers, non-profit as well as for-profit entities, and had a significant impact on slowing the growth of healthcare costs for a short period of time. Lundberg and Stacy (2002) characterize the 1980s era as a time of explosive costs in healthcare in the United States:

By the end of the 1980s, despite the almost heroic attempts to control costs, they had more than doubled in one decade, from approximately $300 billion to $800 billion. (p. 41).

As insurance companies negotiated with healthcare providers promising to deliver large blocks of patients that were "controlled" by HMOs and PPOs, the health insurance premiums began to climb for employer-sponsored plans. The industry was shifting the power base over patients from physicians and hospitals to large, specialized, health insurance corporations. By the 1990s, most private health insurance corporations operated as for-profit entities. During the late 1990s and early 2000s, nearly half of the Blue Cross plans were converted to for-profit plans or were acquired by the mega-insurance companies that reached across the nation: Wellpoint, UnitedHealthcare, CIGNA, and Kaiser Permanente -- these and other giants included hundreds of millions of covered lives.

A 2004 report issued by the federal Agency for Healthcare Research and Quality reviews the trends in employer-sponsored health insurance cost and accessibility in the United States:

In the first half of 2003, the US employer-based health insurance market provided insurance to over 159 million Americans who constitute nearly two-thirds (63.4 percent) of the population under 65. In this voluntary system, employers may choose whether to offer health insurance to their employees and employees may choose to enroll or forgo enrollment. Most employers have chosen to offer health insurance as a fringe benefit to attract employees. It is an attractive option to offer because of the favorable tax treatment to both employer and employee. In addition, employment-based health insurance is likely to be less expensive than individually purchased coverage (for the same set of benefits) and typically provides a broader scope of benefits than is available in individually purchased coverage. The stability of the employer-sponsored insurance system is supported by a tax subsidy that promotes the pooling of risk necessary for the successful functioning of insurance. (p. 2)

Although there were problems with the employer-sponsored, market-based health insurance system in America, it did offer reasonable coverage to a large segment of the population. Since 1987, the percentage of employer-sponsored coverage has been steadily dropping because employers have been shifting more of their healthcare costs to employees -- the average premium per enrolled private-sector employee for single coverage rose 65.2 percent, from $342 to $565 (p. 4). Smaller companies in 2002 had 63.5 percent of their workforce covered by health insurance; larger companies with more than 50 employees had a 97.8 coverage rate. Another phenomenon that occurred with the employer-sponsored insurance system was an increase in the number of underinsured employees and their families. These underinsured families face financial ruination even though they carry minimal health insurance coverage – the burden of large co-pays and deductibles far exceeds the more costly and comprehensive plans. All of these factors have contributed to the growing number of uninsured families in America.

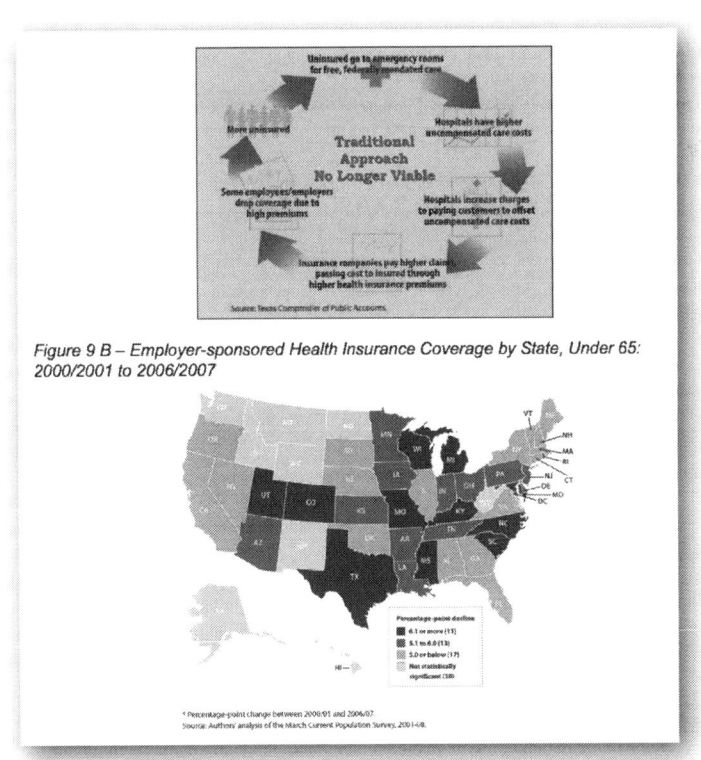

Figure 7 – Cycle of Healthcare Utilization by the Uninsured and Employer-sponsored Health Insurance Coverage by State, Under 65: 2000/2001 to 2006/2007

Since the beginning of the 21st century, the high cost of health insurance premiums forced more companies to increase their employees' share of premiums to reduce overall coverage, and in some cases, discontinue health benefits altogether. The *Economic Policy Institute* reported that most states were presently experiencing large declines in employer-sponsored health coverage because health insurance was taking a bigger bite out of company profits and the fact that the employment market was flooded with qualified candidates, thus making health benefits less of a competitive recruitment item (Gould, 2008, October 9). Researcher Elise Gould found that "forty-one states experienced significant losses in coverage across every region of the United States...no state experienced an increase," during the periods between 2000/2001 and 2006/2007 (relates to the population under 65 only).

States most severely affected by the reduction in employer-sponsored health insurance coverage included Colorado, Kentucky, Michigan, Mississippi, Missouri, North and South Carolina, Texas, Utah, and Wisconsin. The District of Columbia was also among the severely affected areas, with a percentage decline over 6.1. Many of these regions have been hardest hit by layoffs and growing unemployment rates reaching over ten percent (the highest since the Great Depression). Although COBRA[50] health insurance coverage for unemployed workers does help alleviate some of the economic stress during the transition between jobs, the cost of $1,000-plus premiums is unaffordable. Even with federal legislation enacted in January 2009 requiring employers to pay for 65% of the health insurance premium for up to nine months following the layoff of qualified employees, the monthly premium cost is still a major obstacle.

During the 2008 Presidential campaign, both Republican and Democratic candidates debated the financial plight of the middle-class, small owner-operators symbolized by "Joe the Plumber" (Sam Joseph Wurzelbacher, from Ohio), who believed he would be subjected to higher taxation because of business earnings in excess of $250,000. *Joe the Plumber* took issue with presidential candidate Barack Obama about his plan to redistribute wealth and expand services to needy Americans by raising the taxes of wealthier individuals (those with incomes over $250,000 per year). This issue fueled a national debate over the struggle of small businesses to cope with pressures from increasing government taxation, mounting regulations, and diminishing profitability.

Proponents of Obama's *Change* plans argued that the typical business *income* potential for Joe the Plumber and his would-be employees and other American small businesses would be far less than the $250,000 income tax threshold; that was part of the firestorm debate during the 2008 Presidential campaign.

---

50 The Consolidated Omnibus Budget Reconciliation Act (COBRA) gives workers and their families who lose their health benefits the right to choose to continue group health benefits provided by their group health plan for limited periods of time under certain circumstances such as voluntary or involuntary job loss, reduction in the hours worked, transition between jobs, death, divorce, and other life events. Qualified individuals may be required to pay the entire premium for coverage up to 102 percent of the cost to the plan. US Department of Labor website, http://www.dol.gov/dol/topic/health-plans/cobra.htm.

Why The United States Healthcare System Should Be A Limited Human Right For All

What came to light as a result of the 2008 Presidential debates and political rhetoric was the fact that approximately 6 million small businesses, representing nearly half of the US private sector workforce, were subjected to varying degrees of economic pressures resulting from growing taxes on the middle-class. Out of an estimated total of 27.2 million businesses registered in 2007 in the United States, only 17,000 businesses were classified as *large firms* with over 500 employees. Information gleaned from the US Department of Commerce, Bureau of the Census, covering the period from 2003 through 2005, and estimates from the US Small Business Administration Office of Advocacy (SBA) for 2006 and 2007, indicate there were an estimated 637,100 new business start-ups, 560,300 business closures, and 28,322 bankruptcies in the United States during 2007. Economist Brian Headd with the SBA noted in a personal conversation that the latest figures released for 2008 show that the total number of bankruptcies had jumped to a record high of 43,546![51] SCORE lists several key factors contributing to small business failures during the past 5 years, including:

- Limited internal resources and long hours to get the job(s) done.
- Higher operating costs per unit of service than larger companies.
- Employer-based health insurance cost to companies (with growing contributions from employees).
- Cash flow and access to growth capital (operating and plant / equipment).
- Tax and regulatory burdens.

During the economic crisis beginning at the end of 2007, nearly everyone expressed grave concern over the uncontrolled rising costs of healthcare services as well as private health insurance coverage, and the extent to which it impacts the long-term survivability of any business, particularly small owner-operator firms.[52] These small businesses are the backbone of the American workforce. The most significant concerns revolved around the following two issues:

1. In this uncertain economy, low-wage workers are the most vulnerable. How can we protect these low-income families as unemployment rises and wages remain stagnant? How can we help out-of-work Americans update their skills and train for new jobs? What industries are still growing and hiring during this economic downturn?
2. The Urban Institute has tracked job trends for nearly 40 years, following unskilled workers during the 1990s boom, welfare leavers moving into the workforce, and displaced Gulf Coast residents who lost their jobs after Hurricane Katrina.

---

51 Personal phone conversation with Economist Brian Headd, US Small Business Administration Office of Advocacy, Washington, DC, March 25, 2009.
52 Personal phone conversation with Economist Jules Lichtenstein, US Small Business Administration Office of Advocacy, Washington, DC, March 25, 2009.

While unemployment rates continue to escalate in 2009, private insurance companies substantially raised premiums across the board for businesses and individual policy holders. Except for the mid-1990s, The Commonwealth Fund found that annual increases in health insurance rates have exceeded workers' earnings growth and overall US inflation. The escalation in health insurance premiums has directly contributed to a bleak picture for health insurance coverage for adults and children across the nation

Headd confirmed that government analysts were projecting that the overall unemployment rate would exceed 10% in many US states by the beginning of 2010.[53] Today's national unemployment rate is definitely contributing to a growing subclass of unemployed and underemployed Americans who are unable to afford the high cost of COBRA coverage after losing their jobs.[54] The Commonwealth Fund estimated that being uninsured in 2004 was the 6th leading cause of death in the United States among persons 24-64 years of age (higher than diabetes or HIV / AIDS). The Institute of Medicine (IOM) also determined that individuals without health insurance were 25% more likely to become sicker and die sooner than those who had adequate health insurance coverage (IOM, 2002). Undoubtedly, the problem has escalated in 2009.

In the January 2009 report, *The Budget and Economic Outlook: Fiscal Years 2009 to 2019* issued by the Congressional Budget Office (CBO), this panel of expert economic advisors believe that the trillion-dollar Congressional *Bailout and Economic Stimulus Package* created by the Troubled Asset Relief Program of 2008 (TARP) will be able to turn the tide on housing mortgage foreclosures, general inflation, and institutional banking failures that fueled the present deep recession cycle (CBO, 2009). The biggest challenge for our nation, the economists cautioned, relates to the health insurance coverage conundrum that persists in spite of TARP -- this situation must be controlled through immediate and aggressive measures in order to avert a greater national economic collapse over the next decade. The CBO report finds:

High deficits in the near term may be inevitable in the face of the financial crisis and severe economic weakness. However, once the nation gets past this downturn, it will still face significant fiscal challenges posed by rising health care costs and the aging of the population...The rate of growth of spending on health care is the single greatest threat to budget balance over the long run, and such spending will have to be controlled in order for the fiscal situation to be sustainable in future decades. Together, outlays for

---

[53] Personal phone conversation, March 25, 2009, (202) 205-6533; and *News Release* issued by Susan Houston, President of the New England Economic Partnership, (781) 489-6262, November 20, 2008.

[54] The Consolidated Omnibus Budget Reconciliation Act of 1986, referred to as COBRA, is a federally mandated requirement of businesses with over 20 number of employees to continue offering health insurance coverage at their cost, plus 2 percent for administrative fees. Congress recently amended the rules to allow employees who lose their job between September 1, 2008 and January 1, 2010 to keep COBRA coverage for 35 percent of the regular premium for up to nine months, while the employer subsidizes the remainder of the cost and receives a tax credit for its 65 percent share.

Why The United States Healthcare System Should Be A Limited Human Right For All

Medicare and Medicaid (not including offsetting receipts) currently account for about 5 percent of GDP. Spending for those programs is expected to rise at a rapid pace over the next 10 years, outstripping the growth of GDP. By 2019, spending for those programs combined is projected to total about 6.3 percent of the GDP. By 2050, it could reach 12 percent. Without changes to federal fiscal policy, those rising costs would drive the amount of debt held by the public significantly higher as a percentage of GDP than it is today. (CBO, 2002, p. 31)

The contemporary debate over affordable health insurance coverage has drawn strong opposition from conservatives who claim that developing a government-subsidized insurance alternative to compete with private companies (mostly for-profit) will move the country in the direction of "socialized medicine." A *Reuters News* article describes President Obama's uphill battle to pass new healthcare reform legislation by the end of 2009:

Obama aims to sign a [legislative] bill this year making sweeping changes in the healthcare system, which is the world's most expensive even as 46 million Americans have no health insurance and the United States lags other nations in important health measures, such as life expectancy and infant mortality.

Most Americans -- about 170 million -- get private health coverage through an employer, although some buy their own private insurance. Others are eligible for public programs that offer coverage to the elderly and disabled (Medicare), the poor (Medicaid) and low-income children (State Children's Health Insurance Program).

But many go without coverage, paying instead out of their own pockets for care if they get sick, or trying to do without medical attention. A new public insurance program would be intended to offer coverage to those who currently do not have it or who want an alternative to private insurance.

Obama last year proposed "a new public plan based on benefits available to members of Congress that will allow individuals and small businesses to buy affordable health coverage." It is part of an initiative to cut the number of uninsured while improving healthcare quality and controlling costs that are forecast to reach $2.5 trillion this year.

Leading congressional Democrats have embraced the idea but the specifics are still being worked out.

'There are, obviously, different ways of designing a public plan that would have different effects,' White House budget director Peter Orszag told a Senate hearing this week.

Robert Moffit, a health policy expert at the conservative Heritage Foundation think tank, said he believes some proponents of a new public program see it as a first step toward a full government takeover of the healthcare system. 'It's a Trojan Horse for national health insurance where you basically rig the competition against private health insurance and you set up the economic incentives to encourage employers to dump people into the public plan,' Moffit said. (Dunham, 2009)[55]

Robert Moffit, Ph.D., is a respected health policy leader and long-time conservative authority in the areas of healthcare policy, Medicare, and Social Security (and educational reform) -- he is the Director of the Center for Health Policy Studies at The Heritage Foundation[56] based in Washington, DC. Moffit also served as the Assistant Director of Congressional Relations in the Office of Personal Management and as the Deputy Assistant Secretary at the US Department of Health and Human Services during the Reagan Administration in the 1980s. Moffit is credited with spearheading the design team that helped develop the Massachusetts health insurance reform in 2005 – this plan offers a market-based health insurance alternative to small businesses and employees through the state's "health insurance exchange."

Robert A. Book (2009), Senior Research Fellow in Health Economics in the Center for Data Analysis at The Heritage Foundation, issued a follow-up statement cautioning policymakers on the dangers of moving to a *single-payer* health insurance system in the United States: "the result of 'single / stingy payer' health care will not only be lower incomes for physicians now, but reduce access and lower quality health care for future generations as well." Generally, a parallel government-subsidized health insurance plan would create more competitive pricing than the free market controlled by private insurance companies. A government alternative to cover uninsured and underinsured Americans would also serve as a safety net for millions of individuals who cannot afford employer-based health insurance coverage (much like Massachusetts' market-based program).

The adequacy of US healthcare insurance coverage has been a hotly debated subject for over thirty years, yet little change has occurred. I believe that credible evidence supports the proposition that politicians and policymakers have abdicated their *moral* obligation to insure that all Americans have *reasonable* access to affordable and *basic* healthcare coverage in a fiscally responsible manner. Politicians have been reluctant to address this critical problem and enact meaningful healthcare reform because of resistance from special interest groups dominated by the insurance and provider industries (Daschle, 2008).

---

55 *Trojan Horse* in a business context is an offer made by a business designed to lure customers by seeming like a good deal, but has the ultimate effect of extorting large amounts of money from the customer. *American Heritage Dictionary*, 2000 Edition.

56 Founded in 1973, The Heritage Foundation is the nation's most broadly supported public policy research institute, with more than 410,000 individual, foundation and corporate donors. The Foundation is a research and educational institute--a think tank--whose mission is to formulate and promote conservative public policies based on the principles of free enterprise, limited government, individual freedom, traditional American values, and a strong national defense. It has a staff of 244 and an expense budget of $61 million. Washington, DC, 202.546.4400, http://www.heritage.org

As depicted in the graphs prepared by The Commonwealth Fund[57] research group, the 2006 population under age 65 without health insurance reached 18%, or approximately 47 million adults and children (The Commonwealth Fund Chartbook, 2008, p. 54). The health insurance conundrum in the US has been characterized as an abomination. Will President Obama and Congress (through a bi-partisan initiative) have the courage to forge a workable health reform policy that will establish a morally responsible health insurance system for all Americans?

In his message to Americans on July 29, 2009, President Obama appealed for support of a major transformation of the health insurance system in America. The President laid out eight core consumer protections parameters that must be incorporated into the healthcare reform legislation:

1. No discrimination for pre-existing conditions.
2. No exorbitant out-of-pocket expenses, deductibles or co-pays.
3. No cost-sharing for preventative care.
4. No dropping of coverage if you become seriously ill.
5. No gender discrimination.
6. No annual or lifetime caps on coverage.
7. Extended coverage for young adults.
8. Guaranteed insurance renewal so long as premiums are paid.

He cautioned that "over the next month [during the Congressional break in the summer of 2009], there is going to be an avalanche of misinformation and scare tactics from those seeking to perpetuate the status quo" (Obama, 2009, July 29, p. 1 of 2). According to the President, these core principles are non-negotiable because they will improve accessibility to fair health insurance coverage to nearly all the population in the United States in a cost-effective manner – this is what he referred to as the "moral imperative" for Americans (Obama, 2009, July 1).

9.3 -- Joe the Consultant

Consider the dilemma of "Joe the Consultant," a 57-year-old, self-employed healthcare consultant, who recently received renewal notice from UnitedHealth insurance company that the coverage premium for his two-person consultancy was climbing 12.1% over last year's cost, going from $1,466 to $1,643 per month (Figure 11). During a brief phone conversation, the insurance

---

[57] The Commonwealth Fund is a private non-profit foundation that aims to promote a high performing health care system that achieves better access, improved quality, and greater efficiency, particularly for society's most vulnerable, including low-income people, the uninsured, minority Americans, young children, and elderly adults. The Commonwealth Fund is headquartered in New York. Retrieved March 23, 2009, from http://commonwealthfunf.org/About -US.aspx

representative revealed that the increase was actually *below* average compared to other policy holders, since the typical premium rose around 15% to 18% for the 2009 to 2010 timeframe.

For the small business operator, health insurance costs have mounted to approximately $36,000 per year, which represents more than two-and-a-half months' worth of hard-earned income. The irony of this situation is that the latest renewal notice came in the form of a fancy colorful brochure with a matter-of-fact statement: "To keep your current coverage, no action is required." Really? What about being able to afford a twelve percent increase in the premium for this small business owner-operator?

In order to appreciate the magnitude of the cost differential for healthcare insurance coverage between smaller and larger organizations, consider the example in Table 13 based on a two-person family plan with a moderate benefit package. In this example, the small business employee earned $80,000 post-tax income (before health insurance costs are taken out of the check), and overall annual healthcare expenditures in both situations amounted to approximately $25,000. The healthcare insurance burden for the smaller enterprise is nearly 50% higher than for a larger company. It is not surprising that business bankruptcies in the United States exceeded 43,500 in 2008.

A study conducted by Econometrica, Inc., of Bethesda, Maryland, under contract with the SBA (2007), validated the anecdote above. Their analysis focuses on the economic hardships encountered by smaller firms caused by escalating health insurance overhead. The Econometrica study concludes:

The two most important factors associated with being uninsured are wages and firm size. Individuals who work for smaller firms and who receive lower wages are less likely to have health insurance coverage. Workers at firms of 100 to 249 employees spend the most on healthcare expenses, suggesting that the largest firms may be more likely to self-insure and keep a closer watch on benefits and expenditures. This finding may also suggest that the employees of the medium-size firms with 100 to 249 employees have more generous benefits.

The 2006 survey of small businesses carried out by the National Federation of Independent Business indicated that employer-sponsored health insurance was the most difficult problem owners and managers faced: "more critical than taxes, labor quality, and government red tape" (*Econometrica*, 2007). Another study funded by the SBA released in March 2008 examines the propensity of married couples to enroll both parties and children (if any) in the larger company's health insurance plan since the premium cost tends to be much lower when a spouse works for a smaller firm and the other works for a larger company (Seiber, et al., 2008, pp. 22-23).

According to the April 4, 2009 *Economic News Release* published by the US Labor Department's Bureau of Labor Statistics (BLS), "nonfarm payroll employment continued to decline sharply in

March [a decline of 663,000 jobs], and the unemployment rate rose from 8.1 to 8.5 percent...the number of unemployed persons increased by 694,000 to 13.2 million, and the unemployment rate rose to 8.5 percent." The news release went on to describe that the number of unemployed Americans had reached a 25-year record in the first quarter of 2009. The BLS reported that the group of "long-term unemployed (those jobless for 27 weeks or more) rose to 3.2 million...since the start of the recession in December 2007." African Americans represented the racial group with the highest unemployment rate of 13.3%. The Urban Institute[58] writes:

> *The unemployment rate rose steadily in 2008 and showed no signs of slowing down. Roughly 10.1 million people are out of a job, putting pressure on unemployment insurance and other government safety net programs. More layoffs are expected as the country deals with a financial crisis brought on by the subprime mortgage market collapse, which took down Fannie Mae, Freddie Mac, and blue-chip financial giants in its wake.*

The health insurance crisis has exacerbated the financial troubles for the unemployed, affecting the health status of the nation.

9.4 -- Healthcare is an Economic Issue

Health Care Is an Economic Issue

As more and more people become unemployed, many will lose health insurance benefits for themselves and family members. Every 1 percent increase in the unemployment rate will cause a million people to become uninsured. Health care is as much an economic issue as are job insecurity, mortgage payments, and credit card debt.

BY THE ADVOCACY GROUP DIVIDED WE FAIL

Americans are nearly equally divided on the subject of the healthcare crisis and whether it is perceived primarily as a moral or economic issue. *USA Today* (2009, August 10) ran a front-page article discussing the results of its survey of 3,026 respondents across the country about their support for healthcare reform; surveyors inquired about the perceived urgency for reform and

---

58 The Urban Institute is an independent nonpartisan organization created in 1968 by President Johnson for the purpose of gathering data, conducting research, evaluating problems, and offering technical assistance nationally and abroad on social and economic matters – it is charged with helping to promote sound public policy and effective government. Retrieved March 23, 2009, from http://www.urban.org/about/index.cfm.

whether the urgency related mainly to accessibility problems (moral / ethical) or financial concerns (economic)? The answer varied considerably depending on geographic location, race, and age cohorts (Figures 12 A and B).

The survey results indicate that African Americans and Hispanics favored expanding coverage to the uninsured population, and Whites felt that controlling cost was the priority for healthcare reform. Westerners favored increasing universal access, while Southerners favored controlling the rising cost of healthcare. Among age groups, young adults felt that expanding coverage was more important than controlling costs, perhaps because of the difficulty of obtaining lower-cost health insurance coverage while transitioning from home or colleges to the workplace and employer-sponsored coverage. The respondents who were employed (taxpayers) between ages 30 to 64 were most concerned about the high cost of health insurance premiums (increasing health insurance premiums and greater co-payment and medical deductibles).

Seniors with relatively comprehensive Medicare healthcare coverage were most worried about escalating out-of-pocket costs for medications and high premiums for supplemental plans while the amount of retirement income continued to shrink (stagnant Social Security cost-of-living adjustments, falling value of investment income, pension and retirement funds, higher maintenance costs, etc.).

An informative research study – *the Consumer Bankruptcy Project* -- conducted by David Himmelstein, MD, et al. (2009) investigates the number of medical bankruptcies in the United States in 2007 and compares these figures with a similar analysis completed in 2001. The results published in the *American Journal of Medicine* show how "illness and medical bills contributed to a large and increasing share of US bankruptcies" (p. 741). Himmelstein and his colleagues examined nearly 120,000 US bankruptcy petitions filed between January 25 and April 11, 2007 to determine the main causes for these actions. The court records reviewed were supplemented by about 5,000 questionnaires and 2,314 telephone interviews. The Administrative Office of the US Courts reports that there were a total of 850,912 bankruptcy filings in 2007, up 38% from 2006. This figure includes both individual consumers and businesses, or 822,590 and 28,322, respectively. Historical trends indicate that only 8% of families filing for bankruptcy in 1981 were directly related to serious medical financial problems; in 2001, about 50% of bankruptcies were tied to medical financial crises; and in 2007, the number of medical-related bankruptcies had climbed to 62.1% of all filings. These dramatic results occurred *prior* to the economic crash in 2008, so the present rate is much higher. The study notes that medical-related bankruptcies in America occur every 90 seconds.

The researchers discovered that "most medical debtors were well educated and middle class; three quarters *had* health insurance" (p. 742). The data also shows that the key reasons for bankruptcies were (1) medical bill problems (57.1%) and (2) loss of income due to illness and disabilities resulting from medical conditions (40.3%). Furthermore, 77.9% had insurance coverage at the time of the bankruptcy – 60.3% carried private insurance as their primary coverage.

Why The United States Healthcare System Should Be A Limited Human Right For All

According to the study, hospital bills amounted to the single largest out-of-pocket debt (48% of patients), while prescription drugs, doctors' bills, and premiums amounted to 19%, 15%, and 4%, respectively. Their research concludes:

> *Since 2001, the proportion of all bankruptcies attributed to medical problems has increased 50%. Nearly two thirds of all bankruptcies [in the United States] are now linked to illness...For 92% of the medically bankrupt, high medical bills directly contributed to their bankruptcy. Many families with continuous coverage found themselves under-insured, responsible for thousands of dollars in out-of-pocket costs...Nationally, a quarter of firms cancel coverage immediately when an employee suffers a disabling illness; another quarter do so within a year. Income loss due to illness also was common, but nearly always coupled with high medical bills. (pp. 744-745).*

Dr. Himmelstein and his co-authors stress that "medical impoverishment, although common in poor nations, is almost unheard of in wealthy countries other than the US" (p. 745). These findings reinforced the discussion in Section 9 that the health insurance conundrum in America is as much a problem for the uninsured population as it is a struggle for the *underinsured* population of approximately 30 million. This unfortunate situation makes no sense in a country as wealthy as the United States – this is morally reprehensible.

Elliott Fisher, MD, MPH, Director of The Center for Health Policy Research, and Professor of Medicine and Community and Family Medicine, Dartmouth Medical School, is the senior researcher and co-founder of the *Dartmouth Atlas of Health Care.* His group found that there are wide variations in healthcare utilization and patient outcomes across the United States (the *Atlas* tracks hospital utilization and cost of care for Medicare patients from federal sources). In different regions of the country, the cost of treating a particular ailment at a particular hospital in a particular location was substantially different than the national average, while morbidity and mortality rates varied substantially from expectations; this also means that the cost per patient type varies accordingly. Fisher attributes cost variability to four interrelated factors: (1) the number of hospital beds per 1,000 population; (2) the number of physicians relative to the population and health status, especially the number of specialists; (3) the degree of high-revenue service lines and duplication among hospitals; and (4) the percentage of for-profit providers.

Since hospitals, provider organizations, and physicians are remunerated on the basis of the types of patients treated, the volume of procedures performed, and total units of service rendered, instead of the quality of patient outcomes, there is little incentive to control their utilization and hold costs down. Fisher claims that the *Atlas* indicates that "spending for Medicare would fall by about 20% if everybody practiced medicine the way the lowest-spending fifth of the nation does" (Futrelle, 2009, July 16, pp. 82-86). The data also suggests that the lower-cost providers often had the best outcomes. The Mayo Clinic in Rochester, Minnesota, is a good example of cost-effectiveness and quality results. Medicare and Social Security Insurance (SSI) expenditures in 2006 totaled around $420 billion; so according to Fisher's estimates the potential savings for these programs could amount to approximately $90 billion each year.

In his address to members of the US Congress on September 9, 2009, President Barack Obama talked about the growing cost of healthcare in America. He stressed, "We know we must reform this system; the question is how." The economic burden for American taxpayers is not sustainable in the long run. The president cautioned members of Congress:

> When health care costs grow at the rate they have, it puts greater pressure on programs like Medicare and Medicaid. If we do nothing to slow these skyrocketing costs, we will eventually be spending more on Medicare and Medicaid than every other government program combined. Put simply, our health care problem is our deficit problem. Nothing else comes close.

There is no *magic bullet* for addressing the worsening healthcare cost dilemma. The historical record of treating the *symptoms* of diseases and illnesses (sick care model) rather than modifying the *root causes* of unhealthy life-styles guarantees that US healthcare expenditures will continue to outpace economic prosperity.

> *Make no mistake: The status quo on healthcare is no longer an option for the United States of America. If we step back from this challenge right now, we will leave our children a legacy of debt and a future of crushing costs that bankrupt our families and our businesses. It's because we will have done nothing to bring down the cost of Medicare and Medicaid. It will crush our government.*
>
> BY PRESIDENT BARACK OBAMA, INTRODUCING HIS NOMINEE FOR US SURGEON GENERAL, JULY 13, 2009, IN WASHINGTON, DC

In September 2008, the US economy crashed (Chart 5 B), bringing the global banking industry to its knees (starting with the bankruptcy of Lehman Brothers). Shortly after, the New York Stock Exchange, the car industry (GM and Chrysler), the housing industry, business and retailers of all sizes, also fell into a deep recession reminiscent of the American Great Depression of the 1930s. The stock market on Wall Street plummeted nearly 60% to a rock-bottom figure of close to 7,000 points by February 2009. Millions of American workers lost their jobs during the twelve-month period from September 2008 to 2009, pushing the national unemployment rate to 10 percent -- some states are pushing 14 percent unemployment.

The fragility of today's US economic health has accentuated the problems with our healthcare system, which is reliant on the employer-sponsored health insurance and stability of the economy. The present number of uninsured Americans is far too great for policymakers and the public to ignore. Fortunately, there are encouraging signs that the political climate is more favorable for forging a plan to revitalize the healthcare system that has traditionally not rewarded delivery of quality services and improved patient outcomes, nor have payers placed emphasis on prevention and wellness as a way to control sick care and rising healthcare costs.

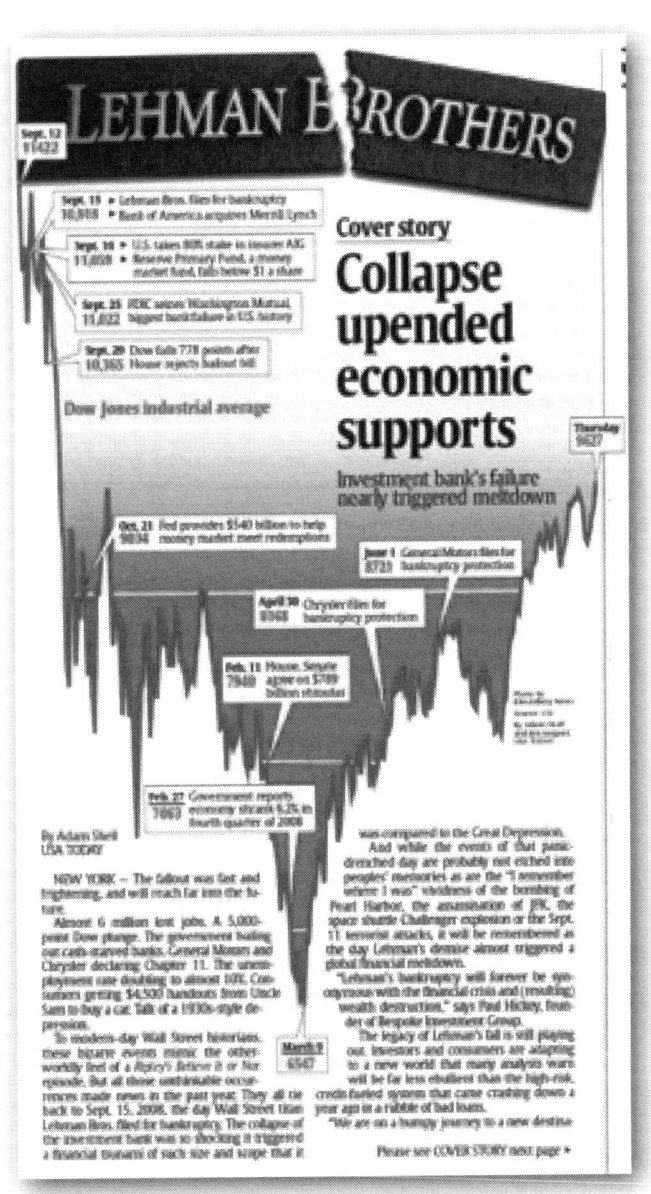

Chart 5 - USA Today Headlines: Economic Collapse -- September 2008 to 2009

Part 3
Foundational Elements of Healthcare

Ten

HEALTH CARE (NOT SICK CARE), A LIMITED HUMAN RIGHT FOR ALL

What's Stronger in Human Life, Rationality or Irrationality?

No contest. Non-rational forces are stronger than rational thought and can cause us sometimes to do very irrational things. But non-rational forces are not themselves irrational. The heart leads us in a way that the mind can't. Emotions are more powerful than reason. And within the realm of the mind, it is the imagination that is much stronger than the logical intellect.

BY TOM MORRIS, PH.D., IN PHILOSOPHY FOR DUMMIES, 1999.

Is there a difference between ethics and morality? How are we able to ascertain when something is morally right or wrong? How does social justice relate to the distribution of healthcare resources? Does culture have a bearing on the development of ethical principles? For example, euthanasia is considered morally right in some societies and not in others. Let's start by examining some basic dictionary definitions that relate to the foundational elements of healthcare in Table 14.

Table 11 – Definition of Key Terms

Definitions

Culture → noun
1. The totality of socially transmitted behavior patterns, arts, beliefs, institutions, and all other products of human work and thought characteristic of a community or population...
2. The act of developing the social, moral, and intellectual faculties through education.

Ethics → noun
1. (u. treated as pl.) moral principles that govern a person's behavior or the conducting of an activity: medical ethics also enter into the question.
2. [in sing.] a set of moral principles, especially one's relation to or affirming a specified group, field, or form of conduct: the puritan ethic was being replaced by the hedonist ethic.

Human right → noun

(u. human rights) a right which is believed to belong to every person: a flagrant disregard for basic human rights.

Morality → noun
1. The relation of conformity or nonconformity to the moral standard or rule; quality of an intention, a character, an action, a principle, or a sentiment, when tried by the standard of right.
2. The quality of an action which renders it good; the conformity of an act to the accepted standard of right.
3. The practice of the moral duties; rectitude of life; conformity to the standard of right; virtue; as, we often admire the politeness of men whose morality we question.
4. The doctrines or rules of moral duties, or the duties of men in their social character; ethics.

Social justice → noun

The notion that society should be organized in a way that allows equal opportunity for all its members (also attributive: social justice issues).

Fair → adjective

Treating people equally without favoritism or discrimination: the group has achieved fair and equal representation for all its members; a fairer distribution of wealth; just or appropriate in the circumstances: to be fair.

Health care → noun

[mass noun] often as modifier the organized provision of medical care to individuals or a community: health-care professionals.

Welfare → noun
1. Health, the state of being well, happiness, wellbeing, or prosperity.
2. Aid in the form of money or necessities for those in need; also the agency through which the aid is given.

Source: **The Oxford Dictionary of English (2008, 2nd ed. rev.)**

The commonality among these terms is that they all pertain to the determination of the "state of wellness" of individuals, groups, communities, or society. Our state of wellness is determined by our perception of the outcomes of these factors. Perception is relative, situational, and subjective. The challenge for any society is to determine how to adequately provide for reasonable access to various determinants of health in a world of intense competition for limited resources. This chapter explores some of the prominent philosophical theories developed to explain and deal with difficult ethical concerns and dilemmas concerning distributive justice and inequities of health and healthcare.

10.1 -- Is Culture the Basis for Healthcare Ethics and Morality?

There are many separate disciplines that are concerned with the study of human behavior and social structures – psychology, religion, sociology, anthropology, political science, biology, philosophy, and others. This section concentrates on the body of knowledge that has evolved from the disciplines of philosophy and human relations, examining the particular aspects of moral and ethical theories that seek to discover why and how humans behave toward each other in society (Rachels, 2003).

Culture is a human attribute. Each society is comprised of unique cultural beliefs, values, customs, and relational exchange mechanisms that are representative of and accepted by its members. Culture is socially transmitted from generation to generation through traditional practices and institutions (i.e., governmental, religious, political, economic, educational and so forth). Culture guides and influences human behavior and shapes the overall determinants of social interaction and the rules of engagement between individuals, groups, communities, states, and nations.

Culture influences moral principles that shape ethical behavior and social exchanges, which in turn govern patterns of social justice and fairness among individuals and groups within society. Locally and regionally, moral principles guide policymakers in the process of determining how to distribute essential services that are considered beneficial for communities they serve. Generally accepted moral principles also govern the protection of liberties, security, goods and services, etc. that are regarded as entitlements and rights of citizens.

T.R. Reid (2009, September 21) shared his experiences while traveling the globe, investigating different nation's healthcare systems and their political and cultural basis for structuring healthcare. Reid found that "a health-care system reflects a nation's basic cultural values (p. 42). What he learned is:

If a nation answers yes to that moral question ['should a rich society provide healthcare to everyone who needs it?'], it will build a health-care system like the ones in Britain, Germany, Canada, France, and Japan, where everybody is covered. If a nation doesn't decide to provide universal coverage, then you're going to end up with a system where some people get the finest medical care on earth in the finest hospitals, and tens of thousands of other are left to die for lack of care. Without the moral commitment, in other words, you end up with a system like America's. (p. 43)

He studied Princeton University economist Uwe Reinhardt's work about how healthcare systems evolve around national values and national character. Reid went on to illustrate that most all wealthier developed countries (with the exception of the US) have developed a strong sense of *solidarity*, and they perceive healthcare as a universal right on equal footing for everyone, regardless of socioeconomic status (following the *permissive* paradigm). Furthermore, the "right to medical care" is protected by most national Constitutions. Although healthcare delivery systems internationally vary considerably, most basic health and preventive services, within reasonable limitations, are guaranteed to all residents. By contrast, the American healthcare system is patterned after the *individualist* paradigm, which is structured around the market-driven distribution approach and considered a commodity that is priced according to supply and demand terms.[59]

> *Healthcare is an ethical issue...If we all agree that healthcare is a right, then it will be easier to move forward with healthcare reform...Until we as a society decide that healthcare is a right, or at least some minimum standard of healthcare that begins to approach equitable, it won't be... regardless, rationing of healthcare services is inevitable (paraphrased).*
>
> NPR Radio Interview with Univ. of Pennsylvania Bioethicist and Prof. Arthur Caplan, December 17, 2008

James Rachels synthesized the current body of philosophical knowledge in his book entitled *The Elements of Moral Philosophy* – it is the "science" of moral judgments backed by good reasoning, and requires impartial consideration of each individual's interests (p. 11). Moral philosophy is *not* a concrete science based on facts and figures about tangible matters, as in the case of scientific chemistry, where there are definite laws governing the formation of H_2O (physical science) or the biology of reproduction (medical science). He makes his point with three interesting anecdotes about moral predicaments:

1. The case of Theresa Ann Campo Pearson, an anencephalic infant (baby born without a brain) known as "Baby Theresa," born in Florida in 1992. Her parents and the physicians agreed to volunteer her organs before her "death," while the organs were still viable, in order to save other infants who could benefit from this *generous act*. The public

---

[59] The descriptions for these three paradigms are found in the text from Brannigan and Boss (2001, pp. 630-634). The free-market approach to healthcare deliver is also called "the individualist paradigm." The equal playing field for all health services similar to the Canadian system is called "the permissive paradigm." Finally, "the puritan paradigm" is characterized by a core set of health services available to all members, with a dual-tiered insurance program – private and public.

controversy arose about the morality of "killing" one infant so that others could live. At that time, ethicists agreed that it was "really a horrendous proposition." (p. 2)
2. The second example involved conjoined twins, known as Mary and Jodie, who were born at St. Mary's Hospital in Manchester, England. The twins were connected at the lower abdomen, where their spines were fused; they also shared a single heart and one set of lungs. The medical consensus was that only one of the twins, Mary, was strong enough to survive the separating surgical procedure – both would die if they were not separated. Here, the parents, who were Catholic, refused to grant permission for the surgery. "We believe that nature should take its course; if it is God's will that both our children should not survive, then so be it," stated the parents, who explained they loved both children. At the request of the hospital, the courts ordered that the operation be performed. Jodie lived and Mary died. (p.6)
3. The third example was the case of the "mercy killing" of Tracy Latimer, a 12-year-old Canadian girl afflicted with advanced stages of cerebral palsy. Her father, in desperation, killed his daughter by confining her in his vehicle and piping the exhaust fumes inside the cab until she was dead. At the time of her death, Tracy had the mental capacity of a three-month-old and weighed less than 40 pounds. The jury convicted the father of second-degree murder but recommended that the judge ignore the mandatory 25-year prison sentence. The trial judge agreed and ordered a one-year sentence in jail, followed by a year confinement to his farm – "However, the Supreme Court of Canada stepped in and ruled that the mandatory sentence must be imposed. Robert Latimer is now in prison, serving the 25-year term." (p. 8)

In each of these difficult and painfully human situations, the parties on both sides of the dilemma acted according to their moral and ethical beliefs. Rachels points out that philosophy demands *reasoning* and *impartiality* to reach an ethical decision. "Our feelings may be irrational; they may be nothing but the products of prejudice, selfishness, or cultural conditioning...At one time, for example, people's feelings told them that members of other races were inferior and that slavery was God's own plan," Rachels states (p. 11). The conclusions deduced from these *morality stories* can be summarized as follows:

> The *minimum conception* may now be stated very briefly: morality is, at the very least, the effort to guide one's conduct by reason – that is, to do what there are the best reasons for doing – while giving equal weight to the interests of each individual who will be affected by what one does (p. 14).

One of the well-established theories pertaining to morality is the concept of *cultural relativism*. Cultural relativists claim that moral codes are culturally biased – different cultures have differing sets of moral codes that determine right from wrong. Anthropologists talk about *ethnocentrism* when one group imposes its moral belief onto another group because they are convinced that their way is the right way to act or treat others (pp. 16-31). If cultural relativism were a perfectly valid theory, Rachels explains, there would be no such thing as *absolute moral codes* or *universal truths* for humans to abide by. This conclusion could lead us to the false assumption that "there is no objective truth" in morality; that right and wrong are only a matter of opinion, and that opinions vary from culture to culture (the cultural differences argument). Such a conclusion does not follow a logical premise within this theoretical framework, asserts Rachels (pp. 20-21).

There is a subtle yet crucial difference between cultural beliefs and cultural values that must be recognized when considering moral and ethical issues. Rachels cites two examples of *foundational moral rules* that exist in all cultures: (1) homicide (taking the life of an innocent person) and (2) intentional deceit (lying). The acceptance of these practices in "society on any large scale would [result in its] collapse," Rachels emphasizes. This is not to infer that there are no special circumstances in which these behaviors are tolerated or even sanctioned under, as in the case of capital punishment for criminals or lying to save another human being from harm's way, but these are exceptions to the general rule.

Professor, philosopher, and prolific writer (of over 30 books), Roger Scruton (1994) comments on the relative abstraction of moral philosophy in his book *Modern Philosophy: An Introduction and Survey*:

> *Philosophy is said to be a priori inquiry, although precisely what this means is a matter of controversy. While science proceeds by experiment, and tests all its theories against evidence, philosophy reaches its results by thought alone, and makes no reference to experience in doing so. (p.11)*

Ethics is concerned with the process of making moral choices and the art of living. Culturally-driven moral imperatives (referred to by President Barack Obama in his July 1, 2009 town hall meeting about healthcare reform) are validated in the mind of the beholder, where they become a perceived reality, in spite of the absence of hard, scientific proof.

So how does culture impact ethical and moral standards in different population groups with regard to the provision of basic health services? Deliberately denying access to healthcare services seems counter-intuitive to the basic moral codes of preserving life and attaining one's maximum potential that ultimately benefit the community-at-large (a basic utilitarian tenet). This brings us to three important questions that are the central focus of this section:

1. Is it reasonable (rationally logical) for a particular culture or society to consider access to basic health and healthcare a universal right for all citizens regardless of socioeconomic

status as morally and ethically justified, while another does not - is one position right and the other wrong?
2. Should health and healthcare be considered a special element of *every* society – or is it merely a market commodity accessible to those who can afford to acquire it?
3. Is reasonable access to basic health and healthcare a culturally determinable factor?

Rachels believes that there *are* rational answers to these important social questions based on sound moral and ethical judgments:

> It is nonsense to say, in the face of all this, that ethical judgments can be nothing more than 'mere opinions.' Nevertheless, the impression that moral judgments are 'unprovable' is remarkably persistent. Why do people believe this? Three points might be mentioned.
> First, when proof is demanded, people often have in mind an inappropriate standard. They are thinking about observations and experiments in science; and when there are no comparable observations and experiments in ethics, they surmise that there is no proof. But in the [realm] of ethics, rational thinking consists in providing reasons, analyzing arguments, setting limits and justifying principles, and the like. The fact that ethical reasoning differs from reasoning in science does not make it deficient. Second, when we think of 'proving our ethical opinions to be correct,' we tend to think automatically of the most difficult issues [like the ethical dilemmas provided above or scientific concerns that perplex physicists]… But of course, there are many simpler matters about which all competent physicists agree. Similarly, in ethics there are many simpler matters about which all reasonable people agree. (p. 43)

Just because cultures (made up of differing norms, practices, values, beliefs, customs, etc.) vary around the globe, it does not mean that there are no universal moral principles that should apply to all members of the human family, regardless of place or time (p. 200). I have referred to these core issues as the *foundational elements* of society. The inherent value of human life is one such universal tenet.

People do not have the option to choose the location and time where they are born -- race, social class, genetic attributes, family wealth, and so forth are "native endowments." Philosopher John Rawls said that all human beings are subjected equally to the whims of "the natural lottery" of life. Given this fact, society is compelled to provide certain inalienable rights to all its members in order to maximize individual opportunities based on the natural *gifts* each person is allotted at birth – regardless of their cultural basis.

Basic nurturance (affection, care, protection, concern, etc.), sustenance, shelter, education (informal and formal), freedom, respect, safety, ability to participate in the democratic process, and health status (personal and environmental) are all universal and essential necessities of human existence. They are foundational elements of a successful democratic society. The key word in this definition is *basic*. Beyond the basics, inequality will continue to persist because of the natural variation of human, environmental, and economic resources in society. The universal respect for human life and social welfare is what makes our species "superior" to other life forms. It is reasonable to infer from the discussion above that a commitment to healthcare *is* a culturally determinable factor in all societies.

In order to support the rationale for the hypothesis that *the United States healthcare system should be a limited human right for all*, we will review in some detail the exceptional work of notable philosophers who have helped define the unique characteristics of health and healthcare that impact individuals and societies: John Stuart Mill, Immanuel Kant, John Rawls, Norman Daniels, Yroam Amiel and Frank Cowell, and Jonathan Mann. The major theories, principles, axioms, and concepts are identified at the start of each chapter for easy reference.

10.2 -- John Stuart Mill – Utilitarian Theory

Major theories, principles, axioms, and concepts
- *Liberty is the ultimate right*
- *Utilitarian theory is synonymous with the Greatest Happiness Principle – actions are right in proportion to the degree of happiness they promote; wrong actions tend to produce pain, and deprivation of pleasure*
- *Greater goods must not be subjugated to lesser goods*
- *Utilitarianism equals modern liberalism*
- *Morality promotes the greatest good, therefore supporting the Utilitarian principle*
- *Healthcare, the medical art and healing profession, is good because it encourages well-being and health*

Any discussion about *utilitarian theory* guides one to the classical works by John Stuart Mill (1806-1873), originally written in the late 1800s. Mill was taught by his father, James Mill, and Jeremy Bentham (both living during the period from 1750s to 1830s), who were staunch advocates of the utilitarian philosophy that was originally proposed by David Hume (1711-1776). Utilitarianism had a profound impact on British and American political liberal philosophy. Mill's literary contributions are far too numerous to list here; however, two of his famous works center on Liberty and Utilitarianism (republished in 1992). He is regarded as one of the most influential economists and philosophers of his time. A brief discussion of some of the key *Utilitarian* concepts relating to healthcare follows.

Mill's essay on liberty concerns the use, or misuse, of political authority over members of a civilized community:

> *...that the sole end for which mankind are warranted, individually or collectively, in interfering with the liberty of action of any of their number, is self-protection. That the only purpose for which power can be rightfully exercised over any member of a civilized community, against his will, is to prevent harm to others. His own good, either physical or moral, is not a sufficient warrant. He cannot rightfully be compelled to do or forbear because it will be better for him to do so, because it will make him happier, because, in the opinion of others to do so would be wise or even right... (pp. 12-13)*

In essence, Mill believed that the state does not have a right to encroach on an individual's independence, "over himself, over his own body and mind, the individual is sovereign" (p. 13). As discussed further on in this section, the concept of absolute individual liberty has an intrinsic relationship between the freedom to treat one's body and health as we choose, and the right to a healthy existence and access to healthcare when the consequences of our choices result in illness and disease (e.g., trauma due to accidents, cancer due to cigarette smoking, brain injury due to drug abuse, etc.).

> *Each is the proper guardian of his own health, whether bodily, or mental or spiritual. Mankind are greater gainers by suffering each other to live as seems good themselves, than by compelling each to live as seems good to the rest.*
>
> JOHN STUART MILL, ON LIBERTY

Moving to the specific concepts of utilitarianism, Mill argues that the utilitarian standard is to seek happiness, not only for oneself, but for the community-at-large. Mill cites the doctrine of Jesus of Nazareth as the perfect example of impartial and disinterested *benevolence* – "To do as you would be done by, and love your neighbor as yourself, constitute the ideal perfection of utilitarian morality" (p. 128). Perhaps we can equate the *Greatest Happiness Principle* with the attainment of a "State of Happiness," where there is the absence (to the extent possible based on environmental and social circumstances) of suffering and pain. Mill (2005) elaborates on this notion of the degree of "righteousness" of certain actions and how it is measured by the degree to which each action contributes to happiness and pleasure. Of course, Mill recognizes, "that some *kinds* of pleasure are more desirable and more valuable than others;" and that the *quality* of the experience must also be factored into the evaluation process, not only *quantity* (pp. 7-9).

> *The creed which accepts as the foundation of morals, Utility, or the Greatest Happiness Principle, holds that actions are right in proportion as they tend to promote happiness, wrong as they tend to produce the reverse of happiness. By happiness is intended pleasure, and the absence of pain; by*

> *unhappiness, pain, and the privation of pleasure…It is quite compatible with the principle of utility to recognize the fact, that some kinds of pleasure are more desirable and more valuable than others. It would be absurd that while, in estimating all other things, quality is considered as well as quantity, the estimation of pleasures should be supposed to depend on quantity alone.*
>
> JOHN STUART MILL, ON UTILITARIANISM

The pursuit of certain "goods" is a simple *means* to an end, in order to achieve happiness or pleasure; other actions are intrinsically proper and good in and of themselves. Mill also talks about *virtue* being an example of an element of one's desire for happiness by seeking happiness and pleasure for others in need (p.39). The connection between utility (individual freedom) and justice lies within the practice of enforcing what is perceived as the right of an individual – "the idea of justice supposes two things: a rule of conduct, and a sentiment which sanctions the rule" (p. 55). Justice serves as the "checks and balances" in society to preserve individual rights. According to Mill:

> *When we call anything a person's right, we mean that he has a valid claim on society to protect him in the possession of it, either by the force of law, or by that of education and opinion. If he has what we consider a sufficient claim, on whatever account, to have something guaranteed to him by society, we say that he has a right to it. If we desire to prove that anything does not belong to him by right, we think this done as soon as it is admitted that society ought not to take measures for securing it to him, but should leave it to chance, or to his own exertions. (p. 56)*

It is also important to realize that there are many differing conceptions of justice throughout nations and within communities. To put this concept into Mill's terminology: "Justice is a name for certain classes of moral rules, which concern the essentials of human well-being more nearly, and are therefore of more absolute obligation, than any other rules for the guidance of life" (p. 61).

James Rachels (2003) characterizes the Principle of Utility as a radical move away from the contemporary ridged rules established by God or the Divine Order: "The point of morality is seen as the happiness of beings in this world, and nothing more; and we are permitted – even required – to do whatever is necessary to promote happiness" (p. 93). The attitude about the pursuit of happiness as the ultimate goal is what is considered the classical or pure utilitarian doctrine. Critics have stated that Utilitarianism is in conflict with the basic ideals of justice and fairness – justice requires that we treat people fairly, according to their individual needs and merits, states Rachels (p. 106). Although an action infringing on someone's individual rights and liberties might bring about the "greater good" of the community, this act of *injustice* cannot be justified from an ethical standpoint. It is necessary to employ moral common sense in circumstances that call into question a person's rights over the general community benefit. Rachels emphasizes: "Utilitarianism is at odds with the idea that people have *rights* that may not be trampled on merely because one anticipates good results" (p. 107). On the other hand, Rachels notes that supporters of the Principle of Utility claimed that it was meant as a mere guide for choosing rules, not individual acts themselves, giving rise to a newer version of the theory called *Rule-Utilitarianism* (as opposed to the original theory called *Act-Utilitarianism*). This brings us back to the key philosophical question: "Are there absolute moral rules that apply equally to all people across the globe?"

The Utilitarian Model

Morality→Liberty→Happiness & Pleasure→Rights, Duties, and Obligations→Laws →Justice System→Security→Societal Wellbeing

The debate about human happiness has come to the forefront once again as policymakers struggle to measure the economic return-on-investment for *welfare* services in communities and nations and the relative impact on health status, or overall wellbeing. For example, the common measure used internationally is the percentage of GDP spent on healthcare in comparison to key health indicators – infant mortality, hospital admission rate, life expectancy, etc. But how meaningful is this standard for comparing wellbeing in communities and nations? What about the degree of happiness individuals and society enjoy as a result of healthier outcomes?

Lionel Beehner (2009) recently reported in *USA Today* that there is "a new wave of world leaders and progressive economists who insist we are way too obsessed with gross domestic product (GDP) as the be-all, end-all benchmark of measuring economic health" (p. 11A). Beehner notes that globally, there is discussion about considering the so-called "softer" quality-of-life indicators beyond the GDP – e.g., the environment, leisure time, labor protections, and healthcare coverage.

This important topic was first raised by King Jigne Singye Wangchuck of the Himalayan nation of Bhutan back in 1972, writes Beehner. In the context of the 2009 economic summit of the "Group of 20" world leaders meeting in Pittsburg on September 24th, the French President Nicolas Sarkozy raised the issue of coming up with a "gross national happiness" index. Sarkozy's commitment to this end included the commissioning of a study by two of the world's leading economists – Joseph Stiglitz and Aramatya Sen -- to develop new "ways to measure a society's wellbeing." The concept is an interesting one, states Beehner:

> On one level, it is a laudable effort. GDP is a lousy way to measure a society's well-being. It does not capture a country's political stability, much less the health of its citizens or the

sustainability of its environment. Nor does it correlate with a nation's "happiness," studies show. Americans are three times as wealthy as they were 50 years ago, but not much happier…What's more, this new yardstick could prove useful as we look to overhaul our health care system and tackle climate change – both of which would put a sizeable dent in our GDP in the short run, but arguably would provide a boost for our health and happiness in the long run. (p. 11A)

According to Beehner, the happiest nation on earth is Denmark (ranked by the Organization for Economic Cooperation and Development); the US does not even fall in the top 10 ranking. Undoubtedly, it will be difficult for Stiglitz and Sen to identify a universal gauge for happiness, since cultural factors have a lot to do with a society's sense of happiness. Other important factors to examine are the correlations between the degree of health status, the degree of happiness, and the degree of productivity in societies around the world – and of course, the famous *chicken-and-the-egg* question, which of these factors should come first?

The applicability of the utilitarian theory to the contemporary healthcare debate in the US has been extensively explored by Brannigan and Boss (2001) in their text on *Healthcare Ethics in a Diverse Society*. A most salient example of the utilitarian notion in American healthcare was employed by the University of Washington, Seattle, at the Seattle Artificial Kidney Center, in 1967, regarding access to limited hemodialysis services for persons suffering from chronic renal failure. An allocation committee – nicknamed the "God Committee" – evaluated accessibility criteria according to a candidate's social worth; "all things being equal, priority was given to candidates who have dependents, who were stable in their behavior and emotionally mature, and who had a record of public service." The authors explain that "basing moral decisions on a cost / benefit calculation of social worth is an example of the application of utilitarianism (p. 25). Of course, persons who did not qualify for treatment on scarce dialysis machines died. Brannigan and Boss noted:

> The principle of utility is sometimes broken down into two separate principles: the no-harm principle and the duty to promote good. The no-harm principle is also known as *non-maleficence* or, in Eastern ethics, *ahimsa*. The duty to promote good is also known as the principle of beneficence or, in Eastern ethics, *jen*…The application of utilitarian theory to the allocation of scarce healthcare resources is also found in the cost / benefit analysis used in 1993 by the state of Oregon in deciding how to best distribute federal funds [for Medicaid beneficiaries]. Should healthcare resources go to those who can afford to pay for them [market-driven distribution method], as in the American system? Or should they be distributed in a more equitable manner that spreads the benefits over more people, as in Canada and, to some extent, the Oregon Health Plan, even if this means that some people will be denied expensive healthcare treatments? (p. 26)

Again, the major limitation of the utilitarian theory is that it tends to sacrifice individual rights for the sake of the "greater good" for society. The extreme abhorrent consequence of blind adherence to the philosophy of utility was exemplified in the case of Nazi Germany, where human experimentation on what they considered "inferior" Jews was carried out in the name of scientific advancement to support the wellbeing of a "superior" race.

Brannigan and Boss note that rather than throw out the utilitarian theory altogether, ethicists and philosophers have argued that a *combination* of the principles of utility, justice, and respect for autonomy can produce rational and reasonable decisions about the "best" healthcare approaches for society (p. 28). In the final analysis, is health and wellbeing intended to primarily satisfy personal happiness (and maximize individual opportunity realization), or should it be rationed in some equitable fashion as to serve the greatest good for the largest number of people in the community? This foundational concern characterizes the challenging dichotomy between individual rights (human and moral) and social benefits that policymakers must reconcile during the present debate over healthcare reform in the United States.

10.3 -- Immanuel Kant – Principle of the Categorical Imperative

Major theories, principles, axioms, and concepts
- *The difference between theoretical and practical knowledge.*
- *The Categorical Imperative and its components.*
- *Duty and moral vision.*
- *Beneficence and humanity.*
- *Healthcare is an obligatory duty of individuals and nations*

Immanuel Kant[60] is revered as one of Europe's[61] great philosophers of the 18th Century. He profoundly impacted Western thought about the nature of humanity, moral reasoning, ethics, and political structure (elucidated in *Metaphysics of Morals*). His major literary contributions to society are summarized in three of his classical books: (1) *Critique of Pure Reason* – discussing the structure of human reasoning and its limitations, (2) *Critique of Practical Reason* – primarily focused on ethical reasoning, and (3) *Critique of Judgment* – the investigation of aesthetics and

---

[60] Kant's biography indicates that his baptismal name was "Emanuel" Kant, and that he changed his given name to "Immanuel" as an adult.

[61] Immanuel Kant was the son of Johann Georg Kant (1682-1746) and nee Regina Dorothea Reuter (1697-1737), born in the Prussian city of Konigsberg (now Kaliningrad, Russia) in 1724. Kant died February 12, 1804. His thinking and philosophy of life was largely influenced by David Hume, John Locke, George Berkeley and other contemporaries.

teleology.[62] Kant's framework for philosophical inquiry was considered a paradigm shift from 18th Century moral thinking.[63] We will confine our review to Kant's principle of *The Categorical Imperative* and its relationship to mankind's actions and determination of wellbeing.

Kant's conception of the categorical imperative was an outgrowth of the notion that there was a single "supreme" moral obligation stemming from the concept of *duty*. The categorical imperative equates to moral laws that dictate what is good – they must be obeyed without exception. Kant believed that all rational beings were capable of discerning the ethical doctrine that "pleasure, variously conceived of in terms of happiness of the individual or of society, is the principle good and the proper aim of action" (also referred to as *Hedonism*). He also believed that people always act in ways to maximize pleasure and avoid pain (Scruton, 2001). In the 1785 *Grounding for the Metaphysics of Morals*, Kant (1993, translated version) argues that the principles of morality were based on *reasoning* rather than the popular notion of *religious revelation* from God. This non-dogmatic approach was a revolutionary concept in his time and caused immense concern in the Christian community. Kant identifies three tests (what he referred to as formulations or propositions) of his categorical imperative:

- *First*, only an act done from duty has moral worth;
- *Second*, the moral worth of an act is not based on the consequences of the act;
- *Third*, the moral worth of an act comes from the agent's respect for the law.

Kant believed that moral rules are absolute. His theory of ethics professes that all rational people must accept the categorical imperative: "Act only according to the maxim by which you can at the same time will that it should become a universal law" (Rachels, 2003). In essence, categorical imperatives have no "wiggle room;" they cannot be compromised or explained away by our choices or desires, and a violation of a categorical imperative has consequences. For example, telling a lie about someone or something is wrong, no matter what the reason or justification for the lie – it is simply wrong. Lies violate trust and cannot become universally acceptable practices because that would undermine the basis of human interaction. Rachels clarifies Kant's position as follows:

> *Moral reasons, if they are valid at all, are binding on all people at all times [and in all places]. This is a requirement of consistency; and Kant was right to think that no rational*

---

62 *Teleology* [derived from the Greek word *teleos* – an end; and *logy* – the study of] in this particular context is concerned with (1) the study of final causes; (2) the fact or quality of being directed toward a definite end of having an ultimate purpose. *The Oxford Dictionary of English* (2nd ed. rev.).

63 According to Robert Hall, author of An Introduction to Healthcare Organizational Ethics (2000, p. 10), "Morality is thus a pluralistic concept; it exists in our society (as laws and professional codes), in our consciences (as values and commitments), in our minds (as rational principles), and in our hearts (as ideals and personal commitments).

person may deny it. This is the Kantian idea – or; I should say, one of the Kantian ideas – that has been so influential. It implies that a person cannot regard herself as special, from a moral point of view: She cannot consistently think that she is permitted to act in ways that are forbidden to others, or that her interests are more important than other people's interests…If Kant was not the first to recognize this, he was the first to make it the cornerstone of a fully worked-out system of morals. That was his great contribution. (p. 128)

Roger Scruton (2001) underscores this Kantian concept by emphasizing that the categorical imperatives "do not typically contain an 'if'" statement (p. 83). Nicholas Rescher (2000) also summarizes Kant's philosophical premise succinctly -- the "super principle" is to "act always on principles, and make sure that they are rational" (p. 247). To reiterate a popular saying, "what is good for the goose should also be good for the gander." Nonetheless, the rigidity of Kantian philosophy has been challenged by philosophers on the basis that moral duties are *prima facie* duties, which occasionally can be overridden by stronger moral claims (Brannigan and Boss, 2001).

In her book *The Ethics of Leadership*, Joanne Ciulla (2003) compares John Stuart Mill's utilitarian philosophy with Immanuel Kant's theory of ethical reasoning:

Utilitarianism is a very familiar moral theory for Westerners. It is the foundation of democracy and at least on the surface, it bears some resemblance to a major tenet of economics, the cost-benefit analysis [also use in the formulation of the Oregon Health Plan described in Section 7.2, above]. Utilitarianism is the flip side of Kant's theory of ethics. Ethical theories based on duty are called deontic theories (from the Greek word for duty, deon). They are concerned with the moral intent of an act. Utilitarian theory is teleological (from the Greek word telos, which means purpose of end). Kant's theory is based on human reason; utilitarianism is based on reason and experience. Unlike Kant, John Stuart Mill believes that we know enough about causation from experience to influence outcomes. Acting to bring about the greatest happiness or good is a rational and empirical calculation. (p. 141)

Cuilla's comparison helps discern the subtle, yet critical, distinction between fundamentally utilitarian or Kantian-oriented societies and their respective moral codes, social structures, and political systems in different parts of the world (e.g., The Netherlands versus the United States).

Kant's deontological (duty) focus is useful in understanding how individuals go beyond themselves in the quest for happiness (Kant referred to this concept as *own-happiness*). Duty is a moral obligation – or moral law (Herman, 2001). There are different perspectives of duty for promoting wellbeing, for instance: (1) own-interest, (2) other-interest – as in the case of distant relationships with country-men, (3) concern for persons we have a special and close relationship with – family, friends, co-workers, group memberships, etc., (4) the duty to rescue those in danger or high risk, (5) goodwill toward others, and (6) beneficence,[64] the expression of kindness, compassion, and charity for others who may be suffering because of inequities of life. In her analysis of Kant's concept of beneficence, Barbara Herman (2001) notes:

> *We do not normally think of Kantian theory as having morally positive things to say about own-happiness. This should strike us as paradoxical, in Kant, or in any non-consequentialist theory that extends beneficence beyond rescue. Why would we have moral concern for each others' happiness when our own happiness lacks moral significance for each of us, except insofar as it is the object of restriction and constraint, a cause of temptation, and the like? Rights and perfect duties protect liberty, not happiness. This may be part of the reason why, beyond rescue, negative tasks and small efforts tend to be the focus of attention in many non-consequentialist discussions of aid and why any more substantial engagement with the happiness of others is frequently located in the space of supererogatory actions, though even that makes little sense in moral theory that does not give own-happiness a place. (p. 237)*

Kant argues that beneficence is a natural attribute of rational human beings. Furthermore, from the time of birth, parents and loved ones give of themselves freely to ensure the child's protection and happiness. We are taught to treat others as we would care to be treated ourselves – "Kant concludes that we must take the fact that happiness is the natural end of human beings as a reason to strive, as much as we can, to further the ends of others" (p. 234).

> *We have different and perhaps special obligations to persons in need who are in one sense or another local to us – friends, family, or coworkers – than we do to those at a distance; we also recognize a continuum of need to which we seem obligated to respond impartially, regardless of relation or locale.*
>
> Barbara Herman, The Scope of Moral Requirement

How much should we strive to ensure the happiness of others? This duty is limited by our particular circumstances in life, our willingness to give of ourselves and our resources (freewill), and our "learned" cultural norms (Kant talks about our *cultural space* as directing effective moral agency). Herman illustrates: "The happiness of others matters morally for the same reason that my happiness matters – the pursuit of happiness is the organizing principle of our [human

---

[64] *Beneficence* (derived from the Latin word *beneficentia*); (1) the fact or quality of being kind or doing good; (2) a charitable act or generous gift. *The Oxford Dictionary of English* (2nd ed. rev.).

beings'] kind of agency" (p. 244). Perhaps this is the fundamental connection with our moral obligation to tend to the health and welfare of all citizens. Healthcare is a means of reducing suffering and improving wellbeing of others and contributing to our collective happiness. Herman elaborates:

> *In the Kantian account of beneficence, the point of the help we may be required to give, in both emergency and normal cases, in not to alleviate suffering per se, but to alleviate suffering because of what suffering signifies for beings like us. In the face of unnecessary suffering one naturally thinks: how could it not be better that it ceases? And if someone can easily make it stop, what good reason does one have not to do so? There is no reason to deny that. Nor to deny that relief of suffering per se is the proper object of our kindness and compassion. (p. 244)*

If Kant's theories are as solid as he purported them to be, then human beings have an obligation – a *natural obligation* – to care for each others' wellbeing. In this context, universal healthcare is an obligatory duty of society (through moral support) and governments (through taxation and institutional structures) to provide adequate health measures according to their natural abilities and limitations. Why? Because, if we apply the Kantian framework of the categorical imperative to the current healthcare reform debate in the United States and consider that healthcare is an essential *good* for some (those fortunate enough to have sufficient health insurance coverage), it stands to reason (from a human intellectual and rational perspective) that collectively, we must also have a *duty* to provide basic health services for all Americans.

> *People are bound by moral laws, which articulate the idea of a community of rational beings, living in mutual respect, and resolving their disputes by negotiation and agreement…The ideas of freedom, responsibility, right and duty contain a tacit assumption that every player in the moral game counts for one, and no player for more than one… If this were not so, the 'moral law', as Kant calls it, would cease to fulfill its purpose, of reconciling individuals in a society of strangers.*
>
> Roger Scruton, Morality, in Philosophy: Principles and Problems

The United States has the necessary resources to meet the imperative of providing *basic* health services to all Americans, regardless of their circumstances of wealth, social status, employment, race, education, etc. It behooves the American people to insist that policymakers develop a healthcare system that affords universal access to all who need basic health services because it ultimately benefits society as a whole. The current employer-sponsored and market-driven healthcare system is *exclusionary* in its foundational structure; therefore, it is contrary to the notion of duty and beneficence outlined by Kant.

10.4 -- John Rawls – Distributive Justice Theory

Major theories, principles, axioms, and concepts
- *The first and second principles of justice.*
- *Stability of justice as fairness in a well-ordered society.*
- *Basic liberties.*
- *Opportunity for attainment of one's rational plan of life.*
- *Morality is a normal feature of human life.*

Most scholars regard John Rawls as the most influential modern-day *distributive justice* philosopher in the United States.[65] In this section, it is necessary to confine our examination of Rawls' work to the narrower subject of *justice as fairness* and its application to an individual's attainment of a rational plan of life within a democratic society. His original 600+ page book A Theory of Justice (1971) was intended to captivate the attention of political leaders of his time, sway them away from the dominant tendency toward a philosophy of utilitarianism, and reorient them to the theory of justice [righteousness] as fairness – "What I have attempted to do is to generalize and carry to a higher order of abstraction the traditional theory of social contract as represented by Locke, Rousseau, and Kant" (Rawls, 1971). In the preface of A Theory of Justice, Rawls lays down his vision for his groundbreaking work:

> *…to organize them [referring to the contemporary social contract theories] into a general framework by using certain simplifying devices so that their full force can be appreciated. My ambitions for the book will be completely realized if it enables one to see more clearly the chief structural features of the alternative conception of justice that is implicit in the contract tradition and point the way to its further elaboration. Of the traditional views, it is this conception, I believe, which best approximates our considered judgments of justice and constitutes the most appropriate moral basis for a Democratic society. (p. xviii)*

---

[65] John Rawls (1921-2002) was regarded as one of the most important political philosophers of the 20th century. He wrote a series of highly influential articles in the 1950s and '60s that helped refocus Anglo-American moral and political philosophy on substantive problems about what we ought to do. His first book, A Theory of Justice [TJ] (1971), revitalized the social-contract tradition, using it to articulate and defend a detailed vision of egalitarian liberalism. In *Political Liberalism* [PL] (1993), he recast the role of political philosophy, accommodating it to the effectively permanent "reasonable pluralism" of religious, philosophical, and other comprehensive doctrines or worldviews that characterize modern societies. He explains how philosophers can characterize public justification and the legitimate, Democratic use of collective coercive power while accepting that pluralism (excerpted from John Rawls' biography).

Rawls developed his theory of justice as fairness in society around his belief that it is essential to treat everyone fairly and equally, while being impartial about the deliberative process of how to distribute necessary and desirable goods to individuals and social groups. Rawls later argued that "moral feelings are a normal feature of human life," in his revised edition he called simply *Theory* (Rawls, 1999, p. 427). He reiterates the two fundamental principles that provide the moral structure of justice as fairness:

> **First Principle** – each person is to have equal right to the most extensive total system of equal basic liberties compatible with a similar system of liberty for all.
> **Second Principle** – social and economic inequalities are to be arranged so that they are both:
>
> (a) To the greatest benefit of the least advantaged, consistent with the just savings principle, and
> (b) Attached to offices and positions open to all under conditions of fair equality of opportunity.

Rawls' fundamental premise for his theory of justice as fairness was that "social cooperation makes possible a better life for all," and that it is necessary to promote a political structure for ensuring that the *fruits* of a successful community accrue to the *common good* of its members. In order for individuals to partake in these fruits of society, each must share rights and duties in the basic institutions of society. Furthermore, Rawls believed that individuals (adults, after the age of reason) are capable of deciding what constitutes their "good" and "just" actions through a process of rational reflection; that "the theory of justice is a part, perhaps most significant part, of the theory of rational choice" (p. 10-15). In the pursuit of goodness and justice in a democratic society, individuals seek to realize their *most rational plan of life*, which is dependent on each person's capabilities and endowments derived from the natural lottery of life process (something no one has control over). In his final remarks in *Theory*, Rawls reaffirms that justice as fairness is a logical outgrowth of the *moral nature of humankind* (p. 508).

A compendium of scholarly critiques of *Theory* edited by Norman Daniels (1989) challenges many of Rawls' assumptions on distributive justice. As expressed by welfare economist-philosopher and Nobel Prize winner Amartya Kumar Sen (1989) in his essay on "Rawls versus Bentham,"[66] the utilitarian procedure (offered by Bentham) "is based on comparing gains and losses of different persons…and is completely insensitive to comparisons of levels of welfare; the Rawlsian procedure does exactly the opposite and is based on comparison levels only without making essential use of comparisons of gains and losses…each approach must be recognized to be

---

[66] For more information about Amartya Sen, see http://homepage.newschool.edu/het//profiles/sen.htm

essentially incomplete" (p. 289). The key difference between these two sociopolitical theories is summarized below:

Utilitarian rule – is intended to maximize the *sum* of individual welfares (the greater good approach).
Rawlsian rule – is to maximize the welfare level of the *worst off person* (and allowing for the opportunity to achieve one's rational plan of life, whatever that might be).

In 2001, Rawls published *Justice as Fairness: A Restatement*, which addresses many of the criticisms of his original *Theory*, and he elaborates on some of the vaguer or more ambiguous assertions found in his 1971 landmark work without abandoning his fundamental premises. He starts out by explaining that his original justice theory was not intended to be a comprehensive moral doctrine – "This restatement removes that ambiguity: justice as fairness is now presented as a *political conception of justice*" (p. xvii). *Restatement* seems to be a much easier book to understand Rawls' fundamental ideas concerning the nature of justice and social cooperation in Democratic society (in conjunction with *Theory*).

For starters, Rawls introduces the concept of *reasonable pluralism* to describe the interplay of divergent and multiple free institutions – religious and philosophical conceptions of the world – that make up a truly democratic society. Rawls emphasizes the distinction between a democratic society and communities:

It is a serious error not to distinguish between the idea of a Democratic political society and the idea of a community. Of course, a Democratic society is hospitable to many communities within it, and indeed tries to be a social world within which diversity can flourish in amity and concord; but it is not itself a community, nor can it be in view of the fact of reasonable pluralism. For that would require the oppressive use of government power which is incompatible with basic Democratic liberties. From the start, then, we view a Democratic society as a political society that excludes a confessional or an aristocratic state, not to mention a caste, slave, or a racist one. This exclusion is a consequence of taking the moral powers as the basis of political equality. (p. 21)

Rawls elaborates on the definitions of the *original* principles of justice and expands the concepts as follows:

First Principle – each person has the same indefeasible claim to a fully adequate scheme of equal basic liberties, which scheme is compatible with the same scheme of liberties for all; and

Second Principle – social and economic inequalities are to satisfy two conditions: first, they are to be attached to offices and positions open to all under conditions of fair equality of opportunity; and second, they are to be to the greatest benefit of the least-advantaged members of society (the difference principle).

Rawls also discusses the concept of *primary goods* to relate the basic necessities of life to enable all members of different communities to achieve their maximum potentiality in a democratic society (p. 58). The primary goods include (1) freedom of thought, (2) freedom of movement and choice of occupation, (3) powers and prerogatives of offices, (4) income and wealth, and (5) social basis of self-respect. He believed that primary goods should be available to free and equal citizens in a democracy, even though relative differences (inequalities) will continue to exist among individuals, as long as the overall goal improves the lot of the least-advantaged in a rational manner and complies with the two principles of justice. According to Rawls, there is an important differentiation between the theory of justice as fairness (based on the two principles of justice – equality of basic rights, liberties, and fair opportunities) and utilitarian theory that stresses the principle of average utility as the sole principle of justice (p. 96).

The crux of Rawls' *Restatement* clarifies his key reasons for balancing economic and social inequalities:

1. In the absence of special circumstances, it seems wrong that some or much of society should be amply provided for, while many, or even a few, suffer hardship, not to mention hunger and *treatable illness*… Unless there is real scarcity, all should have at least enough to meet their basic needs.
2. Controlling economic and social inequality is to prevent one part of society from dominating the rest. When those two kinds of inequalities are large, they tend to support political inequality.
3. Significant political and economic inequalities are often associated with inequalities of social status that encourage those of lower status to be viewed both by themselves and by others as inferior – this violates the concept that humans are fundamentally equal.
4. Inequality can be wrong or unjust in itself whenever society makes use of fair procedures…Monopoly and its kindred are to be avoided, not simply for their bad effects, among them inefficiency, but also because without a special justification they make markets unfair. (pp. 130-132)

Rawls' arguments support the general notion that basic needs, including healthcare, are part of individual rights rather than market-driven *commodities* that are dispensed primarily according to socioeconomic considerations. The monumental challenge is to ensure that the social regime does not tilt too far to one side or the other – for example, support of *laissez-faire capitalism* on the one hand, or *liberal (democratic) socialism* on the other extreme (p. 136). Rawls contends that *property-owning democracy* is the fairest "system of cooperation between citizens regarded as free and equal" (p. 140). The other two social systems referenced by Rawls were *welfare-state capitalism* and *state socialism* within a command economy.

This brings us to Rawls' definition of the *difference principle* that is complementary to the two original principles cited in *Theory*:

Our native endowments are ours and not society's – namely, that we cannot be subject to a head tax to equalize the advantages our endowments might confer. That would violate our basic liberties. The difference principle does not penalize the more able for being fortunately endowed. Rather, it says that to benefit still further from that good fortune, we must train and educate our endowments and put them to work in socially useful ways that contribute to the advantages of those who have less.

Rawls' concluding remarks about *Theory* express his contention that "those who grow up in a society well ordered by justice as fairness, who have a rational plan of life, and who also know, or reasonably believe, that everyone else has an effective sense of justice, have sufficient reason founded on their good (rather than on justice) to comply with just institutions" (p. 202). This certainly is an idealistic position, even utopian (192). From a practical perspective, it is critical to provide incentives for individuals to pursue their maximum potentiality, especially when the political system offers support for basic necessities such as unemployment benefits, educational grants, emergency healthcare services (EMTALA), food banks, disaster relief (FEMA), and other guaranteed rights to its citizens.

Unfortunately, there are those who are unwilling to engage in meaningful and productive work and contribute very little back to society. These individuals simply prefer to take advantage of the safety-net system, assuming that they are entitled to these "*free*" services and support without giving back to their community in accordance with their natural abilities. There is no such thing as a "free ride" in any society, and this kind of "taking" attitude creates a sense of hostility and ill-will on the part of the *haves* toward the *have-nots*. Welfare dependency is a complex social concern that must be guarded against – each human being has the *responsibility* along with the *opportunity* to maximize her potential in order for society to reap the ultimate benefits from social cooperation and justice-as-fairness proposed by Rawls.

Consider these key elements of a balanced Democratic societal structure and control system:

Figure 8 – Elements of a Balanced Democratic Social Structure

Intellect – *knowledge and ability to rationalize decisions that maximize positive outcomes*
Wealth – *accumulation of desirable resources, income, goods, and services that provide economic advantages*

Strength – *personal or group (large numbers of individuals or strategic devices) power necessary to change the direction of undesirable conditions*
Influence – *political, legislative or regulatory authority entrusted by members of the community or state*

As long as there is a reasonable balance and functional interrelationship between these four key elements -- intellect, wealth, strength, and influence – society as a whole can enjoy progress in spite of prevailing inequities. Once any one of these elements becomes substantially unbalanced, the other elements will seek to equalize the situation as much as possible through evolution or revolution (consider the African American civil rights movement and riots during the 1950s and 1960s). Perhaps this is why Rawls felt that the difference principle relating to social and economic inequalities must ultimately benefit the *least-advantaged* members of society so that a careful balance of political power can be maintained from generation to generation.

Toward a Healthier, More Fair America

Perhaps the most important reason to act now is the shared American ideal of fair opportunity for all to pursue life, liberty and happiness – all of which depend on good health. This is a timely moment to seek better ways to help people choose health – to strengthen individuals' abilities and resources to make healthy choices and to remove the avoidable obstacles that deter too many Americans on the road leading to long, healthy productive and fulfilling lives.

By Risa Lavizzo-Mourey, MD, President and CEO, Robert Wood Johnson Foundation (to members of the Commission to Build a Healthier America).

Rawls intended to push beyond the prevailing utilitarian philosophy of his time. He also knew that *Theory* was not the perfect answer to the question about how individuals in any society (or community) should conduct themselves toward one another. It appears that Rawls attained his goal for writing his masterpiece and his belief that "purity of heart, if one could attain it, would be to see clearly and to act with grace and self-command from this point of view" (p. 514).

Rawls' *A Theory of Justice*'s principles have been applied to the concerns about equitable distribution of healthcare resources by various scholars – Norman Daniels, John Dunn, Colin Farrelly, and Amartya Sen, to name a few of the prominent philosophers and economists. In the next section, we examine Norman Daniels's theories for health and healthcare based on *equality of opportunity*, which ties to the earlier work of John Rawls.

10.5 -- Norman Daniels – Equality of Opportunity Theory

Major theories, principles, axioms, and concepts
- *Healthcare is special because it protects the individual's fair share of the normal opportunity range (NOR).*
- *Need for criteria to determine reasonable allocation of limited health resources.*
- *Theory of health needs versus wants.*
- *Intergenerational equity of health distribution.*
- *The Prudential Lifespan Account.*
- *Accountability for reasonableness and access to basic healthcare.*
- *Just Health – the connection of a population's health status to the broad issues of social justice and the expanded focus for bioethics as a field.*

Norman Daniels devoted much of his 30-year career in philosophy to the topic of healthcare justice and health policy development.[67] He was a prolific writer and major contributor to the subject of health and healthcare and the achievement of human opportunity. In his original work, Daniels, along with Bayer and Caplan (1983) tackled the controversial topic of the need for healthcare *rationing* head-on, weaving innovative theories into the theoretical framework of distributive justice and justice-as-fairness originally published by philosopher John Rawls (1971). One of Daniels's goals was to demonstrate how his "theory of health care needs" helps explain the special consideration healthcare deserved in society and "that it should be treated differently from other social goods" (Daniels, 1985).[68] He also emphasized why certain kinds of healthcare needs to take priority over other social needs because of their intrinsic link to achieving

---

[67] Norman Daniels is Mary B. Saltonstall Professor and Professor of Ethics and Population Health at Harvard School of Public Health. Formerly Goldthwaite Professor, Chair of the Tufts Philosophy Department, and Professor of Medical Ethics at Tufts Medical School, where he taught from 1969 until 2002, he has degrees from Wesleyan (B.A. Summa, 1964), Balliol College, Oxford (B.A., First Honors, 1966), and Harvard (Ph.D., Plympton Dissertation Prize, 1971). He has published over 150 articles and numerous books - his *Just Health: Meeting Health Needs Fairly* (2008) is a sequel to *Just Health Care* and integrates his work into a comprehensive theory of justice for health. A member of the Institute of Medicine, a Fellow of the Hastings Center, a Founding Member of the National Academy of Social Insurance and of the International Society for Equity in Health, he has consulted with organizations, commissions, and governments in the US and abroad on issues of justice and health policy, including for the United Nations, WHO, and the President's Commission for the Study of Ethical Problems in Medicine. He has held Fellowships and Grants from the National Endowment for the Humanities, the National Science Foundation, the National Institutes of Health, the National Library of Medicine, the Robert Wood Johnson Foundation, the Retirement Research Foundation, the Greenwall Foundation, and others. He held a Robert Wood Johnson Investigator's Award for the period 1998-2001, as well as a Rockefeller Foundation grant for the international adaptation of the benchmarks (excerpted from Norman Daniels' biography).

[68] Norman Daniels outlined his healthcare theory in an essay – Health Care Needs and Distributive Justice – contained in Chapter 1 of *In Search of Equity*, which was excerpted from his book *Just Health Care*, that was being prepared for publication in 1985, by Cambridge University Press.

and maintaining "normal species functioning" and ultimately optimizing an individual's range of opportunities (which is the attainment of human potentiality).

Daniels's theory is predicated on a "connection to opportunity [that] helps clarify the kind of social good health care is and provides the basis for subsuming health care institutions under principles of distributive justice" (p. 2). His conviction was that healthcare is a foundational aspect of society, since it enhances opportunity for individuals and empowers them to attain their natural potential. Healthcare also protects the individual's fair share of the normal opportunity range (NOR), "to the exclusion of other reasons," commonly held by other philosophers – i.e., that healthcare's special role in society is to reduce pain, suffering and social disadvantage, as advocated by Thomas Schramme and his contemporaries. Daniels responded to his fervent critics concerning his position on the special moral role of healthcare by arguing that "for purposes of justice, the relationship between health and opportunity is central, though other values, such as beneficence or compassion, may come into play in cases where opportunity cannot be an issue" (Daniels, 2009, p. xx).

Daniels's stance about the special relationship of healthcare and attainment of opportunity does not necessarily mean that individuals are *de facto* entitled to unlimited access to health resources. He goes on to enumerate many of the perceived inadequacies of the employer-sponsored, market-based health insurance coverage in the United States, which does not provide all citizens with a reasonable package or fair share of basic healthcare services, unless one has the financial wherewithal to purchase sufficient health insurance or qualify for government-funded safety-net programs (Medicaid, charity care, disability coverage). Without adequately defining what exactly constitutes reasonable and fair access to necessary health services, policymakers are at risk of diverting limited health resources away from the most needy, simply because of the "excess" and "unregulated" consumption of health services by individuals who can afford whatever healthcare they desire (and do not actually need to restore or maintain their health potentiality). This is the basis of the argument in favor of universal healthcare.

In his classic essay, *Just Health Care*, Norman Daniels (1985) introduces the concept of *discernable differences* between assuring a *state of health* to individuals (which is influenced by vast external socioeconomic conditions), and providing equal access to healthcare services:

> *My working assumption in this essay is that the appeal to a right to health care is not an appropriate starting point for an inquiry into just health care. Rights are not moral fruits that spring up from bare earth, fully ripened, without cultivation. Rather we are justified in claiming a right to health care only if it can be harvested from an acceptable, general theory of distributive justice, or, more particularly, from a theory of justice for health care. Such a theory would tell us which kinds of right claims are legitimately viewed as rights; it would also help us specify the scope and limits of justified right claims. (p. 5)*

In other words, the main concern should be confined to the question of one's moral right to certain critical health services such as the formal system of providing, restoring, or maintaining positive health status through appropriate health measures and interventions offered on an equitable basis to all members of a social group.

Furthermore, Daniels evaluates the ramifications (and negative publicity and bad press) of limiting all individuals, regardless of income status, to only the necessary and efficacious health services in order to make sure that basic health resources are readily available and accessible to the most needy individuals (reallocating health resources accessible the more wealthy as a means to serve the less fortunate). This type of system is referred to as the *single-payer* healthcare plan – e.g., the Canadian healthcare system. These concerns lead Daniels to develop a *theory of needs* to better address mal-distribution of limited health resources throughout society. His theory of needs helps clarify the difference between personal needs and preferences for healthcare resources, since "not all preferences are created equal." In order for a distributive justice theory to thrive, Daniels postulated, there needs to be objective criteria to prevent the subjective consumption of (and perhaps wasteful) limited health services.

Objective criteria for distributing limited healthcare resources can be based on "those things we need in order to maintain, restore, or provide the functional equivalent (whenever possible) to *normal species functioning*," asserts Daniels. He offers several examples:

- Adequate nutrition and shelter.
- Sanitary, safe, unpolluted living and working conditions.
- Exercise, rest, and other features of healthy lifestyles.
- Preventive, curative, and rehabilitative personal medical services.
- Nonmedical personal (and social) support services.

The notion of opportunity maximization is certainly different among individuals and diverse groups, since they are society-dependent, explains Daniels. Health status must be considered in the context of the normal range of effective opportunity, which is dependent on many factors (a so-called *truncated scale* as opposed to a *satisfaction scale* for measuring well-being) such as age (stages of life), hereditary and genetic predisposition to diseases, employment circumstances (ranging from mild to severe risk), community expectations (performance and aesthetics), social structure (income inequalities), etc. Daniels concludes:

> *I shall urge a normative claim – we ought to subsume health care under a principle of justice guaranteeing fair equality of opportunity. Actually, since I cannot here defend such a general principle without going too deeply into the general theory of distributive justice, I shall urge a weaker claim: if an acceptable theory of justice includes a principle providing for fair equality of opportunity, then health care institutions should be among*

those governed by it...Rawls urges that we hold society responsible for guaranteeing the individual a fair share of basic liberties, opportunity, and all-purpose means, like income and wealth, needed for pursuing individuals conceptions of the good. But the individual is responsible for choosing ends in such a way that there is a reasonable chance of satisfying them under such just arrangement...But individuals remain responsible for the choice of their ends, so there is no injustice in not having sufficient means to reach extravagant ends. (pp. 19-21)

The fundamental concept for prioritizing healthcare in society presented by Daniels -- maximizing *equality of opportunity* -- should be tempered by the reality that individuals tend to exercise their (excessive) right of free will. And in doing so, each individual shapes his own dimensions of opportunities to pursue in life. Additionally, there is a serious problem when addressing risky choices that result in catastrophic or cost-prohibitive health consequences (e.g., lung cancer caused by cigarette smoking; traumatic brain injury caused by reckless motorcycle driving without protective helmet; or a failed suicide attempt). How should these circumstances be included in the evaluation criteria for deciding how to fairly distribute and pay for limited healthcare services? Should risky life-style consequences be equally covered by market-driven health insurance coverage premiums, extraordinary taxation, or all-out rationing?

Daniels' theory of the importance of healthcare to society seems to lead to a morally acceptable *tiered-healthcare system* involving (1) basic health services available to all and funded by public sources in order to maximize opportunity and productivity of the social group, and (2) market-based health services that are distributed on the basis of preference and ability to pay for such services by individuals with means. The philosophical premise argued by Daniels about the need for prioritization criteria concerning fair allocation or re-distribution of limited and necessary health resources has major implications for policymakers in the United States and the global society in three foundational areas:

- What constitutes basic acute care treatment and rehabilitative services that are the responsibility of governmental entities, and how should public and private funding be allocated in relationship to other recognized human needs and rights (education, safety, environmental protection, infrastructure, etc.)?
- What constitutes an appropriate funding level for preventive, public health, and primary care services, and how should individual responsibility mesh with governmental initiatives and requirements (compulsory vaccination for children, control of the spread of HIV / AIDS among high-risk groups, etc.)?
- What moral obligations does our society have for caring for the less fortunate individuals who suffer from progressive and / or permanent disabilities that cannot be cured by traditional medicine (this includes the increasing number of frail elderly) – how do we account

for these precious individuals in a prioritization scheme that emphasizes maximization of opportunity?

Daniels warns that these types of healthcare challenges are tough, complex, and persistent – they require careful and deliberative societal judgment along with a reasonable balance of moral justice and economic investment.

Daniels (1988) wrote a sequel to his famous 1985 work, *Am I My Parents' Keeper: An Essay on Justice Between the Young and the Old*, where he concentrated on a unique aspect of healthcare relating to the importance of establishing fair allocation methodology to deal with the special health needs of our aging population. He was touched by a personal experience with an aged relative suffering from multiple chronic complications and dealing with vastly different moral attitudes from younger relative-caretakers who were torn by decisions on how to handle extraordinary life-extending measures versus allowing nature to take its course (death).

His earlier position about the moral priority of healthcare in society is based heavily on the special requirements for protecting equality of opportunity for individuals. Daniels later recognized and accounts for the unique problems of distributive justice at the end-stage of life for the aged. The over-65 (arbitrary retirement age in America) population typically consumes the majority of their entire life's healthcare resources during the last 2 to 3 years of life – and nearly three times the average healthcare consumption of persons age 17 to 64. The disproportionate consumption of health resources by older cohorts poses special challenges for society because of the substantial economic investment in traditional medical care that has little or no impact on improving potential opportunity for older persons (at this stage, the body is declining and death is a certain outcome in the near future). The marvels of modern medicine have indeed successfully extended the average lifespan of White American women to 78 years of age, and for men to 75. It is also a fact that thousands of seniors are living into their 80s, 90s, and even 100s; therefore, it is possible for someone reaching retirement age to live another 30 years – almost as long as the work-life period.

Nevertheless, the treatment objectives of healthcare professionals and providers caring for seniors are not necessarily curative, recuperative, or even restorative in nature, as is the case for younger patients. For older persons, the major benefits healthcare provides is to improve the quality of living and alleviate pain and suffering caused by declining bodily capacities, and to enhance certain mobility constraints characteristic of the natural aging process (joint deterioration, congestive heart disease, long-term consequences of diabetes, etc.). In many cases, care is also provided for palliative reasons, or to postpone inevitable death.

This realization lead Daniels to develop a new theory of "generational equity" to accommodate the special challenges common to different *age cohorts* and the appropriate degree of opportunity enhancement that relates to different age groups: infancy (birth to 17 years of age); working age (16 to 64 years); post-working generation (retirees eligible for Social Security and

Medicare benefits) or the young-old (age 65 to 74 years); and the old-old generation, who are often cared for by younger family members or patients bound to nursing home care (over 75 years of age). According to Daniels' *intergenerational* health theory:

> *I have suggested that we face a 'new' question of justice, 'How should we distribute social resources among the different age groups competing for them?' It is this question that must be answered if we are to solve the problems posed by the aging society. Yet this question about justice between age groups is not really a new problem, even if it suddenly seems urgent and even if it has been little discussed. Moreover, it does not arise merely because of the recent aging of society. Rather, the just distribution of resources between the old and the young is a problem for every society, past and present. (p. 11)*

The significance of this concern for intergenerational health parameters is depicted vividly in Chart 6 that shows the steepness of the population growth curve for older citizens projected by the US Census Bureau for 2020. The age cohort over 65 is projected to nearly double by the year 2020, while the younger age cohort is projected to increase by a modest 10% during the same horizon.

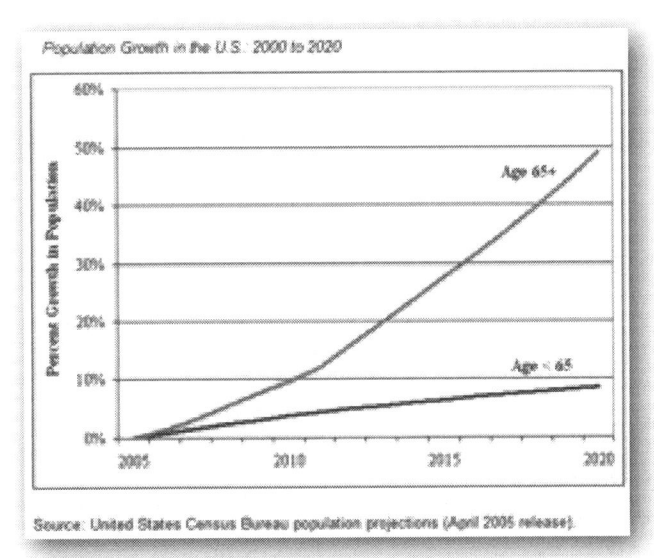

Chart 6 – Population Growth in the US: 2000-2020

Medical innovation, socioeconomic improvements, and governmental efforts to expand access to healthcare services for citizens represent a two-edged sword for society. The greater the number of younger lives that the nation is able to save on the front end from the grips of health disasters and premature deaths due to traumatic injuries, cardiovascular disease, cancer, and other dreaded kills, the larger the over-65 population will become on the back-end of the population curve. This has been especially true for the very-old age cohort; there are more persons alive today over age 85 than any other generation in American history – the generation of super seniors.

As people live longer and survive medical problems and health issues that formerly resulted in premature death or permanent disabilities, these new survivors will inevitably require additional medical resources during their lifetime for treatment of chronic impairments and debilitating illnesses that affect quality-of-life and opportunity attainment discussed by Rawls. It also becomes necessary to ask the sensitive and difficult question: "At what point in one's life does it make sense to gracefully accept the inevitability of death and regard it as a natural consequence of living without demanding extraordinary healthcare measures?" Is it morally justified to expend huge sums of money and consume scarce healthcare resources in order to prolong the life expectancy of the aged by six months, one year, two years…? Perhaps the quick and simple answer is, of course, especially if it is one's own life or the life of a loved one! Medical ethics will continue to drive healthcare decisions as the US and world population ages.

Another complex dilemma common to physicians who are trained and expected to administer every reasonable and available measure to conquer diseases, illnesses, save lives, and reduce suffering in light of the *Hippocratic Oath*, "do no harm." Deciding when to administer and when to withhold care is an awesome responsibility of the caregiver. Is society obligated to provide equal opportunity to each age cohort equally? What should be the size of each citizen's healthcare "bank account" in American society? These are the sort of challenging questions which Daniels attempts to reconcile in *Am I My Parents' Keeper* – "That problems in our aging society are the result of the success, not the failure, of longstanding social policy does not make them easier to tackle" (p. 10).

The challenge with the aging dilemma, Daniels notes, is that there are basic healthcare needs that *differ* from cohort to cohort, which in turn result in inherent conflicts between these age groups over limited healthcare resources. He suggests that the answer partially lies with what he called *The Prudential Lifespan Account*, where society develops "rational choices regarding how to prudently allocate the fair shares of basic social goods [during a normal person's] lifespan" (p. 66). Aside from the fact that each individual is subject to the effects of a natural lottery at the time of birth that randomly assigns social advantages and disadvantages, genetic predisposition to health issues, and environmental circumstances beyond one's control, Daniels argues that society has the responsibility to ensure basic resources and tools to assist its members to achieve individual potentiality and to maximize productivity (within the normal opportunity age-ranges) for the ultimate benefit of self and the community-at-large (pp. 66-82). The prudential lifespan account, according to Daniels, would help determine what types of health resources are most appropriate for each distinctive phase of life, in accordance with morally and socially relevant distributive criteria.

In the final analysis, the middle-aged working populace is the one that generates the bulk of economic wealth and support for healthcare services through taxation of labor, goods, and services that benefit primarily the very young and the older members of society. This is how our socioeconomic "system transfers resources from stages of our lives in which we have relatively little need for them into stages in which we do," emphasized Daniels. Consequently, it is reasonable to deduce, as Daniels did:

> A healthcare system that treats age groups unequally does not generate inequalities between persons over time. If prudently designed, it can benefit each person. A healthcare system that treats blacks and whites, or women and men, unequally will generate inequalities between persons over time. It will not benefit each person; it will be open to the objection that it takes benefits away from some people in order to help others (and for morally irrelevant reasons) … The difference between the race [or other criteria that can be construed as discriminatory] and age cases should by now be clear. Distributive schemes that take age into account look like cases in which we cross boundaries between persons only if we adopt the perspective of a moment or time-slice…The shift in perspective I urge is thus rooted in a real, distinctive, and morally important fact about age. It is not philosophical sleight-of-hand. (pp. 45-46)

This bold approach for distinguishing the theories of *generational equity*, *intergenerational justice*, and the *prudent life span account* from other distributive criteria opened Daniels to numerous attacks from academics and scientists (Daniels, 2009, pp. 36-41). In response to the challenges from other scholars regarding his *variable* fairness allocation theories about healthcare for the aged, Daniels elaborates on why he chose to single out this particular cohort for special theoretical discussion – it was because of the unique ethical considerations affecting older persons. Daniels believed that it is morally wrong to arbitrarily lump the older cohort into the more generic rationing methodology that was intended to deal with gender and race bias along with the civil rights movement issues of the 1980s. After all, everyone ages regardless of socioeconomic class, sex and race. Also, Daniels was convinced that *quality-of-life*, *wellbeing*, or *attainment-of-opportunity* is not any more or less important for older citizens. Rather, the unique health concerns and needs of seniors deserve special attention that would shield them from potential discriminatory considerations.

Daniels notes that his theory of intergenerational justice (prudential framework) turned out to be much more complex than he originally anticipated during his 1988 work; he expresses reservations about the applicability of the theory of intergenerational justice to resolve disputes about prudential healthcare resource utilization during a lifetime in his later years. This realization gave rise to Daniels' theory of *accountability for reasonableness*, a deliberative fairness process, as a way to practically resolve disparities associated with rationing across age cohorts.

As Daniels exchanges one theory for another, he reasons that "theory should guide practice, and if it cannot, that is a problem for the theory" (pp. 39-40).

It seems like the intergenerational justice theory holds together rather nicely as long as there was reasonable equity between age cohorts in terms of contributions for financial support of the healthcare system and disproportionate consumption (not necessarily need) of limited resources in later years of one's life. Once this delicate balance was disrupted by a significant reduction in the number of financial contributors (i.e., the number of working-age individuals paying into Social Security, Medicare and Medicaid), or a substantial rise in the amount of health resources consumed by younger or older cohorts due to technological advances or longevity way beyond normal retirement age, then the necessity of rationing limited healthcare resources raises its ugly head. The salient message from Daniels to his readers is the absolute imperative of connecting sound philosophical theory about distributive justice with public policy pertaining to the creation and maintenance of a just healthcare system in any society.

The United States is beginning to feel pressure associated with the dramatic impact of escalating consumption of limited healthcare resources and skyrocketing costs associated with the aging of America. The Baby Boom generation will only exacerbate the problems as this age wave makes its way into the golden age; at the same time, the number of working contributors (tax payers) will drop from 16 workers per retiree back in the 1950s, to only approximately 2 tax payers per retiree in 2050 (Graph 24). The struggle to morally and fairly apportion limited healthcare resources for the aging generation of Americans is the key to the Congressional debates about healthcare reform. The economic crisis generated by out-of-control healthcare costs seems to demand the implementation of a new regulatory approach embracing accountability for reasonableness in order for the United States to effectively and rationally limit healthcare utilization while encouraging greater personal responsibility for healthier behavior by all citizens who wish to partake in the reformed healthcare system (based on prevention, public health services and medical services).

In Daniels' (2008) book *Setting Limits Fairly: Learning to Share Resources for Health* with co-author and practicing psychiatrist James Sabin, they expound on the practical requirements for implementing the theory of *accountability and reasonableness* (pp. viii and 22). Daniels and Sabin discuss the necessity of first developing specific criteria for determining fair healthcare resource distribution *before* a workable plan for universal healthcare can actually be implemented. They also state that unfortunately, no democratic society we are aware of has achieved consensus on such distributive principles for health care (p. 2).

There are four main opposition groups to Daniels's and Sabin's idea of public accountability for limiting health resource consumption, which include (1) the *health-is-priceless advocates*, (2) the *scarcity skeptics*, (3) the *market hawks*, and (4) the *implicit rationers*. Each of these groups expresses disdain for any rationing schemes for different yet related reasons. These oppositions mainly apply to the conviction that healthcare is an inalienable (and perhaps unlimited) human right. The theory of public accountability for limiting healthcare resource consumption, in their estimation, contradicts this premise.

According to Daniels and Sabin, the reason society should hold health and healthcare in high esteem is that it enables individuals and the community at-large to attain its full potential:

First, health care is of special moral importance because of its central (if limited) contribution to protecting our opportunities or capabilities. Our social obligations to protect opportunity – our rights to equal opportunity – give us claims on others for appropriate forms of health care. A right to health care is thus a special case of a right to equal opportunity. A second shared feature is the fact that society has to set limits to health care, despite its special moral importance. (p. 43)

This dual notion by Daniels and Sabin seems particularly valid since health is only one of many important goods and services that societies must offer to its citizens to maximize the community's success (consider for example other valuable human rights such as education, public safety, community infrastructure, etc.).

The preeminent challenge for any society, the authors comment, is to enact an equitable means for deciding (1) how much healthcare to offer its citizens and (2) what kinds of services should be curtailed or restricted based on morally acceptable criteria. This is why public accountability must be a central feature of such a process, assert Daniels and Sabin. There are two main forms of public accountability to consider (pp. 44-46):

Market Accountability -- In this instance, purchasers (consumers) are afforded the opportunity to choose among various provider options, and by voting with their wallets, providers compete for healthcare business. These market forces do not necessarily ensure that the best choices are available on a fair and equitable manner to consumers. The existing mixed private-public health system in the United States is a good example of the challenges and failures (rising costs, millions of uninsured, wasteful performance, etc.) inherent in the market accountability process.

Accountability for Reasonableness -- Under this scenario, the key rationale for distributing limited healthcare resources is to exercise transparent judgment by *fair-minded* people in public forums. In essence, accountability for reasonableness is Daniels's way of achieving consensus when difficult decisions must be made about scarce resources for the greater good of the community. This type of public discourse about allocation of health resources and intrinsic valuation process of various service options encourages society to take an active interest in the healthcare system and participate in priority-setting initiatives. In many respects, the *Oregon Health Plan* (discussed in Section 7.2) is an example of accountability for reasonableness at work relative to the community's participation in the decision-making process, and it values determination for a *rationing methodology* that apportions finite Medicaid financial resources in the context of growing statewide demand for health resources.

An organization praised by Daniels and Sabin in *Setting Limits Fairly* is the Group Health Cooperative of Puget Sound, which is an HMO based in Seattle, Washington, that is cooperatively owned by its members. The authors also note that accountability for reasonableness is a much broader form of accountability in healthcare than market accountability and is dependent on four main conditions:

Publicity *condition* – direct and indirect limits for healthcare must be publicly accessible
Relevance *condition* – the rationale for limiting healthcare must be based on evidence, reasoning, and principles (values) that fair-minded individuals would find acceptable
Revision and appeals *condition* – there must be a (fair) process for challenging and dispute resolution regarding healthcare limiting decisions
Regulative *condition* – there must be a public or voluntary regulatory mechanism to ensure that the aforementioned conditions are met (p. 45)

Daniels and Sabin state that although they believed that consumer participation is not essential to reach a state of accountability for reasonableness, "our field work, however, convinces us that appropriately conducted stakeholder participation will enhance accountability and leads us to proposing an alternative view…consumer participation can increase the legitimacy of limit-setting decisions by increasing accountability of reasonableness" (p. 62). Their point seems to hinge on the interrelationship between meaningful consumer participation and the impact on public accountability regarding healthcare limiting-decisions. To the extent that the democratic process can serve to motivate society to get closer to the decision-making process and enforcement of *right and moral decisions* about healthcare rationing, that is positive. It can be thought of as a constructive and beneficial approach for attaining accountability for reasonableness.

It is difficult to establish a universally acceptable framework of values to prioritize decisions about appropriate allocation of limited health resources, no matter which communities are chosen to be evaluated in Europe, Asia, the Americas, or any of the developing nations. These are some of the more salient moral dilemmas concerning questions about how limited (and costly) healthcare services should be distributed: (1) to the sickest patients, the ones most likely to benefit the most from health services; (2) to health systems that are the most efficient and can demonstrate better outcomes; (3) to patients that can contribute the most to society and overall economic wellbeing; (4) to the youth, which have the greatest opportunity to affect the future of the nation; (5) to those who can pay the most; or (6) to those who "deserve" the best care because of social status, and so forth.

Perhaps the process of accountability for reasonableness suggested by Daniels and Sabin could assist policymakers in determining the necessary parameters for establishing a basic healthcare package that would benefit most Americans, while simultaneously providing for fair and equitable limitations of medical resources on the basis of efficacy and affordability -- not just for the poor, but for all citizens.

In wrapping up their discussion about the theory of accountability for reasonableness as a fundamental aspect of improving decision-making and increasing public acceptance of healthcare priority-setting, Daniels and Sabin conclude:

> *We can only hope that in the United States, where the climate may be favorable for launching another effort at a universal insurance coverage system, better evidence that accountability for reasonableness…will make it more likely that insurance reform will incorporate a fair process for limit setting. (p. 232)*

It is important to appreciate the distinction Daniels (2008) makes between *healthcare* and *health*, which is a central theme in his book, *Just Health: Meeting Health Needs Fairly*. In his early work during the 1980s, Daniels stresses the special function of healthcare systems designed to provide necessary services to patients who needed medical attention and restorative treatment in order to maximize each individual's well-being and opportunities in life planning. In *Just Health*, Daniels broadens his focus by emphasizing the implications that health has not only on the individual's wellbeing, but also its impact on the socioeconomic and environmental circumstances that have a direct and indirect bearing on the entire human community. From this more global perspective of health, different cultures have developed multiple views on how to prioritize individual rights to healthcare services as well as developed practical judgments about what constitutes just health.

> *Though health care has special moral importance, justice still requires that we set limits on its provision. The fact of non-ideal conditions does not exempt us from the task of learning to set limits fairly… We should try to correct these problems as best we can, but we should not use the fact that they exist to evade the need to address the long-term problem of setting limits fairly. That is the task we must face regardless of the design of our system, its degree of efficiency, and its method of financing.*
>
> By Norman Daniels and James E. Sabin in Setting Limits Fairly (2002; 2008, 2nd edition)

Politicians and policymakers often ask, "How do we meet needs fairly when we can't meet them all?" Daniels replies with the following statement:

> *Knowing that health is of special moral importance because of its impact on opportunity gives us general guidance in the design of systems that meet health needs. Similarly,*

knowing that achieving equity in health requires broader achievement of social justice gives us general guidance about social policy that impacts health. Unfortunately, this general guidance falls short of telling us how to meet health needs fairly when we cannot meet them all…The moral controversy that surrounds the creation of winners and losers in resource allocation decisions results in a legitimacy problem: Under what conditions do decision-makers have the moral authority to set limits they impose? … Our characterization of fair process must be general enough to apply in both developed and developing countries and in health systems with public, private, and mixed organizational forms, though, of course, details will have to fit the institutional context. (p. xx)

To reach culturally sound health and healthcare decisions that are recognized as just and fair in the minds and hearts of society, Daniels (2001) urges more transparent deliberation and consensus building on three integrated fundamental questions of justice, or what he called the *focal questions* (pp. 24-28):

1. Is health, and therefore health care and other factors that affect health, of special moral importance?
2. When are health inequalities unjust?
3. How can we meet health needs fairly under resource constraints?

His answer to the first question is, "The special moral importance of health derives from its [implicit] impact on our [individual] opportunities…As members of a society seeking fair terms of cooperation to protect each other's health, we owe it to each other to design institutions that do that and create a collective space to protect opportunity in this way." Opportunities are limited by the respective talents and skills available to each individual that determines the inherent range of normal opportunity. In *Just Health*, Daniels expands his concept of opportunity maximization beyond *Just Health Care*, whereby all health needs are included in the social obligation context instead of only in healthcare institutions (Chapter 2).

Daniels' response to the second question is "that a health inequality is unjust when it derives from an unjust distribution of the socially controllable factors affecting population health and its distribution…To answer this Focal Question, we must identify the sources of health inequality in populations and learn to correct them." Daniels further details that the state of economic development of any nation is a central, but not exactly a fixed indicator, of the relative level of health of the population. This is because other important human ecological variables such as culture, social organization, education, legal system, and governmental policies each have differing degrees of influence on the administration of social justice throughout communities (Hawley, 1950; and Bryan, 2007). This approach helps researchers and policymakers pay particular attention to those controllable socioeconomic variables and healthcare services that ensure a minimum threshold of health-promoting conditions are accessible to all citizens. Daniels cautions that it is shortsighted to look only at medical services and interventions [curative medicine] as the major way of improving health status of a population -- it remains important to point to the broader ways in which social justice underlies public health (Chapter 3).

Daniels offers a practical approach for answering the third and perhaps most perplexing dilemma for health planners, economists, social scientists, policymakers, politicians, etc. charged with the responsibility of helping to shape the health delivery system in the United States: "We must supplement guidance from general principles with a fair deliberative process [in cases where reasonable people disagree on legitimate claims on scarce resources for meeting population health needs]." In circumstances where resources are limited, should healthcare resources be allocated mainly on an equal basis, regardless of the measurable degree of need or likelihood of success; by using cost-effectiveness / return-on-investment scores; on the basis of majority rule (democratic process); or by concentrating disproportionately on situations that provide probable assurance that the greatest good can be realized for the greatest number of people? Daniels argues that the approach of accountability for reasonableness contributes to the fairness of limit-setting decisions. In other words, there are no magic formulas or perfect theoretical principles for reaching the *morally correct* answer to distributive justice concerns in healthcare and health in general – a deliberative and public process "allows organizations and society itself to increase their skill at reaching justifiable conclusions" (p. 139).

Finally, Daniels outlines the analogy between *moral rights* and *human rights* to health and healthcare. Moral rights are rooted in philosophical theory about an individual's attainment of reasonable opportunity to attain one's life plan and protection of normal functioning. Human rights pertain to agreed-upon universal standards and entitlements for all human beings that are upheld by international law.

> *Moral rights to health and healthcare – the special importance vested in healthcare in society stems from a philosophical premise that healthcare promotes health (or normal functioning), and since health contributes to protecting opportunity, then healthcare protects opportunity. If justice requires society to protect opportunity, then justice attributes special importance to healthcare (adapted from Daniels, 1985). Furthermore, healthcare is one of several contributors to [the] overall health status of a population – therefore the broad concept of health and all of the influential components are foundational elements of distributive justice in meeting health needs of individuals (Daniels, 2008).*
>
> *Human rights to health and healthcare – leaders of the international community recognize the legal imperative to respect, protect, and fulfill human rights relevant to health and to the delivery of health care. A broad cluster of rights is related to health, including rights to non-discrimination, education, security, basic liberties, and political participation. A rights-based approach thus reaches beyond the health sector to emphasize the*

responsibility of a government in securing the health and well-being of its population (Daniels, 2008).

Daniels explains that the legal framework concerned with human rights is primarily derived from "natural law," which is the foundation for at least some of the human rights embodied in international law (p. 313). The United Nations (UN) adopted international rules that affirm certain inalienable rights of entitlement to people of all nations (regardless of their active participation in the UN) in 1946. Health is considered a human right. The UN doctrine sets a "progressive realization to specific human rights" based on realistic capabilities of a nation and the resources it has to offer to its members (allocation process). Policymakers must prioritize how to best protect the human rights of individuals and balance the distribution of goods and services along a continuum of defined rights (housing, food, education, freedom, health, etc.). Daniels writes:

> *In a human rights approach to health, negotiation among various stakeholders, with particular responsibility on the part of government officials, is necessary to determine which interventions may have the biggest impact on health or meet the most important health needs, thereby moving a system closer to providing what a right to health or health care requires. There will be reasonable disagreements about how resources can most effectively be used and about what kinds of partial improvements – for example, in access to care – should be emphasized. Decisions about these issues will create winners and losers. Consequently, it is important to establish that all are being treated fairly and that the outcome of the negotiation is perceived as legitimate. (p. 319)*

Daniels further claims that his theory of accountability for reasonableness works just as well with human rights as it does for the moral rights dilemma: "In both contexts, we face underlying ethical disagreements, not just a lack of information or complex empirical considerations" (p. 326).

In striving to improve global human health, it seems necessary to broaden one's horizons beyond considerations about the distribution and access to healthcare services and to encourage more socioeconomic systems that foster personal responsibility in healthy decisions, prevention and public health, and medical care that enhances wellbeing. The right (human or moral) to healthcare cannot be unlimited; resources are scarce, and the capabilities of individuals, groups, communities, states, nations, and continents differ dramatically in quantity, quality, and level of development. These realities and shortcomings result in health inequalities between developed and developing nations, and in many cases foster *unjust* healthcare systems (as is the case of employer-sponsored, market-driven healthcare in the United States). According to Daniels, there are three main categories of international health inequalities that persist:

1. Those that result from domestic injustice in distributing the socially controllable factors determining population health and its distribution;
2. Those that result from international inequalities in other conditions that affect health; and
3. Those that result from international practices -- institutions, rule-making bodies, treaties – that cause harm to the health status of some countries.

The key ingredients for improving the health status of a population group and developing its healthcare institutions are (1) the quality of healthcare policies, (2) the level of commitment of policymakers to the principles of distributive justice and accountability for reasonableness, and (3) the ethical behavior of regulators and providers in rendering healthcare services. Daniels cautions policymakers:

In short, good health policy even in poor countries can yield excellent population health, and poor health policy even in wealthy countries, like the United States, can produce worse-than-expected performance…Primary responsibility for realizing rights to health and health care in a population should rest with each state. The fact that some poor states can and do produce excellent population health makes this point dramatically. (p. 344)

Some say Americans use too much healthcare, that even if reform is achieved, universal access should not mean unlimited access. Tough choices must be made. Others worry that the neediest or least able to fight for they will be left waiting. Should healthcare be rationed?

By Michael Tanner, "Not Enough Care to Go Around," in US News & World Report, August 2009.

Daniels's masterful work in the field of philosophy of health and healthcare, along with the efforts of many others seeking a more equitable and healthier solution for mankind, remains a work in progress.

10.6 -- Yroam Amiel and Frank Cowell – Income Inequality Theory

Major theories, principles, axioms, and concepts
- *There is a recognized correlation between decreasing health status and increasing level of poverty – the socioeconomic conditions (SEC).*
- *Acceptable level of inequity in society is variable.*
- *The threshold between income sufficiency and poverty are culturally defined.*

- *Society determines when and how to level the playing field between the haves and have-nots.*
- *Income redistribution is a fundamental democratic process.*

In *Thinking About Inequality* (1999), Amiel and Cowell extensively explore the economist's view, the cross-cultural perspective, and the income and poverty perspectives. The literature reviewed for this section seems to indicate a strong correlation between higher levels of poverty and a corresponding decrease in overall health status. Comparing various key health indicators, lower-income individuals tend to experience significant disparities in access to healthcare services and quality care, resulting in higher mortality rates, higher utilization rates of emergency room visits, lower infant birth weights, less frequent visits to primary and preventive care providers, higher HIV / AIDS rates, etc.[69]

If income and health status are inextricably related, then a succinct definition of the way one evaluates income distribution and inequality is very important to policymakers. Amiel and Cowell suggest the following building blocks for analyzing income distribution within a society (p. 2):

> The **definition of income** – We need to specify carefully, or to be told clearly, what the thing called 'income' is
> The **income recipient** – We also need to be clear about the nature of the entities – persons, families, households, or whatever – that receive those incomes
> The **reference group** – We should explicitly define the universe: the collection of persons or groups within which inequality comparisons are to be made
> The **calibration system** – The 'inequality thermometer' – the inequality measurement tool has to be precisely specified

It is also important to realize that *income* and *poverty* mean different things to different population groups and nationalities. For example, to the *Yanomamo* indigenous tribe of the Amazon jungle in South America, wealth and poverty are measured by social status and the relative abundance of "goods" available to tribal leaders and their families.[70] In the United States, the government sets the poverty level at a certain dollar threshold depending on the national average income of individuals and family size. The poverty threshold is adjusted annually to reflect changes in the economy and overall wealth of the population.

Essentially, extreme poverty in modern society is considered a state of inequality that jeopardizes the social welfare of affected individuals and groups. "Income inequality is a subject that has been vulnerable to the whim of fashion within the domain of economic thought," state

---

69 Mark Tozzio and Willie V. Bryan, (2008, June 25), Understanding cultural diversity and the interplay with health status of the population in Southeast District of Columbia, *Unpublished White Paper*, prepared for United Medical Center, Washington, DC.
70 Mark Tozzio, (1975), Human Ecological Studies on the Tropics, University of Washington, Seattle, Washington: *Unpublished Thesis*; see also Amiel and Cowan, 1999, pp. 114-126.

Amiel and Cowell, because cultural perceptions and economic resources have a direct bearing on the determination of the prevailing national sentiment from time to time (pp. 133-134).

According to Amiel and Cowell, social welfare defined by income distribution is to be regarded as a *good thing*, and inequality is to be regarded as a *bad thing* (p. 55). These are moral and ethical standards adopted by society. There is a point where society agrees to level the playing field and share resources through a means of redistribution from those that have to those that do not. The usual methodology for redistribution of wealth in the United States is through taxation formulas established by federal and state governments. To put this into proper perspective, the US Census Bureau reports that the average family income for all households combined in the United States in 2007 was $50,233, up from $49,568 in 2006; 37.3 million, or 12.5% of all Americans, were classified as living in poverty; the federal poverty line in 2009 for a family of four was $22,050 (Census Bureau, 2008, August).

By moving the line of poverty up and down the scale, government officials irrationally change the eligibility criteria for entitlement to necessary human and health services of millions of needy people to meet budgetary constraints and shortfalls every year. The problem with this approach is that there is no reasonable correlation between individual needs and the availability of necessary services that affect the health and welfare of affected cohorts.

Table 12 – Federal Poverty Guidelines: 2009

Persons in Family / Household	Poverty Line -- 48 Contiguous States and DC
1	$10,830
2	$14,570
3	$18,310
4	$22,050
5	$25,790
6	$29,530
7	$33,270
8	$37,010

$3,740 added for each person above 8

Source: Federal Register Vol. 74, No. 14, January 23, 2009. Covering Health Issues 5th Edition: A Resource for Journalists, 2009 (5th Edition), Alliance for Health Reform, Washington DC.[71]

---

71 Retrieved June 20, 2009, from http://www.allhealth.org.

In the final analysis, questions about what constitutes fairness and equality in America are tied to our system of beliefs, moral values, and ethical practices regarding the entitlement of certain human rights that are universally protected by members of society, and particularly to those individuals (policymakers and regulators) responsible for controlling and redistributing finite healthcare resources in a just manner.

10.7 -- Jonathan M. Mann, et al. – Health and Human Rights Theory

Major theories, principles, axioms, and concepts
- *Human rights and public health are two complementary approaches and languages to address and advance human wellbeing.*
- *Public health can be defined as "ensuring the conditions in which people can be healthy."*
- *Public health deals with populations and prevention.*
- *From a human rights perspective, interest in health has primarily focused on governmental actions taken in the name of public health and their impact on the rights, as enshrined in international human rights law.*
- *The connection between health and human rights is predicated on three relationships or linkages: (1) H → HR, the potential impacts of health policies, programs, and practices on human rights; (2) H ← HR, violations or lack of fulfillment of any and all human rights have negative effects on physical, mental, and social well-being (health); and (3) H ←→ HR, conveys the theory that the health and human rights movements have an inextricable connection and act in synergy.*
- *The challenge of the gradient relating to socioeconomic status and health.*

Jonathan Mann[72] and his co-authors (1999) compiled a collection of contemporary articles relating to the emerging study of health and human rights. In the opening chapter of *Health and Human Rights: A Reader*, Mann et al., outline their hypothesis:

Explanations for the dearth of communication between the fields of health and human rights include differing philosophical perspectives, vocabularies, professional recruitment and training, societal roles, and methods of work. In addition, modern concepts of both health and human rights are complex and steadily evolving. On a practical level, health workers may wonder about the applicability or utility ("added value"), let alone necessity, of incorporating human rights perspectives into their work, and vice versa…Yet health

---

[72] Jonathan Mann died prematurely in a plane crash on September 2, 1998, prior to the publication of their book. Sofia Gruskin, Michael Grodin, and George Annas dedicated this anthology to Mann for his major contribution to the body of knowledge concerning health and human rights.

and human rights are both powerful, modern approaches to defining and advancing human well-being. Attention to the intersection of health and human rights may provide practical benefits to those engaged in health or human rights work, may help reorient thinking about major global health challenges, and may contribute to broadening human rights thinking and practice. (p. 7).

Although the healthcare system is mainly preoccupied with medicine and public health (distinct yet related disciplines), and the human rights discipline is founded on universal beliefs, standards, and international laws (including public policies and legislation) protecting the inalienable rights of members of our global society, these two schools are intrinsically linked because they both encourage and promote human well-being in the modern world (p. 18). The *basic principles* of human rights are:

1. People have rights simply because they are human.
2. Human rights are universal.
3. Human rights treat all people equally.
4. These rights are primarily the rights of individuals – human rights address directly the relationship between governments and individuals.
5. Human rights encompass the fundamental principles of humanity.
6. The promotion and protection of human rights is not bound by the frontiers of national states. (pp. 21-22)

In 1948, the United Nations (UN) members adopted the Universal Declaration of Human Rights (UDHR), which stipulates the "basic rights for all people and all nations."[73] This historic document includes an important reference to the rights to protect health (Article 25). The health-arm of the UN, the World Health Organization (WHO), defined health as a state of complete physical, mental, and social well-being, and not merely the absence of disease or infirmity, at the International Health Conference in 1946. This definition of health was incorporated into the UDHR in 1948. In 1966, the UN reinforced its commitment to recognize "the right of everyone to the enjoyment of the highest attainable standard of physical and mental health" by adopting the International Covenant on Economic, Social, and Cultural Rights. This Covenant spells out specific steps for governments (states) to take in order to achieve the highest attainable standards:

- The provision for the reduction of the stillbirth rate and of infant mortality and for the healthy development of the child;
- The improvement of all aspects of environmental and industrial hygiene;

---

[73] Originally there were 51 members of the United Nations Assembly (UN) in 1945. Today there are 192 participating *states* that make up the UN. See the UN declaration at http://www.un.org/en/documents/udhr/

- The prevention, treatment and control of epidemic, endemic, occupational, and other diseases; and
- The creation of conditions which would assure to all medical services and medical attention in the event of sickness.

First Lady Eleanor Roosevelt served as the United States representative to the United Nations and chaired the Human Rights Commission that authored the International Bill of Rights in 1947. The UN's declaration does not leave much room for an argument why health should *not* be dispensed on the basis of a market-driven approach for those who are fortunate enough to have adequate health insurance coverage to avail themselves of necessary health services. Yet this is exactly how one of its many founders treats the national healthcare system. Ironically, America is the only remaining industrialized nation in the world that has not implemented a universal healthcare policy (Vladeck, 2003).

The qualification written into the International Covenant adopted in 1966 was that the human right to health is *limited* to the highest attainable standard, in recognition of the reality (and tempering the extent of the obligation) that varying economic circumstances and resource limitations would obviously impact the level of health and healthcare differently among developed and developing nations around the globe. According to the International Federation of Red Cross and Red Crescent Societies and the Francois-Xavier Bagnoud Center for Health and Human Rights, there is an implicit responsibility and obligation for governmental agencies to "provide resources for health promotion and disease prevention along with an adequate health care system" (Mann, 1999, p. 28). Furthermore, governments are also expected to curtail individual human rights whenever there is a threat to the public health (an example is when an individual transmits a communicable disease that poses a threat to unsuspecting partners while exercising her right to sexual freedom).

Figure 9 – United Nation's Protection of the Right to Health

United Nations Protection of the Right to Health
Universal Declaration of Human Rights

Adopted and proclaimed by General Assembly resolution 217 A (III) of 10 December 1948

On December 10, 1948 the General Assembly of the United Nations adopted and proclaimed the Universal Declaration of Human Rights.

PREAMBLE

Whereas recognition of the inherent dignity and of the equal and inalienable rights of all members of the human family is the foundation of freedom, justice and peace in the world,

Why The United States Healthcare System Should Be A Limited Human Right For All

Whereas disregard and contempt for human rights have resulted in barbarous acts which have outraged the conscience of mankind, and the advent of a world in which human beings shall enjoy freedom of speech and belief and freedom from fear and want has been proclaimed as the highest aspiration of the common people,

Whereas it is essential, if man is not to be compelled to have recourse, as a last resort, to rebellion against tyranny and oppression, that human rights should be protected by the rule of law,

Whereas it is essential to promote the development of friendly relations between nations,

Whereas the peoples of the United Nations have in the Charter reaffirmed their faith in fundamental human rights, in the dignity and worth of the human person and in the equal rights of men and women and have determined to promote social progress and better standards of life in larger freedom,

Whereas Member States have pledged themselves to achieve, in co-operation with the United Nations, the promotion of universal respect for and observance of human rights and fundamental freedoms,

Whereas a common understanding of these rights and freedoms is of the greatest importance for the full realization of this pledge,

Now, therefore, the General Assembly Proclaims this Universal Declaration of Human Rights as a common standard of achievement for all peoples and all nations, to the end that every individual and every organ of society, keeping this Declaration constantly in mind, shall strive by teaching and education to promote respect for these rights and freedoms and by progressive measures, national and international, to secure their universal and effective recognition and observance, both among the peoples of Member States themselves and among the peoples of territories under their jurisdiction.

The Right to Health was affirmed at the international level in the Universal Declaration of Human Rights, Article 25 in 1948.

Article 25
(1) Everyone has the right to a standard of living adequate for the health and well-being of himself and of his family, including food, clothing, housing, and medical care and necessary social services, and the right to security in the event of unemployment, sickness, disability, widowhood, old age or other lack of livelihood in circumstances beyond his control.

(2) Motherhood and childhood are entitled to special care and assistance. All children, whether born in or out of wedlock, shall enjoy the same social protection.

The Preamble to the WHO constitution also affirms that it is one of the fundamental rights of every human being to enjoy "the highest attainable standard of health." Inherent in the right to health is the right to the underlying conditions of health as well as medical care. The United Nations expanded upon the "Right to Health" in Article 12 of the International Covenant in Economic, Social and Cultural Rights in 1966. Not only did this document guarantee the "right of everyone to the enjoyment of the highest attainable standard of health", but it also specifically called for the "provision for the reductions of . . . infant mortality and for the healthy development of the child; the improvement of all aspects of environmental and industrial hygiene; the prevention, treatment and control of epidemic, endemic, occupational, and other diseases; and the creation of conditions which could assure to all medical service and medical attention in the event of sickness."

The Right to Health

Article 12 of the Covenant recognizes the right of everyone to "the enjoyment of the highest attainable standard of physical and mental health."[40] "Health" is understood not just as a right to be healthy, but as a right to control one's own health and body (including reproduction), and be free from interference such as torture or medical experimentation. [41] States must protect this right by ensuring that everyone within their jurisdiction has access to the underlying determinants of health, such as clean water, sanitation, food, nutrition and housing, and through a comprehensive system of healthcare, which is available to everyone without discrimination, and economically accessible to all.[42]

Article 12.2 requires parties to take specific steps to improve the health of their citizens, including reducing infant mortality and improving child health, improving environmental and workplace health, preventing, controlling and treating epidemic diseases, and creating conditions to ensure equal and timely access to medical services for all. These are considered to be "illustrative, non-exhaustive examples", rather than a complete statement of parties' obligations. [43]

The right to health is interpreted as requiring parties to respect women's' reproductive rights, by not limiting access to contraception or "censoring, withholding or intentionally misrepresenting" information about sexual health. [44] They must also ensure that women are protected from harmful traditional practices such as female genital mutilation. [45]
In 2000, the United Nations further expanded upon the "Right to Health" with General Comment No. 14. This document expanded upon the original ideas from 1966 by

exploring the historical context of this right, further defining the meaning of an adequate health care system, detailing obligations of states, and defining violations, and discussing the basics of implementation.

World Health Organization's (WHO) Definition of Health

Preamble to the Constitution of the World Health Organization as adopted by the International Health Conference, New York, on 19 June, 1946; signed on 22 July 1946 by the representatives of 61 States (Official Records of the World Health Organization, no. 2, p. 100) and entered into force on 7 April 1948.

Health is a state of complete physical, mental and social well-being and not merely the absence of disease or infirmity.

Note: This Definition has not been amended since 1948.

Stephen Marks (1999) summarizes the main goal for the movement of establishing the field of health and human rights as an organized scientific endeavor – to move the rights discussion from theory to practice and action. Right or wrong, the realistic solution to health improvement is heavily controlled by political and governmental leaders who are charged with the responsibility of allocating available and necessary funding and adopting regulatory mechanisms and structures to promote wellness and health strategies and programs. Just because theoretical and historical trends validate the soundness of supporting human rights-sensitive health policies, it does not necessarily result in affirmative healthcare reform and universal access to basic health services. For *remarkable* change to occur, Marks notes:

> *…with a call to action addressed to everyone [all the healthcare providers, policymakers, and consumer stakeholders], so that we will not remain bystanders while millions of children, women, and men continue to live in ignorance, poverty, and deprivation of their fundamental dignity and integrity. Ideas do change the world, and the linkage of human rights and health work is one of those ideas. (p. 403)*

Other human rights contributors affiliated with the US-based Physicians for Human Rights (PHR) have called for a return to the original healing covenant relationship between physician (provider) and patient outlined in the Hippocratic Oath, and a departure from pressures associated with corporatization of medicine (Hannibal & Lawrence, 1999, pp. 404-416). PHR volunteers were engaged in several human rights violations cases (with health and medical consequences) investigated by the United Nations in Cambodia, El Salvador, Israel, Mozambique, Rwanda, Turkey, Venezuela, and Yugoslavia over the past couple of decades.

Having personally worked with hundreds of physicians and provider organizations in urban and rural settings throughout the United States over the past 32 years, there is no doubt in my mind that most physicians enter the profession with a commitment to help alleviate pain and suffering as well as to treat patients as best they can without regard to socioeconomic factors. Unfortunately, the current health system in the US is poorly designed to encourage humanitarianism and does not incentivize providers to keep patients from getting sick. The American healthcare system is in the sick care business, where increasing utilization of resources is the measure of payment for services. However, there are also countless examples in which physicians and provider institutions offer free care and donate their time, talents, and resources to charitable missions in this country and abroad.

Nancy Adler, et al. (1999, pp. 181-201), contributors to the *Health and Human Rights* reader, note in their article the correlation between socioeconomic status (SES) and health status. They discuss how SES directly affects health status all along the "gradient," rather than simply at the threshold of poverty (at the very bottom of the economic scale in society). They clarify:

Socioeconomic status is 'a composite measure that typically incorporates economic status, measured by income; social status, measured by education; and work status, measured by occupation.' The three indicators are interrelated but not fully overlapping variables.

These researchers found evidence of variability along the gradient of morbidity and mortality incidence rates and risks within four distinct levels of socioeconomic status. The causal relationship of SES and health status has been the subject of longstanding debate in the social sciences realm. Considerable analysis has been devoted to understanding the implications of access, genetics, socioeconomics, environment, and behavior on health status. There is also alternative evidence supporting the notion that illness has an influence on socioeconomic status – for example, schizophrenics and mentally-challenged individuals are nearly always found to be part of the lowest economic status of society (from a productivity standpoint). None of these factors have been found to be *the* single determinant of health status. Rather, the evidence suggests that there is a continuum of interrelated factors that are responsible for health status; these factors are changing and interacting along a gradient within major groups in society (pp. 185-186). Adler, et al. offer the following psychological and behavioral model showing important determinants of health status:

Health behaviors – smoking, physical activity, and alcohol consumption
Psychological characteristics – depression and hostility
Psychological stressors – life events, fear, and emotional distress
Social ordering – social class and position in the hierarchy of the clan, community, and society (dominance and control factors).

The strongest link appears to be the association between lower social status and higher rates of morbidity and mortality in society, according to Adler, et al. However, they caution that there are several reasonable explanations affecting health status that must be carefully evaluated. Their review of the literature indicates that the variability in health status clearly "is not simply a threshold effect in which morbidity and mortality increase only at severe levels of deprivation, but is a graded relationship occurring at all levels with the spectrum of social position" (p. 182). Preventive measures to improve health status must be widely available (and adopted) to enhance the overall wellbeing of the population and affect the social gradient, not just members of the lower SES.

The representation in Figure 17 shows the interrelationship of the foundational dimensions of human life that combine to establish and reinforce dignity, morality, and rights within a typical society. These dimensions are (1) spiritual and religious beliefs; (2) social, cultural, and economic structures; and (3) philosophical and scientific knowledge. The degree of health status for any population is tightly intertwined with each of these foundational dimensions -- the triangle is tilted purposefully to indicate that none of the groupings on the three points is superior to the other; instead, each grouping contributes to progress along the whole continuum of society.

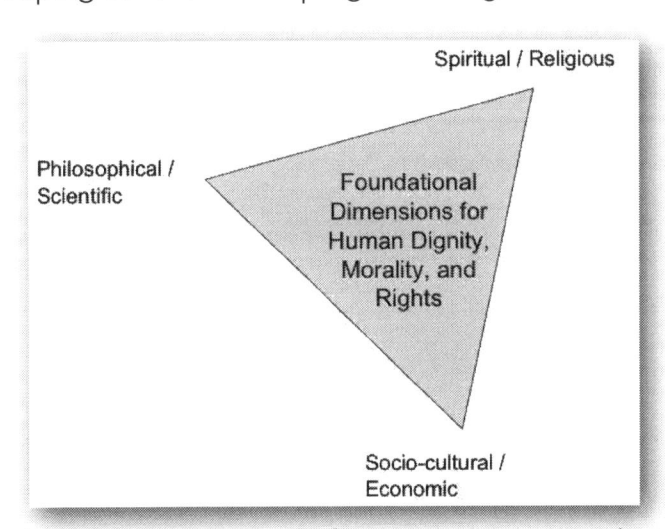

Figure 10 – Foundational Dimensions for Human Dignity, Morality, and Rights

Perhaps this is the reason it is so difficult to pinpoint why health and healthcare play such an important role for individuals and society, and why it requires an interdisciplinary perspective to determine the proper allocation of resources methodology.

10.8 -- Should Healthcare in the United States Be Considered a Right or a Commodity?

When one considers *human rights* issues, they typically refer to the legal, contractual, or moral human entitlements. Rights pertain to individuals and social groups. The domain of human rights falls into two main categories: (1) legal and (2) moral. These categories are sub-divided into distinct theoretical frameworks that help describe various methods for dealing with complex human situations. For instance, economic, social, and cultural rights, liberty rights, property rights, natural rights, and so forth. A *commodity*, on the other hand, is something that is valued or considered useful (economically or sentimentally) by individuals and social groups, and is the subject of exchange or commerce within the marketplace. The monetary exchange rate typically is dependent on the availability of, and demand for, a particular commodity. Commodities are traded at a particular time, location, and price.[74] This section discusses the special aspects of healthcare that relate to human rights and market commodities concerns in the US

Amnesty International (AI) was founded in 1961 and is a worldwide organization that advocates human rights issues and prevention of abuses toward human beings. AI is a multi-national policymaking body with some 2.2 million supporters governed by the International Council, which upholds the Universal Declaration of Human Rights UDHR). AI issued an official statement in 2008 regarding its position on universal access to healthcare: "We believe that health care is a right, not a privilege or a commodity."

The basic principles to achieve a human right to healthcare, according to Amnesty International, include:

> **Universality** – this means that everyone in the United States has the human right to healthcare; every person should have access to comprehensive, quality healthcare and should not be discriminated against on the basis of income, health status, gender, race, age, immigration status or other [socioeconomic] factors
>
> **Equity** – this means that benefits and contributions should be shared fairly to create a system that works for everyone: (1) healthcare is regarded as a public good, not a commodity; (2) gaps in the healthcare system should be eliminated so that all communities, rich and poor, have access to comprehensive, quality treatment and services; and (3) publically financed and administered healthcare should be expanded as the strongest vehicle for making healthcare accessible and accountable
>
> **Accountability** – this means that the US government has a responsibility to ensure that care comes first; all stakeholders in the healthcare system, whether public or private, have human rights obligations, and must be accountable to the people, and furthermore, the government is ultimately responsible for ensuring that both public agencies and private companies make healthcare decisions based on health needs, not on profit margins or other factors

These are worthy principles. What seems to be missing is a working definition of the *scope* of health services that should be included as a part of a human rights charter. Another shortcoming

---

74 Paraphrased from the *Merriam-Webster's Dictionary and Thesaurus*, 2006.

of the AI statement is that there is no mention of how universal healthcare will be funded. Governments have limited funds to pay for healthcare demands from their people. To suggest that any government can guarantee unlimited access to healthcare is illogical. Lastly, AI does not carefully lay out its moral basis for claiming that healthcare must be a human right for all, other than referencing the UDHR document.

Religious leaders entrenched in the healthcare delivery in the US have urged the 2009 Congressional delegation to act swiftly and address the present inequities of our system. The most vocal group on this issue is the United States Conference of Catholic Bishops (USCCB). The USCCB issued their official statement in February 2009: "The bishops have consistently insisted that access to decent health care is a basic safeguard of human life and an affirmation of human dignity from conception until natural death." The statement goes on to state: "Health care is not just another issue for the Church. It is a fundamental issue of human life and dignity." This position statement closely follows the theological doctrine and philosophical teachings of great religious philosophers of the Catholic Church -- St. Augustine of Hippo and St. Thomas Aquinas. The USCCB has been practicing what it preaches: one out of six patients in the United States is cared for in Catholic hospitals, which are the largest non-profit health system in the country. The USCCB defines their concept of universal healthcare:

All people need and should have access to comprehensive, quality health care that they can afford. Access to health care should not depend on a person's stage of life, where or whether one works, how much one earns, where one lives, or where one was born. Health care is a social good, and accessible and affordable health care for everyone benefits both individuals and society as a whole. The moral measure of any health care reform proposal is whether it protects human life and dignity and offers affordable and accessible health care to all.

The USCCB acknowledges the importance of fiscal responsibility and claims that the reformed healthcare system must restrain the rapid growth of overall health costs so that sufficient resources will be available to cover all people, without sacrificing quality or accessibility. The group also recognizes that health resources should be allocated according to a rational methodology of distributive justice. So how should US policymakers attempt to *eat* this philosophical healthcare elephant (the question posed at the start of this section)? The practical answer is: one healthy bite at a time.

Daniels (2008) makes an excellent point that healthcare services (the individual bites of the metaphorical elephant) command special moral importance in our society because they impact human opportunity, which is the fundamental argument by Rawls (1971), according to his theory of *justice as fairness*. The problem with trying to eat the entire healthcare elephant by tackling the full range of human inequities impacting health status as well as the multi-faceted social injustices that are tolerated in this country is that it will *choke* the policymakers with the infinite range of resources that are necessary to address a myriad of socioeconomic problems. Americans have come to terms with the vast income chasm that exists between the wealthy and the poor. This might help reveal why we have been so complacent about the inequities built into the employer-sponsored, market-driven health insurance system in the United States.

Humanity has little tolerance for *blatant* access restrictions to necessary healthcare services for the youngest and oldest members of society. The American culture does not condone denying care to persons in extreme pain and suffering that could result in premature death or permanent disability, at least in principle. However, the present healthcare system does deprive millions of citizens from obtaining basic healthcare because of the structure of health insurance coverage – our nation does not dispense healthcare services on the basis of need or *moral* standards.

Michael Porter is a leading professor of economics and competitive strategy in business and teaches at the Harvard Business School. He has authored sixteen books and over 100 articles relating to national and international concerns including healthcare delivery. Porter's (2004) essay, *Solving the Health Care Conundrum*, discusses why healthcare does not follow the normal patterns of a market-driven commodity. He details:

> *The US health care industry is unique in that despite the presence of significant competition, which usually drives increased value through decreased costs and improved quality, the nature of the competition in health care has been 'zero sum.' Behaving as if health care were a commodity, the major actors have focused primarily on lowering and shifting costs, increasing their bargaining power, and restricting services. Providers have offered and undifferentiated services, competing based on convenience and historical reputation in their local market.*

A critical factor affecting the economics of healthcare in the US that is often mentioned by healthcare planners is the difficultly for patients to differentiate the actual quality of care they are "buying" from providers. Hospital satisfaction scores usually reflect "creature comforts" and degree of interpersonal relations that patients experience during the encounter rather than measure quantifiable healthcare outcomes and benefits of care. There is little understanding of or concern for *evidenced-based medicine* on the part of consumers, supporting personnel, and even insurance payers. Evidence-based performance indicators would be part and parcel of a true commodity exchange process. Porter cites five key features that are lacking in most valuation transactions in healthcare:

1. The US health care system is a paradox in that it has competition, yet fails to deliver improving value.
2. The root cause of these problems is that the competition taking place has been the wrong kind.

3. The key to addressing these problems is moving to value-based, positive-sum competition.
4. Moving to value-based competition has important implications for providers as well as health plans and employers.
5. Public policy can serve as an important catalyst to accelerate change. However, policy changes are not necessary to initiate migration to value-based competition.

There needs to be greater transparency in price comparison, service-valuation (what advantages to the patient are generated by a particular provider, services, or technology option), quality outcomes reporting, compliance with standards of care, and other performance indicators in order for patients to be able to determine price-value considerations. Furthermore, "access to care must be addressed through mandatory health insurance coverage with subsidies for low-income citizens not covered by programs such as Medicaid and Medicare" (Porter, 2004, p.3). These factors are essential to creating healthcare equity. Universal participation in the healthcare system is the best way to stimulate value and lower the per-unit cost of care, notes Porter.

Donna Coffman, MD (2004) offers a practicing physician's perspective, commenting that there is a stronger sentiment in America that healthcare is becoming a *right* for citizens rather than a commodity. She cites the federal law regarding the Emergency Medical Treatment and Active Labor Act of 1986 (EMTALA), which mandated equal treatment of patients seeking care at any hospital emergency department, regardless of ability to pay, as an indication that society and policymakers consider some types of healthcare as entitlements, thus reconciling "our need for autonomy with our often-unspoken feeling that health care is a right" (p. 2). This movement toward healthcare becoming a human right must also demand personal and societal responsibility to carefully manage limited health resources, cautions Coffman, or the system cannot work.

In a critique of Norman Daniels's work, T. Schramme (2009) argues that his concentration on the moral importance healthcare, associated with its impact on the *normal opportunity range* (NOR) for individuals – pathological conditions involve comparative disadvantage – detracts from the critical nature of *personal responsibility* for health (and healthy decision-making). Schramme points out regulators in Western societies are usually hesitant to interfere with health problems that are the result of personal lifestyle choices. He cites examples of pathological conditions that result in "bodily harm" or physical limitation in health status that definitely result in opportunity disadvantages (socio-economic conditions) for these individuals. For instance:

> *Someone who breaks a leg in a test of courage [i.e., trying to help a child in distress] might still be treated, though he is also clearly causally responsible [for voluntarily risking personal well-being in the act]. We would treat him, I submit, not because a broken leg is disadvantageous, but because it is non-comparatively harmful. So I believe that when we assess responsibility for health we distinguish between pathological conditions that involve harm and pathological conditions that merely cause disadvantage...the moral*

significance of disease and disability, and the moral point of healthcare, are not only found in their relation to disadvantage but also, and probably more importantly, in their relation to suffering and absolute harm.

Schramme reasons that self-inflicted *harm* seems to be more of a basic moral condition affecting personal wellbeing than the degree of health or healthcare *disadvantage* or deprivation (p. 18). This assumption contradicts Daniels's theory that healthcare *deprivation* results in opportunity disadvantage (normal opportunity range), justifying the recognition of health and healthcare as special moral agents in society (Table 16).

Table 13 – Reasons Why Health and Healthcare Are Special Elements of Society

Reasons Why Health and Healthcare Are Special Elements of Society

Cause	Effect
Improving individual opportunity	Enhanced human potentiality
Maximizing human potentiality	Stronger and more productive community
Healthier individuals	Greater overall opportunity realization
Healthier society	Increased human-wellbeing and productivity / Gross domestic product growth
Higher GDP	**More resources available for rational allocation to members of society on the basis of fairness and justice**

A practical alternative to this philosophical argument might be to concentrate on the manageable *bite-sized* aspects of the healthcare system, with an emphasis on (1) personal responsibility for health improvement and maintenance, (2) creation of a basic universal system for rationally treating acute and chronic diseases, and (3) a strong public health program for (pathological illnesses and communicable diseases) preventive and wellness services accessible to all citizens. Unfortunately, the abundance of competing social and economic inequities prevalent in the US is a constant distraction for politicians and policymakers from having to face the challenges within our healthcare system and tackle meaningful healthcare reform initiatives. Moreover, the monumental social and economic distractions make the addition of the *healthcare elephant* (a $2.3 trillion system with tough special interest groups) simply too big to eat in one reform bite!

Bernard Baumrin (2002, p. 79) presents an intriguing theory on why he believes there is no implicit human right to health care. He explains that for healthcare to be an entitlement, it must be

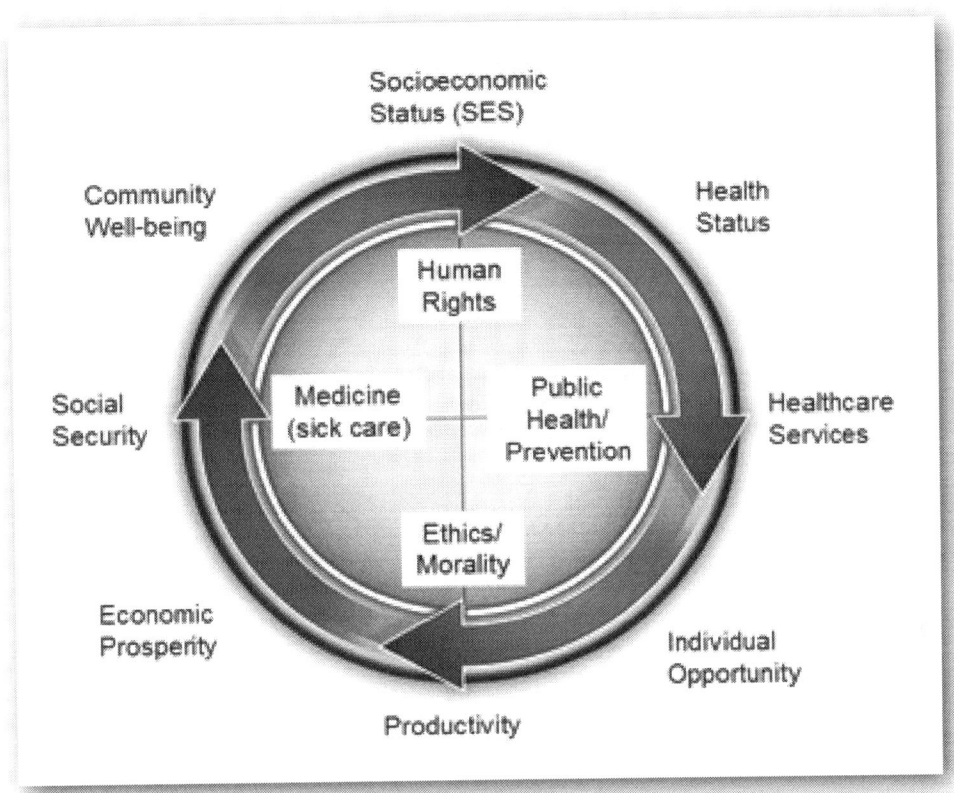

Figure 11 – Cycle of Health and Healthcare

grounded through one of three recognized societal frameworks: (1) *naturally*, as in the right to life; (2) *contractually*, as in the right to property or repayment of debt; or (3) *legislatively*, as in the right to exercise free speech. Baumrin contends that even if the *duty* to provide healthcare existed (as outlined by the United Nations UDHR discussed in section 10.7), it is also necessary that the *means* be available to provide healthcare services to all citizens. Simply talking about human rights does not create real duties; it takes much more, writes Baumrin (p. 81). There needs to be *substance* behind the claim to a human right to healthcare, either naturally, legislatively or contractually. An empty assertion that a group has the right to healthcare does not carry any weight.

According to Baumrin, if policymakers actually specified what types of healthcare services belong to the entitlement, and if there is a feasible mechanism to pay for these specific services, then it is reasonable to declare that these *limited* health services are truly human rights. For instance, Baumrin suggests that the following services should be part of a prioritized list of healthcare entitlements – what he called List 1:

- Emergency trauma care
- Epidemic disease treatment and prevention services (public health)
- Acute illness treatment and recuperative facilities
- Obstetrics

Everything else beyond the prioritized list would not be part of the *right* to healthcare and would only be supplied to patients if resources (either private or public) were available. Interestingly, this was the approach used by the Oregon legislature to fund its Medicaid program over 20 years ago (see Section 7.2). The OHP is an explicit form of healthcare rationing. "In some nations (e.g., the United States) there is no general legislation, hence no right of this sort," concludes Baumrin (p. 82). His argument is logical.

I feel that it is a matter of *theoretical semantics* to argue about *moral* or *human* rights to healthcare unless Americans are willing to accept the notion that a predetermined set of *basic* healthcare services (not only sick care) should be a *limited* right for all because of its direct impact on the potentiality and productivity of individuals, and ultimately the nation (an economic benefit to society as a whole). Universal healthcare is not the same thing as *free and unlimited* healthcare services available to meet everyone's desired and perceived needs.

The principles of *justice as fairness* relating to healthcare in the US should be conditioned upon the personal and communal responsibility for *accountable and reasonable* resource allocation, as suggested by Daniels and Sabin (2007). In other words, we must also develop a workable public forum for *rational* rationing (the dreaded "R" word) of limited resources.

> *Is Health Care a Right or a Commodity? Like it or not, health care has become a right for citizens in this country...Since both health care and the money to pay for it are limited, we must control the usage and the cost of health care to society. This is where we have failed. We don't like imposing limits on health care...*
>
> *We must accept the responsibility for managing that right in a reasonable and affordable way.*
>
> BY DR. DONNA COFFMAN, FP, UNIQUE OPPORTUNITIES –
> THE PHYSICIAN'S RESOURCE, JAN/FEB, 2004

Governments are expected to provide for all of the necessary health and human services to its citizens in order to fulfill their moral and legal obligations (depending on fluctuating tax revenues). In extreme cases, this brings about economic disaster, like in the situation of California – a $50 billion shortfall! Rights, moral or human, can only exist if there is a rational process for allocating scarce resources on the basis of a prioritization methodology that ensures people with the greatest and most appropriate needs are cared for, regardless of socioeconomic status. This would mean that if we as a nation chose to consider healthcare a human right, it is important to qualify such a right as *limited* to the economic ability of society, relative to all other human necessities.

Eleven

THE PUSH FOR UNIVERSAL HEALTHCARE COVERAGE

11.1 -- Public Health Plan, a Realistic Part of Universal Healthcare Coverage?

The Oregon Health Plan is not a panacea for either (1) achieving universal health coverage or (2) containment of healthcare costs. The most recent analysis of the effectiveness of the OHP was published by the Department of Human Services, Office for Oregon Health Policy and Research (OHPPR) in 2009 (OHPPR Report, 2009, pp. 71 and 84). The OHPPR trended data indicates that following a significant drop in the percentage of uninsured in Oregon between 1994 and 1996, the number of children and adults 18-64 years of age without health insurance coverage actually climbed steadily through 2004; the hospital utilization rate in the state between 2005 and 2007 continued to grow in most all areas (Graph 26 and Table 17). This does not mean that the OHP failed to accomplish its original goals. Oregon's allocation mechanism remains in place and has enabled the Oregon legislature and government officials to rationally adjust funding for the *Prioritized List* when the state faces an unsustainable imbalance between revenues and the cost of demand for healthcare services.

Rational allocation of limited health resources in the United States (and globally) is not an option; it is necessary to accomplish universal healthcare coverage in the United States. Alternative healthcare insurance options being explored by the US Congress must include an affordable and basic health services package that improves the health status of all Americans (Senate Finance Committee, 2009, April). Furthermore, universal healthcare coverage is not a commitment to a *single-payer system* run by the government, as has been falsely promoted by the health insurance industry and opponents to healthcare reform. This *red herring* is an attempt to once again derail reform initiatives and preserve the status quo. David May, Assistant Managing Editor of *Modern Healthcare*, emphasizes the irony of the private health insurance industry's position:

> *The insurance lobby, notably America's Health Insurance Plans, has called the inclusion of such a plan a deal-breaker in its support of reform, saying it would create an unfair*

playing field in favor of the public plan. It presumes lower payment rates that would harm providers and would be the first step toward a single-payer system...This is about providing one more choice [option] for struggling Americans in an unquestionably troubled healthcare system. Without a public option, any systematic healthcare restructuring will be more status quo than reform. (Modern Healthcare, 2009, May 25, p. 18)

The health insurance industry also claimed that a public health option would be *unfair competition*. How do these health insurance leaders *ethically* justify 70 million Americans who are uninsured or underinsured because they cannot afford to buy adequate healthcare coverage from the *disadvantaged* health insurance companies? There is a popular saying that goes something like this: "If they say it is *not* about the money, it really *is* about the money."

The Lewin Group's Vice President, John Sheils, testified before the US Senate Ways and Means Committee on April 29, 2009 about "The Cost and Coverage Impacts of a Public Plan" that is being advanced by Democratic members of Congress and President Obama.[75] Sheils noted that the potential impact of a public health option on the private health insurance industry could amount to a reduction of 119 million enrollees. According to the Lewin Group's calculations, that would amount to 70 percent of all people switching from their private health insurance plans (excluding supplemental coverage for Medicare beneficiaries) to a public plan by the government. How could this possibly happen if the government-run plan was such a terrible alternative? Table 18 summarizes the major assumptions published by The Lewin Group.

Table 14 – Potential Impact of a Proposed Public Health Plan on the Traditional Health Insurance Industry Utilization in the US

Potential Impact of a Proposed Public Health Plan on Traditional Health Insurance Industry Utilization in the US

Impact Area	Projected Consequence
• Estimated number of Americans who would enroll in a Medicare-style Public Health Insurance Program if available	$131 Million
• Estimated number of Americans who would drop private coverage in favor of a Public Health Insurance Program	$119 Million

---

75 The Lewin Group self-disclosure included in the printed version of the April 29, 2009 testimony by John Sheils stated: "In keeping with our [25 year] tradition of objectivity, The Lewin Group is not an advocate for or against any legislation. The Lewin Group is part of Ingenix, Inc., which is a wholly owned subsidiary of the UnitedHealth Group. To assure the independence of its work, The Lewin Group has editorial control over all of its work products."

Why The United States Healthcare System Should Be A Limited Human Right For All

- *Estimated uninsured Americans who would obtain coverage with a Public Health Plan* — *$28.2 Million*
- *Estimated reduction in physician net income (6.8%) if the Public Health Insurance Plan reimbursed at current Medicare payment levels* — *$33 Billion*
- *Estimated reduction in physician net income (3.1%) if Public Plan's reimbursement levels were between Medicare and average private payer levels* — *$16.8 Billion*

Source: Medical Economics, May 22, 2009, p. 12 (original research prepared by The Lewin Group, a healthcare and human services policy research consulting firm)

By reducing the customary administrative costs associated with private health insurance plans, Sheils noted that there could be an estimated decrease in family coverage premiums under the public option to an average of $761 per month. This is about 22% less than the current average family premium of $970 per month charged by the traditional private insurance companies.

Essentially, The Lewin Group found that the creation of a public health option could virtually annihilate the private health insurance industry. Because of lower payment schedules used by the government to reimburse hospitals and physicians for their services, Sheils explained that total hospital margins could drop by as much as $36 billion, and physician incomes could fall by $33 billion from current levels, or by a decline of 4.6% and 6.8%, respectively. The key variable affecting the magnitude of the impact relating to the "successful" implementation of the proposed public option is whether or not Congress would allow large employer groups to participate in the government-run plan. The Lewin Group predicted that 28.2 million uninsured Americans would also obtain health insurance coverage through a new public plan (which is probably close to the total number of *chronically* uninsured Americans).

> 'Never before has the healthcare system come under legislative review such that reform may finally be achieved…This moment's urgency is matched only by the opportunity for united faith voices to make a profound and positive impact…' Whether you're a creationist or Darwinist, it's clear that no one wants a survival of the fittest approach to healthcare anymore. Hallelujah.

By Linda Walling, Executive Director of Faithful Reform in Health Care, Modern Healthcare, May 25, 2009

Although there is no simple solution to the existing employer-sponsored, market-driven health insurance conundrum in the United States, the problem has become too great a national concern to ignore. Americans from all walks of life are demanding that their representatives in Washington, D.C. approve legislation that deals with healthcare inequities and mitigates the financial crisis resulting from a broken healthcare system.

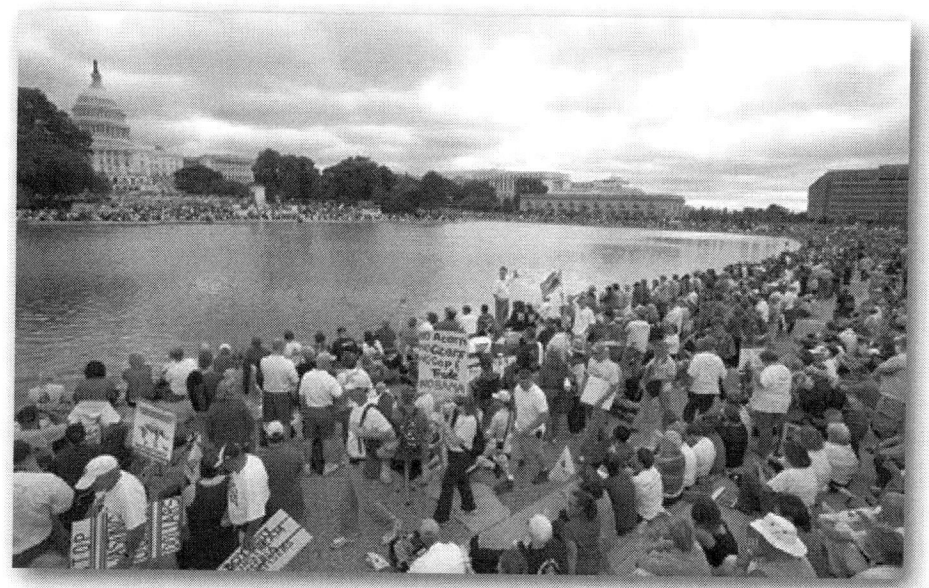

Figure 12 – Washington, D.C. Health Reform Demonstration
Source: Photo by Raoul LeBlanc, September 12, 2009, Washington, DC.

11.2 -- What Constitutes Basic Health Services?

To reiterate the main premise for ensuring equal opportunity and access to healthcare advanced by Norman Daniels, fairness does not necessarily equate to *equal* or *limitless* access to health services for all members of society. Daniels wrote in 1988:

> The fair equality of opportunity account has several important implications for the issue of access to health care. First, the account is compatible with, though it does not imply, a multitier health-care system. The basic tier would include health-care services that meet health-care needs, or at least important needs, as judged by their impact on opportunity range. Other tiers might involve the use of health-care services to meet less important needs or other preferences, for example, cosmetic surgery. Second, the basic tier, which we might think of as a "decent basic minimum," is characterized in a principled way, by reference to its impact on opportunity. Third, there should be no obstacles – financial,

racial, and geographical – to access the basic tier. (The account is silent about what inequities are permissible for higher tiers within the system). Social obligations are focused on the basic tier. (pp. 71-72)

Daniels makes a strong case for justifying multiple venues for healthcare delivery as long as society ensures that a *basic threshold* of health services is available to all citizens, regardless of their status in life. This approach is necessary because health and healthcare impact the normal opportunity range (NOR) for individuals – the golden rule for achieving *Justice in Health Care*. Therefore, a political goal for offering unlimited access to the *full range* of health services nationally is not prudent, fiscally responsible, or morally justifiable. Daniels suggests that a just healthcare system include a *basic* range of services that (p. 72):

- Impact on NOR.
- Foster preventive measures that make the distribution of risk of disease more equitable.
- Regulate [ration] consumption of personal medical services [sick care], weighed against other forms of health and healthcare.

An important question on the mind of observers of the healthcare reform debates in Washington, D.C. is the appropriate level of coverage that should be included in the universal healthcare plan being crafted by the Senate and the House on Capitol Hill (Figure 20). Gainer Pillsbury, Chief Medical Officer for Long Beach Memorial Medical Center in California, shares his thoughts in a letter to the editor of *Modern Healthcare* on July 27, 2009:

No system on earth can provide for all of the treatments and technology now available to everyone, much less all of the new technology and pharmacology being developed. Some treatments can cost $1 million per month. There must be some prioritization of services if any plan of universal coverage is to be successful. Coverage in the new public plan should perhaps include only evidence-based cost effective treatments, and if patients want more, they should be allowed to buy them or obtain excess coverage insurance to defray the increased expense. (p. 26)

Pillsbury also discusses his concern about the government incorporating the (stingy) prospective payment system used by Medicare and Medicaid in the new public plan, and how that might further limit the number of providers willing to participate in government-run programs.

The results of an opinion poll conducted by *Commonwealth Fund* and *Modern Healthcare* published late July 2009 and administered to healthcare leaders indicates that they ardently support the comprehensive overhaul of the United States healthcare system in four main areas:

1. Universal healthcare coverage including an employer mandate.
2. Cost controls with limitations on excessive profits.
3. Heavy taxation on alcohol, cigarettes, and soft-drinks with high sugar content.
4. Addition of a new publicly funded health option to compete with private (for-profit) insurance companies.

Not surprising, their focus remains on shoring up the existing sick care system rather than embracing expansion of preventive and public health services and programs aimed at keeping people healthy and improving the health status of the nation. The tendency of protecting the hospital industry is a matter of self-preservation and perpetuation of the economic engine that drives the present healthcare system. There are very few financial incentives to motivate providers to work to reduce the amount of sick care rendered by our system. The reality is that sick people pay the bills and generate profit margins.

Figure 13 – Health Insurance Coverage Schemes

*Seven of 10 respondents to the survey, conducted by Harris Interactive, support the creation of a national health insurance exchange with the authority to enforce standards of participation by carriers, standardize benefits, set rating rules, and review or negotiate premiums. Two-thirds (65%) say that the exchange should offer a **public plan** that incorporates innovative payment methods, **moving away from traditional fee-for-service and toward bundled payments**. Half of opinion leaders (51%) support setting provider payment rates in a public insurance plan either at Medicare levels or between Medicare and commercial plan levels. Other findings from the survey include:*

- *Fifty-six percent of respondents believe that, in designing an individual mandate, the required benefit package should be similar to the standard BlueCross/BlueShield option offered in the Federal Employees Health Benefit Program.*
- *In considering strategies to reduce health costs, opinion leaders express substantial support for new insurance reporting requirements (78%), joint negotiation of pharmaceutical prices (72%) and provider payment rates (61%), and limits to high cost providers and overvalued services (71%).*
- *Forty-five percent of respondents believe provider participation in the public plan should be linked to Medicare, while 43 percent believe it should not, with the strongest opposition among those working in health care delivery.*
- *Nearly three quarters of opinion leaders (72%) support ending the two-year Medicare waiting period for the disabled.*

Why The United States Healthcare System Should Be A Limited Human Right For All

- *When asked to indicate their support for a variety of approaches to financing coverage expansion, more than three-fourths of survey respondents (79%) support increasing the federal excise tax on alcohol, cigarettes, and sugar-sweetened drinks, and 77% support requiring employers to offer coverage or pay a percentage of payroll to finance coverage (pay or play).*

Source: Commonwealth Fund / Modern Healthcare Opinion Leaders Survey, July 2009; this survey included 208 respondents from various roles in the health system across the United States.

The discussion in this section begs for an answer to several excellent and important questions. A few of the most salient issues for which Americans must demand answers from their Congressional representatives are enumerated below:

1. Who will be in charge of deciding how to ration the allocation process of distributing limited healthcare resources in the US? Will it be Congress, physicians, other providers, a new Healthcare Board, citizens, a lottery process, philosophers, scientists, etc.?
2. Who should pay for the fair distribution of healthcare services on a universal basis – should healthcare (prevention and wellness services) or sick care be *the* number one priority in the reformed US healthcare system?
3. Should healthcare be limited to non-profit providers, or is there a benefit to maintaining a mixed competitive model with greater governmental price regulation?
4. Should the *individual healthcare account* described by Daniels (1988) in *Am I My Parents' Keeper* become the standard approach for determining who has exceeded her / his allotment of health services during a lifetime?
5. How should healthcare be valued in the United States in the future – should it be regarded as a right (moral and human) or a commodity?

The underlying conclusion of this book is that none of these important and complex questions can be resolved until a rational and public decision is reached about the *foundational* relevance of health and healthcare in society. Once our society reaches a *contemporary*[76] consensus about the foundational elements of healthcare, then we can effectively begin to design and develop viable solutions that meet society's expectations for a reformed healthcare system in America. If the general public and policymakers decide that healthcare *is* a limited human right because

---

[76] For the past century, health and healthcare have been treated as a commodity in the United States as attested by the employer-sponsored market-driven system that dominates the health insurance industry. The voice of Americans clamoring for change is growing louder these days and President Barack Obama is leading the charge to reform the US healthcare system in Washington, DC and is calling on Congress to adopt legislation to that effect in 2009.

health and financial resources are finite and contribute to a healthier and more productive society, it seems logical that certain *basic* health services and institutional processes (the foundational elements) would be incorporated into a reformed US healthcare system, including:

1. Substantial emphasis and incentives placed on *primary care, prevention, and wellness services* – PCPWS -- the suggested minimum amount of investment on PCPWS should approximate 30 percent of the total expenditures on healthcare in the US, or about $800 billion annually, in order to make a noticeable impact.
2. All Americans must have ready access to quality preventive and wellness services, regardless of socioeconomic circumstances – i.e., public health surveillance, STD prevention, vaccinations, immunizations, health screenings (colonoscopy, blood analysis, mammograms, etc.), wellness checks, health education, weight management, chronic disease management, exercise programs, food and nutrition programs, stress control, etc. These foundational elements of healthcare would be paid for on the basis of first-dollar coverage.
3. Sick care services must incorporate evidence-based, cost-effective diagnostic and treatment modalities with an emphasis on *need* (not want) and demonstrable positive outcomes. An *accountability for reasonableness* process must be part of the decision making process to ensure *just* allocation of limited resources.
4. There should be a comprehensive range of alternatives for ensuring access to healthcare and sick care – public and private healthcare insurance options could bring the nation closer to universal healthcare coverage and reduce inherent inequities due to socioeconomic circumstances. Pre-existing bias must be prohibited.
5. Profits resulting from the provision of healthcare and sick care services (providers and insurers) should be regulated to control the flow of financial resources throughout the system and maintain progressive development and quality services. I believe that provider profits or excess margins should average six to eight percent over a three-year period.
6. The current fee-for-service reimbursement model tied to volume and utilization increases must be revamped to reward prudent use of appropriate resources. There should be adequate provisions to care for the spectrum of human limitations and suffering due to disability, sickness and pain. At the same time, it is critical to reduce wasteful healthcare costs caused by unnecessary duplication and overutilization of services and treatment modalities, and to promote collaboration and coordination of care along the continuum (including extra global payment systems that reward these efforts).
7. Greater reimbursement for primary care providers is needed to reverse the trend of increased sub-specialization in medicine at the expense of prevention and wellness initiatives.

A newly-adopted universal healthcare plan, referred to as the Essential Benefit Package (EBP), is being implemented by the Oregon Health Fund Board (OHFB); it includes a *foundational* level of coverage for all government employees and their families. The universal healthcare program will run parallel to the private insurance sector and will be offered within the proposed Health Exchange that will regulate all health plans operating in Oregon. The EBP is part of the "minimum cost" array of preventive and wellness services such as *integrated home health services.* Other higher-intensity treatment services will be provided on a "cost sharing" basis according to specifications within four distinctive *tiers* that have graduated co-payment and deductible levels tied to each participant's income level. The guiding principles used to develop the EBP are:

- *Rational redesign* of the healthcare system to incentivize participants to utilize preventive, primary care, and wellness services to mitigate expensive inpatient utilization (sick care).
- *Innovation* that incorporates value-based (also called evidence-based) services to reduce unnecessary and unproven care and control costs while at the same time encouraging outpatient services; these services include substantial incentives for enhancing personal responsibility for one's wellbeing.
- *Affordability* for beneficiaries, including variable deductibles and out-of-pocket maximums to protect individuals and families from financial ruination due to catastrophic illness or injury.
- *Foundational level of health care coverage* below which no individual's coverage should fall – a safety net – (1) allowing private insurance companies to supplement the package, (2) prohibiting disease-specific plans that do not serve the overall health of an individual or insured population, and (3) general access to coverage that is compliant with the OHP Plus benefit package with "nominal" co-pays.

The OHFB's principles for developing the EBP are compatible and consistent with moral doctrines that advocate (1) justice as fairness and personal as well as society responsibility for wellbeing (Rawls), (2) accountability for reasonableness (Daniels), (3) limited basic healthcare as a human right (WHO), (4) transparency and evidence-based decision making (AHA / AMA), (5) maximization of human potential and social productivity, and (6) equal access to affordable health services, regardless of socioeconomic status (human right instead of commodity).

According to examples offered by the OHFB (p.10), value-based services are grouped according to six broad categories (see Exhibit B for Checklist, p. 235):

- **Preventive care** – immunizations, Pap smears, mammograms and colorectal cancer screening, etc.
- **Chronic disease management** – provider visits, selected medications, self-treatment education, care coordination, etc.
- **Maternity care** – pregnant women would have no cost sharing for prenatal care.

- **Dental services** – preventive dental exams, cleanings, and fillings for dental cares would be fully covered.
- **Vision services** – regular vision exams for specified age groups.
- **End-of-life care** – patients with advanced directives could access emergency services and hospitalization with reduced co-pays.

Plan participants who abide by the value-based service guidelines (weighted to the outpatient setting) accrue "points" that help reduce out-of-pocket expenses for more serious care, if necessary. The Oregon concept rewards enrollees to seek preventive care services early on in order to mitigate more serious and costly acute care in hospital settings. Oregon's emphasis on *healthcare* rather than *sick care* instills a sense of individual and societal responsibility for wellbeing.

Table 15 – Oregon Evidence-Based and Community Driven Essential Benefits Package Proposal (Framework)

Service Tiers and Services and Conditions Covered

Basic
Tier 1
Preventive and Wellness Care, Primary Care, and Chronic Disease Management with Very Effective Treatment
- *Preventive services*
- *Pregnancy and delivery*
- *Alcohol and drug treatment*
- *Life-threatening newborn conditions (e.g., very low birth weight or serious birth trauma)*
- *Life-threatening chronic diseases (e.g., treatment for asthma, diabetes, congestive heart failure, and HIV disease)*
- *Life-threatening mental health disorders (e.g., major depression, bipolar disorder, schizophrenia)*
- *Imminently life-threatening trauma (e.g., internal injuries, severe head injuries, major wounds)*
- *Imminently life-threatening acute illness (e.g., meningitis, appendicitis, intestinal obstruction, heart attack)*
- *Conditions of public health concern (e.g., tuberculosis, STD)*

Tier 2
Common Chronic and Disease / Conditions with Less Impact on Overall Health Status with Effective Treatment
- *Potentially life-threatening trauma*

- Cancers with effective treatment
- Chronic diseases with less impact on health or less effective treatment
- Potentially life-threatening acute illness

Extended
Tier 3
Generally, Non Life-Threatening Trauma and Chronic Conditions with Less Effective Treatments
- Non life-threatening trauma (e.g., severe sprains and strains)
- Non life-threatening mental health disorders (e.g., acute stress disorder, dysthymia)
- Non life-threatening acute and chronic disease (e.g., gout, migraines, kidney stones, miscarriage, tooth loss)
- Cancers with less effective treatments (e.g., pancreatic, esophageal and liver cancers)

Not Covered
Tier 4
Non life-threatening infections (e.g., sinusitis, otitis media, acute bronchitis)
- Self-Limiting Conditions, Conditions with No Effective Treatments, and Problems with Limited Effects on Overall Health Conditions with no effective treatment or no treatment necessary (e.g., rib fractures, benign cysts and growths, non-venereal warts)
- Self-limited conditions (e.g., clods, minor burns, cold sores)
- Conditions with limited effect on health (e.g., seasonal allergies, acne, diaper rash)
- Cosmetic Surgery, Infertility Services, Services Shown to Result in Harm, Experimental Treatments
- Conditions and Treatments Not Covered on the Prioritized List

Source: Adapted from the Essential Benefit Package (EBP) implemented by the Oregon Health Fund, June 20, 2008.
Note: Base premiums for Universal Health Insurance (proposed mandatory coverage for all Americans) would be the same for all enrollees; no one would be turned down for coverage, regardless of pre-existing conditions. Coverage levels would fall according to the tiered program proposed above.

The OHFB recommends that the HSC (with over 20 years of experience operating Oregon's Medicaid program) oversee the EBP process and correlate the classifications within the prioritized list of health services and proven evidence-based schemes, including the Drug Effectiveness Review Project (DERP), Oregon Evidence-Based Practice Center (PEPC), and Medical Evidence-Based

Decisions (MED). There are two safeguards built into the program for exceptional cases: (1) the Discretionary Services and (2) Appeals Process. The Oregon health plan is also tied to the proposed federal Health Insurance Exchange centers that are designed to broker various plans and supplemental packages that can extend coverage beyond the basic package for higher premiums. Oregon is leading the way for bringing rationality to the state's healthcare system and encouraging individuals to assume greater responsibility for managing their own healthcare destiny.

Janice Simmons (2009), a political journalist for *HealthLeaders Media*, published a commentary entitled "Making the Jump to Value," where she discusses the notable clamor in the halls of Congress for encouraging a *values-driven healthcare system in America*. The traditional fee-for-service and volume-based reimbursement system has done little to curtail the growth in the overall healthcare budget and has minimal impact on producing a healthier nation. Quoting Mayo Clinic's leader, Denis Cortese, MD, Simmons summarizes the typical attributes depicted by high-performance health systems across America:

- A higher level of a cultural focus is aimed at the needs of the patient.
- A higher level of physician or provider engagement, leadership, and change is found among those taking care of patients.
- A higher level of coordinated care is found where the teams use integration and coordination in managing the patients themselves.
- A higher rate of sharing of medical records and information is found from one place to another.
- Greater focus is placed on "the science of healthcare delivery."

Simmons points out that there is an inclination for policymakers to support incentivizing value-oriented performance, and a heightened awareness that Medicare, being the largest single payer for seniors, could trigger a paradigm shift in the reimbursement philosophy through healthcare reform initiatives. In fact, the Senate Finance Committee's draft version of its healthcare reform bill proposes implementing a values-based scheme for Medicare reimbursement starting in 2015. The big question is whether or not Congress will ultimately pass landmark legislation with such a radical transformation for the US healthcare system in the current session.

There is a unique opportunity to implement a values-based reimbursement system as long as all the healthcare players share in the collaborative assessment and treatment process of patients from start to finish. The experimental *bundled payment* (also referred to as global reimbursement) program being piloted at a few health systems across the country is validating the difficulties associated with the equitable distribution of funds to all participating providers according to their individual and system-wide contributions. For fully integrated health systems like the Mayo Clinic, this type of payment method could work well because most of their physicians (who drive the care delivery process) are employed by the system. However, the vast majority of providers in America are not part of vertically integrated healthcare systems, which will hinder implementation of innovative risk-sharing payment arrangements. The sentiment in Congress seems to be leaning in the right direction for creating positive incentives for providers who are committed to quality outcomes and values-based care.

11.3 -- Transitioning to the Next Generation of Healthcare in the United States

In his 2009 commentary, David Knowlton, the former Deputy Commissioner of Health for New Jersey and current president and CEO of the New Jersey Healthcare Quality Institute, calls upon government officials to change the incentives inherent in the US *sick care* system and confront the threats of the projected unabated healthcare cost increases. "By following a course of action that provides both incentives and investments in chronic-disease prevention," Knowlton states, "we can save lives and dollars at the same time." Education will pay off in the long run – it is estimated that the US could save about $300 billion annually by instituting universal health insurance coverage, increasing preventive and wellness services, expanding primary care, employing better health information technology, establishing integrated health networks, and improving life-style practices, explains Knowlton.

The crude mortality rate in the United States has remained rather steady at approximately 873 deaths per 100,000 people over the past decade. A systematic analysis of 2.4 million deaths in the United States, as recorded by the CDC in 2000, was conducted by Ali H. Mokdad, et al. (2004). The results of this study appeared in the *Journal of the American Medical Association* (JAMA) and identified the main causes of American mortality. They validated the general perception that "modifiable behavioral risk factors are leading causes of mortality in the United States." Specifically, tobacco smoking, nutritional and exercise inadequacies, and alcohol consumption were responsible for 38.2% (920,000) of all deaths in this country in 2000. The other major preventable causes of death in the United States in 2000 (239,000) in descending order were microbial agents, toxic agents, automotive accidents, firearms incidents, sexual behaviors, and drug abuse. One of the most tragic and dramatic increases in preventable deaths between 1990 and 2000, according to the authors, was caused by obesity – an increase of 100,000 cases in ten years (p. 1240). Mokdad and his group found that poor diet and lack of exercise caused a modern-day epidemic of overweight persons in this country. "It is clear that if the increasing trend of overweight [persons] is not reversed over the next few years… [they] will likely overtake tobacco as the leading preventable cause of mortality," the report boldly states (p. 1242). The combined number of deaths in the United States from tobacco and nutrition/fitness-related problems accounted for almost one-third of all deaths, according to Mokdad's 2004 report, and they urge policymakers to place greater emphasis on a "preventive orientation in health care and public health systems in the United States" (p. 1243).

Of the 2.4 million deaths that occurred in the United States in 2004, heart disease (27%) and cancer (22%) continued to be the two top killers, according to the US Centers for Disease Control and Prevention (Table 20). These are deplorable statistics for a country that is consuming $2.4 trillion and nearly 18% of the GDP for healthcare in the United States.

Table 16 – Causes of Death in the US: 2003-2004

Source: CDC, National Vital Statistics Reports, Deaths: Preliminary Data for 2004, Vol. 54, No. 19, p.4.

Oklahoma (in the center of the United States) ranked 12th worst among all 50 states and the District of Columbia regarding the highest percentage of overweight and obese adults (*HealthLeaders*, April 2007) in the United States.[77] The main culprits for the obesity epidemic are the general lack of physical activity, poor eating habits, and excessive food portions (super-sized fast food meals), lack of aerobic exercise, and excessive sugar, salt, and fat in diets. These issues contribute to the following health conditions: hypertension, osteoarthritis, dyslipidemia (high cholesterol and triglycerides), type 2 diabetes, coronary heart disease, stroke, gallbladder disease, sleep apnea, respiratory problems, and some cancers (endometrial, breast, and colon) (p. 2).

Andrew Weil, MD blames our general state of poor health on *blind faith* in professional medicine. In his book, *Health and Healing* (2004), Dr. Weil illustrates the limitations and dangers of total reliance on traditional (allopathic) medicine and presents several kinds of proven alternatives, or complementary medicine techniques that can improve health status. The *instant gratification* mentality of our society encourages high utilization of sick care, which perpetuates the growth of the healthcare system rather than encouraging preventive care and wellness. Seldom do Americans seek proactive ways to remain healthy – it is much easier to visit the doctor or take

---

[77] According to the annual state-wide health status assessment published by The Commonwealth Fund in November 2009, Oklahoma ranked second to last among all states and Washington, D.C. See "Sickly State," by Kim Archer, *Tulsa World*, November 5, 2009, A1.

pills for illness rather than modify poor life-style habits or adverse behavior. President Barack Obama campaigned (2007 and 2008) on the issue of *change* for the United States and promised to implement an aggressive agenda for the economy, *healthcare*, and social responsibility. His healthcare agenda was especially ambitious in light of numerous powerful special interest groups that have succeeded in toppling healthcare reform attempts for decades.

In his recent compilation of contemporary social essays, *The Covenant with Black America* (2006a) and *The Covenant in Action* (2006b), Tavis Smiley, an African American national commentator and human rights activist, outlines several crucial promises – covenants -- made by politicians to get elected that remain unfulfilled. Smiley speaks about the goals of the *Covenant* to "secure the right to health care and well-being" for all Americans, regardless of socioeconomic circumstances. Smiley notes that accountability of leaders is only half the equation. In his book, Smiley stresses that individuals should lead by personal example, and must assume greater responsibility for their own wellbeing by following a prescription for self-care. Smiley's call-to-action is loud and clear -- a healthier society is the by-product of public, private, and personal partnerships and joint community initiatives; it is not only the responsibility of governmental entities.

Tavis Smiley and Stephanie Robinson (2009) concentrate on social inequities of minorities and the poor in their call-to-action and demand that newly elected President Obama must uphold his *health covenant* with the nation. Smiley urges the public to remain actively engaged in the political process and to constantly evaluate progress on campaign promises. President Obama's key 2008 campaign promises pertaining to healthcare reform were:

- Deliver a new healthcare plan that will be available to all Americans with guaranteed eligibility, comprehensive benefits, affordable health insurance coverage, simplified paperwork, easier enrollment procedures, increased portability between jobs, and a greater choice of plans.
- Lower the cost of health insurance and drugs by offering more competition in the healthcare market (e.g., public health plan, cooperative exchanges, and other creative non-for-profit options).
- Provide relief for businesses, especially hard-hit smaller businesses, from the constant price increases for employer-sponsored health insurance that affect the viability for these employers. Universal coverage legislation should also require all employers to offer some minimum level of health insurance coverage to all employees (employer mandated healthcare coverage).
- Offer subsidies for the lower-income families to access insurance coverage.
- Support the already-insured and provide economic relief for those devastated by healthcare debt -- protect individuals from catastrophic illness and economic perils (bankruptcy).
- Expand existing [health insurance] plans and make them affordable to families caught in between the safety-net.

- Greater focus on prevention.
- Establish a National Health Insurance Exchange.
- Mandate payroll contributions for all workers so the burden of healthcare cost is spread over the largest possible group.
- Make child [health insurance] coverage mandatory.
- Support legislative reform for malpractice insurance limits.
- Reform bankruptcy laws to protect families facing medical crises.
- End insurance company 'cherry-picking' and other discriminatory practices.

For Black Americans and other minority populations, poor health status remains undeniably correlated with social, economic and environmental inequities that have plagued this cohort for centuries, especially in urban ghettos and mega-metropolitan cities like New York, Chicago, Detroit, and other crowded centers. "There is no quick fix for healthcare inequities that have persisted (and worsened in many cases) in this great democracy," asserts Smiley, "but the time has come for Americans to take a definitive stand and tackle these difficult social issues by demanding accountability from our political leaders." In his contributing essay in *The Covenant*, author and physician David Satcher summarizes the healthcare dichotomy in America as he sees it from the African American perspective:

The health of African Americans has suffered greatly because of social disparities that rendered us, and therefore our treatment, less than equal in quality and access. There are major disparities in healthcare and health outcomes. For example, if we had eliminated disparities in health in the last century, there would have been 85,000 fewer black deaths overall in 2000...In addition to health outcomes, disparities in health also relate to access to care. Access to healthcare is determined by many factors, i.e., insurance status, living in underserved communities, being underrepresented in the healthcare professionals, being uniformed about healthcare services and need, and feeling insecure about or untrusting of the healthcare system. These are major barriers to access. (Smiley, 2006, The Covenant, p. 3)

Nowhere in America is this unfortunate scenario more blatant than at the doorstep of the United States Capitol located in Southeast Washington, DC. By every health status measure, Southeast DC ranks poorly compared with the rest of DC and other major cities around the nation (Tozzio, unpublished paper, 2008).

The most important factors impacting the health status of Southeast DC residents, beyond the obvious extremely high level of poverty, are the unique impediments associated with the *ethnicity* of the African American population, which have a direct bearing on healthcare practices and medical utilization patterns. Willie V. Bryan (2007, pp. 148-150) studied the dynamic nature of African American families and the dominant role that the matriarch, or mother-figure (sometimes this is the real mother, or it is an adopted "mother" who takes over the care of related and unrelated children), has over healthcare delivery. There are complex culturally-based barriers that accentuate *distrust* of healthcare professionals, particularly non-African American physicians, and prevent early primary care intervention, which leads to higher emergency care utilization and unnecessary or inappropriate hospitalization in Black communities like Southeast Washington, DC.

Bryan describes the critical role that local community leaders play in the orientation process for medical providers regarding the importance of incorporating culturally competent practices into ordinary treatment protocols. This approach instills heightened sensitivity to African American ethnic beliefs and practice patterns about healthcare prevention and treatment. Cultural influences (African American, Hispanic, Asian, European, etc.) present complex and multifaceted challenges for providers to improve healthcare service delivery to high-risk populations; they require an interdisciplinary approach and ethnically-based solutions, not just the infusion of extra money and health resources.

Part 4

Critical Findings, Conclusions, and Epilogue

There seems to be a strong likelihood that healthcare will be recognized as more than a commodity in the United States. Perhaps our economic crisis and double-digit unemployment have put the spotlight on the importance of healthcare as a *foundational* element of our society because it directly contributes to our wellbeing and productivity. The problem is not that we do not invest heavily in the healthcare system...$2.3 trillion is a huge chunk of America's wealth! The issue is how we spend approximately $8,000 per citizen in this country. It used to be that the 47 million uninsured were hidden from mainstream America. Today, everyone has a relative, friend, or neighbor who is unemployed, underinsured and on the verge of bankruptcy, or flat uninsured. The challenges of the healthcare system in the US are at everybody's doorstep, not just the United States capitol!

Over half of Americans believe the US healthcare system is broken. President Obama and the Democrats in Congress also feel strongly that the healthcare system is failing to carry out its mission for at least 70 million Americans. Even the majority of healthcare providers sense that a major change in the employer-sponsored, market-driven insurance industry is necessary to equalize the burden of indigent care more equitably. Finally, we must come to grips with the reality that the present trend in healthcare spending will eventually bankrupt the nation – perhaps the healthcare tab will settle in at around $4 trillion, or 20% of the US GDP. So how should the American people and their local, state, and federal representatives proceed with the implementation of healthcare reform?

This book covered a lot of ground and many different aspects of the healthcare system's dilemma we face as a society. In Part 4, I will highlight key findings and conclusions of this research. The epilogue is where I begin to develop recommendations aimed at policymakers, providers, and consumers as we continue the journey to refine the United States healthcare system and prepare for the 21st century and beyond.

Twelve

CRITICAL FINDINGS

- It is not my goal to demonstrate that the US healthcare system is a total failure. The level of innovation and technological sophistication in this country is unmatched around the world. However, the time has come to explore new and innovative options that address the needs of 70 million uninsured and underinsured Americans who have limited access to this marvelous healthcare system due to the shortcomings of the employer-sponsored, market-driven health insurance industry that has controlled our delivery system for the past half-century.
- All United States citizens should have reasonable access to *basic* health services that are allocated in a fair and equitable manner. Basic healthcare services should entail, at a minimum, the promotion of primary and preventive care, public health services and education, as well as appropriate *sick care* services that ensure "treatments according to their overall medical effectiveness, and draw... a cut-off line essentially determined by fiscal realities within a market-oriented health system" (Brannigan, 1993).
- The key elements of Oregon's *basic* universal healthcare system are defined in the *Essential Benefit Package* (EBP)[78] advanced in 1994:

  ✓ Improve the overall health of the community
  ✓ Incentivize a rational redesign of the healthcare system
  ✓ Reward personal responsibility
  ✓ Reduce overall health care costs (on a per unit of service and outcome)
  ✓ Be innovative
  ✓ Provide a social safety net (to those persons with special needs)

---

78 *The Essential Benefit Package* (EBP), developed by the Oregon Health Fund Board's Benefits Committee, Oregon Health Services Commission, June 20, 2008. Retrieved April 22, 2009, from http://www.oregon.gov/ OHPRS/HSC/.

- ✓ Be affordable for the individual and the state
- ✓ Be values-driven (reflective of the moral beliefs of the community)
- ✓ Be evidence-based and outcomes-oriented

- Healthcare should not be regarded as a market-driven commodity available to those fortunate enough to afford employer-based health insurance or poor enough to become eligible for government-sponsored care. In the same manner that Americans believe that offering universal access to basic educational resources is an *ethical* and *moral duty* which benefits our society, likewise investing in healthier Americans and improving the health status of our communities will foster a prosperous nation.
- Universal care does not equate to free and unlimited care for anyone who desires any kind of healthcare services. Healthcare resources are finite, and we cannot consume the nation's economic goods and services (wealth) without a methodology for ensuring rational utilization. Universal care should offer various health insurance options tailored to meet the *basic* healthcare needs of all individuals that comprise our society.
- Healthcare should be treated as a *foundational* element of society; without it, there is a danger of perpetuating a *sickly* society that is less productive and economically draining on the nation as a whole (although the US outspends every other nation in the world on healthcare in real dollars and percentage of GDP, we continue to rank low on the list relating to health status).
- Healthcare (the promotion of wellness, health, primary and preventive care, and public health services and education) in the United States should be a *limited* human right, because as human beings we all share in the ownership of natural resources and communal abilities that maximize our potentiality as a society. In this context, reaching our societal maximum potential ensures each citizen the most beneficial and cost-effective lifestyle -- *fostering the greatest good for the greatest number of people.*
- Evidence supports the notion that *healthcare*, as opposed to *sick care* (curative treatment once individuals are afflicted by illness, injury and chronic diseases) generates a significantly greater return-on-investment (ROI) when it is better balanced in the overall healthcare system.
- Our *humanity* is the result of our unique ability (and perhaps propensity) to concern ourselves with the *social wellbeing* of the community-at-large, rather than merely pursuing *self-preservation and self-gratification*. According to recent national surveys, the fact the about 75 million Americans are uninsured or underinsured is undeniably disturbing to this nation and urges Americans to rectify this inequity.
- "Do onto others, as you would have done onto yourself…" Consider this: under circumstances beyond their control, how would politicians, policymakers, governmental regulators, drug manufacturers, hospital managers, automotive manufacturers, health

insurance executives, and other stakeholders, consider the fairness of their circumstances if they found *themselves* without affordable (employer-sponsored) healthcare coverage because of job loss? (Rachels, 2003, pp. 117-129).

- Economic conditions are forcing more and more states to exclude impoverished families from the Medicaid programs, even though they meet the federal family poverty criteria. Each state establishes its own eligibility criteria, which typically is a percentage *above* the federal family poverty level due to fiscal constraints.
- Oregon is the only state in America that has developed a *rationing* process for eligible medical recipients based on (1) empirical data of medical effectiveness of treatment, (2) effect on the quality of life of the individual, and (3) healthcare values from the community's perspective.
- A healthier society is the by-product of a partnership between public, private, and personal initiatives that extends healthcare rights to all citizens in a responsible and fiscally accountable manner.
- By shifting significant healthcare dollars to support and expand preventive care and public health services and education, the $8 trillion healthcare budget projected by the CBO for 2028 could be cut in half. Approximately 30% of the total healthcare expenditures should be devoted to prevention and public health initiatives in order to make a noticeable impact – this would amount to about $800 billion annually (compared to the present $65 billion level).
- The present trend of escalating healthcare costs in the United States is not sustainable in the near term – *a paradigm shift is inevitable*. Shifting our *foundational* emphasis from the predominant *sick care* model to a more balanced philosophy, including a serious commitment to prevention and wellness with true incentives for healthcare providers to promote a healthier society, is a *moral imperative*.
- Regardless of the type of healthcare reform that is eventually adopted in the United States by policymakers, our healthcare system will be drastically reconfigured over the next decade in comparison to today's health delivery system. The current estimated budget projection for healthcare in the United States will likely settle in at around $4 trillion by 2018, consuming approximately 20% of the GDP. This is twice the size of the 2008 healthcare budget.

Thirteen

Conclusions

There are several good reasons why the United States healthcare system should be considered a *limited human right*, with the government ensuring that all Americans receive *basic health services*. First and foremost, a viable healthcare system can contribute to healthier individuals, and they in turn can build a stronger and more productive society. This premise is hard to dispute. The difficulty is figuring out what should go into a package of basic healthcare services that reinforces a *wellness-oriented* life-style that does not unduly infringe on individual freedom of choice and is affordable to the nation. The large body of research reviewed during the development of this book suggests that the ideal healthcare system should emphasize the following basic healthcare elements: (1) personal responsibility for health, (2) easily accessible preventive care and public health services, (3) health education, and (4) a defined range of sick care services and treatment modalities that are likely to produce favorable outcomes and meet community-based values.[79]

From the perspective of satisfying the *demand* for healthcare services (not necessarily justified by individual healthcare needs), after the basic healthcare elements are met through universal healthcare programs, the system should offer a range of non-profit and for-profit health insurance coverage options to supplement basic health services and address individual's desires based on ability to pay.[80] Reconciling actual healthcare needs with the insatiable demand for services and resources in a cost-conscious manner is a tall order for policymakers. The following

---

[79] The push from multiple regulatory and payer entities is towards a comparative effectiveness, evidence-based medicine, and measurable quality outcomes approach.

[80] Universal healthcare proposals generally include: (1) private health insurance plans (profit and non-profit), (2) government-sponsored health coverage (Medicare, Medicaid, military plans, and Federal Employee Benefits Program), and (3) a new form of public health insurance plan.

conclusions should assist decision-makers to reach *just*, *accountable*, and *rational* solutions for restructuring the US healthcare system over a five-year horizon:

- Healthcare should be considered a *foundational* element of society because all other needs depend on our society's wellbeing.
- Health and healthcare directly contribute to individual and social wellbeing and productivity.
- The current growth in healthcare spending on "sick care" in the United States is unsustainable beyond 2016, when the projected annual budget is anticipated to top $4 trillion; a systemic change in the insurance coverage approach is both an *economic* and *moral imperative*.
- Universal healthcare coverage should provide every citizen with *basic* health services in order to enhance each individual's opportunity for life-plan fulfillment (Daniels, 1985; Daniels and Sabin, 2008).
- The US healthcare system should incorporate a reasonable mechanism for allocating limited resources, involving scientific knowledge that is tempered by community standards and national principles of fairness and justice; the Oregon Health Plan is an example of a rational model to examine closely.
- The main hurdle for reformers to overcome is how to determine healthcare needs and funding mechanisms according to life-rescuing, life-sustaining, life-improving, and prevention priorities. This will require a delicate balance between evidence-based medicine and community-determined valuation.
- Incremental implementation of healthcare reform legislation to enhance the present employer-sponsored, market-driven health insurance system is imperative! Ultimately, a tiered universal healthcare system including public and private options, or the so-called *Puritan Paradigm*, seems most compatible with America's future needs and belief system (Brannigan and Boss, 2001).
- Universal health insurance coverage, with ample freedom of choice, would ensure that basic health needs are met at the lowest per capita cost. This could also reduce inequities experienced by providers with higher indigent patient populations that struggle under the burden of uncompensated care. All Americans must be covered by affordable health insurance programs to spread risk and eliminate the burden of disproportionate indigent care throughout the healthcare system.

Applying the foundational principles explored in this book, I have suggested specific steps in Chart 8 that could further *moralize* healthcare reform in the United States, beginning in 2010:

Chart 7 – Tozzio's Prescription for US Health Reform Based on Principles of Justice

Tozzio's Prescription for Healthcare Reform in the United States Based on the Principles of Justice for Healthcare

CRITICAL SUCCESS FACTORS /
Key Action Steps

1. **Implement aggressive health promotion and prevention programs instead of pouring more money into the "sick care" system**
Shift payment from traditional medical care to prevention by requiring that all providers prove to the IRS and HHS that they are spending real dollars on demonstrable community health promotion programs – at least 30% of all patient care revenue received from all sources (commercial, government, and other)

2. **Limit overall healthcare expenditures to a maximum of 18% of the GDP – statutorily**
Cap national health expenditures at around $4.8 trillion annually by 2028

3. **Create a government-sponsored, universal health insurance program for uninsured, underinsured and small employers – enact federal legislation requiring universal health care for all Americans by 2010**
Through regionally developed / managed cooperatives supported and sanctioned by the federal government, create a competitively priced (and perhaps subsidized) national insurance program, in addition to existing Medicare, Medicaid, Federal Employees, and Military plans

3. **Renew and enhance support for primary care services**
Increase payment to primary care providers substantially, with higher differentials paid to rural providers (physicians, NP, PA, allied health providers) to encourage growth in this sector of healthcare

4. **Implement government regulation of profit levels for proprietary providers (hospital corporations, pharmaceutical companies, etc.) and non-profit healthcare entities**
Limit profit margins (EBITDA) to a three-year average of 6.0% to 8.0%, which will allow reasonable growth and ROI without creating a windfall for providers, commercial insurers, or suppliers of healthcare services (pharmaceutical, equipment manufacturers, etc.)

5. **Motivate health care providers to implement innovative provider-patient health information systems by 2012**
Provide federal grants and subsidies to collaborative healthcare groups and facilitate the development of Community Health Information Networks (CHINs), electronic medical record systems and other proven information management systems

13.1 -- Why Healthcare in the United States Should be a Limited Human Right for All

> *We stand at the threshold of reform. We shall soon see whether this administration and the Congress will confront the abyss of a widely divided electorate, spook at the potential political calamity that awaits, and rear up and retreat in disarray, allowing meltdown to loom ever closer. Or will the political leadership grasp a vision of our future, charge firmly and steadfastly ahead to bridge the abyss with eyes wide open in the interests of patients, the public, and the nation, placing narrow political vistas and rigid ideologies behind them, and plan and act strategically in all our best interests?*
>
> BY GEORGE D. LUNDBERG, MD, IN "THE AURA OF INEVITABILITY BECOMES INCARNATE," JAMA, MAY 19, 1993.

It is interesting to observe how history has repeated itself when it comes to healthcare reform efforts – special interest groups fought vigorously to maintain the status quo. Will the 2009-2010 Congress have the courage to chart a new course for the United States healthcare system, or will political infighting prevent legislators from debating the real philosophical issues affecting health and healthcare? In my opinion, members of Congress on both sides of the aisle must approach the healthcare conundrum from an interdisciplinary perspective and address these *foundational* concerns:

- First and foremost, healthcare (not necessarily the traditional concept of *sick care*) should be perceived as a *limited moral and human right* rather than a market commodity.
- The need to *rationalize* the distribution of *basic health services* is an essential economic reality – there are finite resources to pay for health care.
- We must recognize that a healthier society is more productive, and therefore, more economically viable and supportive of its citizens – this in turn enhances the overall wellbeing of the least fortunate, and mitigates inequalities.
- The *moral fiber* of American society establishes an ethical duty for a special, compassionate attitude and behavior towards those individuals who suffer from congenital, acute, and chronic debilities -- therefore, it is the duty of policymakers to ensure that *basic* health services are universally available to those who truly need healthcare.
- Multiple health insurance venues should be available to accommodate *prioritized* healthcare needs of all citizens -- this should include both public and private health insurance options and a prevention and wellness infrastructure supported by tax payers.

- A *rational* system for allocating limited health resources should incorporate community value-based criteria through a universal healthcare system based on the *accountability for reasonableness* standard suggested by Norman Daniels. This approach does not imply equal access and availability of *all* health services existing throughout the US; *basic health services* should be readily accessible to all citizens on a prioritized basis.
- A *Healthcare* rather *sick care* model will foster and encourage healthier and happier lives and reduce the overall per capita expenditures from private and public sources in the long term. The per capita cost of healthcare in the United States in 1960 was about $146 and consumed 5% of the GDP; today, the overall cost of healthcare is pushing $2.4 trillion, or a per capita expenditure of $7,500, which amounts to 18% of the GDP. This suggested paradigm shift (from sick care to healthcare) for healthcare reform in America is an ethically sound approach that should reap long-term benefits and help reduce the economic burden to society.

Efforts to overhaul the US healthcare system during the past half-century have faced overwhelming resistance from special interest groups committed to preserving the employer-sponsored and market-driven healthcare system. At this juncture, the inequities inherent in the American healthcare system are so blatant that it is impossible to ignore them. As noted by Brannigan and Boss (2001, p. 606), a key reason for the runaway healthcare costs is that our medical philosophy is basically crisis-oriented, with an emphasis on rescuing rather than on preventing illnesses, injuries, and chronic diseases. This shortsightedness concerning the foundational elements (moral standards) of our healthcare system has pushed serious reform efforts to the *back of the political bus*.

The American public and government officials have not seen fit to prioritize basic healthcare as a limited *human right* for all citizens. Instead, policymakers concerned with healthcare reform have concentrated primarily on addressing the economic consequences of America's healthcare structure by *cost containment* approaches instead of a health improvement strategy. Why is this? Perhaps an important difference between other cultures that have adopted universal healthcare as part of their moral structure (i.e., Asian and European countries) and the United States is that Americans view healthcare primarily as a commodity. Americans also have strong individualistic values rather than a philosophy of social solidarity. In European countries, as in the case of The Netherlands reviewed in Section 7.1 above, government-developed programs reinforce *solidarity* and ensure *equity* concerning the allocation of limited health resources. In the United States, healthcare is tied directly to employment status and is controlled by health insurance companies.

In his editorial published in *Health Care Analysis* David Seedhouse (1993) notes that "reformers keen to improve health systems are putting the practical cart before the philosophical horse" (p. 3). Furthermore, Seedhouse reasons:

Why The United States Healthcare System Should Be A Limited Human Right For All

In principle they [politicians and policymakers] have a simple choice. Either, medical services are no different from any other commercial enterprise, in which case the normal laws of capital should apply, and so there is no reason why those unable to pay for such services should be assisted to do so. Or, medical services are morally special since they offer fundamental support which it would be unjust to supply to one person and deny to another. But although the options seem stark, health reformers in the USA [and other nations as well] seem unable to decide which to choose…The most simple view is that many governments are currently concerned solely with the question: 'What measures can we put in place to control and limit financial costs of medical services?' But if the only problem is how to control spending on medicine, and if the governments in question [UK, US, Netherlands, New Zealand, and others] really believe in 'market forces' as much as they say they do, then the obvious policy would be to allow the market to find its own level. But governments too cannot decide whether medicine is special or not and also have in mind the question: 'How do we ensure adequate medical care for all our nation's citizens?' And so they dither. (p. 2)

Unless Americans demand that their representatives act decisively to redefine healthcare as an essential *human right*, there is little hope for achieving meaningful and beneficial healthcare reform. It is not enough for the government to simply offer health insurance coverage options for a privileged segment of the population. Community stakeholders must be intimately involved in the process of deciding what *they* believe constitutes essential health services and be encouraged to participate in the prioritization process that determines which services should be publically funded and who is entitled to healthcare. This type of transparent and participatory *allocation* process must be based on a genuine ethical and moral foundation to succeed.

> *The greatest threat to America's fiscal health is not Social Security. It's not the investments that we've made to rescue our economy during the crisis. By a wide margin, the biggest threat to our nation's balance sheet is the skyrocketing cost of health care. It's not even close.*

By President Barack Obama, in a speech at the White House, 2009

Brannigan and Boss (2001) characterize the United States health system as more of an *individualist paradigm*. In this scenario, health services are treated as "a privilege for those who themselves contribute to the healthcare system [by virtue of employer-based health insurance] and thereby deserve to reap its benefits" (p. 630). Persons outside of the regular employment circle have limited or no access to affordable health insurance coverage in the United States. Some advocates of healthcare reform have concluded that the long-term solution to alleviating the present crisis in the United States is to implement a *single-payer* program run by the national government, similar to the Canadian health system. The single-payer national health insurance approach is considered a *permissive paradigm* (pp. 631-634). This type of health insurance program has also been labeled *socialized medicine* by its critics who believe that the single-payer approach goes against the "moral grain" of the American democratic and capitalist principles.

The major problem with the individualist paradigm is that only those individuals who can afford to *pay* are given the opportunity to *play*. That leaves approximately 70 million Americans at risk who are either uninsured or underinsured and have limited or no access to the health care they need. The permissive paradigm, on the other hand, also has its shortcomings -- the single-payer system lacks a rational methodology to distribute healthcare resources, which often causes access problems and excessive backlogs for receiving important care due to public funding constraints.

A third approach is referred to as the "Puritan paradigm." In this instance, a *core* package of health services is available to all citizens – a basic universal healthcare package. Those who can afford to buy additional or supplemental health insurance coverage at market rates have the freedom to do so. The challenge with the Puritan paradigm, according to Brannigan and Boss, is that it tends to promulgate multiple levels (and possibly differential quality standards) of care, or a *tiered health system* (p. 633). It seems inevitable that our healthcare system will move further away from the exclusionary approach, the individualist paradigm, and adopt a model that offers universal access to *limited* and *basic* medical and preventive health services in this country, regardless of employment status and socioeconomic class. *Universal health coverage* is sometimes confused with a *single-payer health insurance plan* (the dreaded "socialized medicine" threat that is strongly opposed by conservative legislators). The two approaches are vastly different from each other. It has also been suggested that an alternative form of universal healthcare could be developed involving a government-sponsored insurance program similar to the Federal Employee Health Plan, Medicare, and Medicaid programs, which would function alongside the present private insurance sector.

> *The task of health care reform is indeed daunting; for every two hands, there seems to be three corks to hold under the water. Yet we must take immediate steps to control costs and expand coverage, and we must proceed with an eye toward the growing needs of an ageing population. The economic vitality as well as the moral character of our society is at stake as we prepare to enter the twenty-first century.*
>
> By Chris Hackler, Health Care Reform in the United States, Health Care Analysis, 1993

Brannigan and Boss (2001) note that "the United States has the embarrassing distinction of being the only industrialized nation besides South Africa that does not legally provide healthcare coverage for all its citizens" (pp. 633-634). Creation of a *fair* government-subsidized universal health plan would undoubtedly be a major *paradigm shift* for the US healthcare industry to the same degree that the creation of the Medicare and Medicaid programs was a historical breakthrough for seniors and the poor in the 1960s. The real obstacle to change is the perspective that the US healthcare system is a market commodity.

While the AHA reported that operating margins for community hospitals in the United States averaged 3.45% in 2007 (Graph 27), the performance of the private health insurance industry was much stronger. Until the national economic crisis hit at the end of 2007, the private insurance industry was reporting double-digit profit margins (Chart 9). A case in point was UnitedHealth Group Insurance, which had over 70 million covered lives in 2008; they reported a margin of 6.7% on revenues of over $75 billion, according to their Annual Report (Chart 10).[81] This disparity between the average profitability of hospitals (providers) and private insurance companies (payers) has worked to the disadvantage of consumers and exacerbated rising costs on both sides of the healthcare system. [See reference URLs for specific data on these entities: American Hospital Association, *TrendWatch Chart Book 2009;* Retrieved April 27, 2009, from

http://www.aha.org/aha/trendwatch/chartbook/2009/chart3-1.pdf http://www.aha.org/aha/trendwatch/chartbook/2009/chart1-29.pdf https://www.sendd.com/~webdrop/ezproxy/200904/UNH_2008_AR_FINAL.pdf

Perhaps a sound strategy for reforming the United States' healthcare system would be to invest substantially more resources in the development of basic primary care and preventive, public health, and wellness services (defined herein as true *healthcare*) in order to help "bend the cost curve" and restrain the exponential growth of the national debt attributable to traditional acute-care utilization and high-tech equipment (*sick care*). A focus on health maintenance and improvement is more cost-effective and morally justified than profiting from sick care. A more equitable and rational funding balance between healthcare (wellness orientation) and sick care will warrant radical changes to the current fee-for-service reimbursement system in the US -- today's healthcare economic incentives encourage duplication services and wasteful consumption of limited resources.

Unless the pace of healthcare spending in America is slowed down or eventually reversed, the projected annual expenditures for healthcare could reach $8.5 trillion by 2028. That figure would represent over 22% of the GDP! This size of a healthcare budget is not economically sustainable since the percentage of tax-paying Americans will continue to decline in relation to the growing number of retirees that are enjoying their golden years and demanding a larger share of healthcare resources. Posner (2007) warns policymakers that unless there is a major shift from

---

81 UnitedHealth Group is a diversified health and well-being company dedicated to making health care work better. Headquartered in Minneapolis, Minn., UnitedHealth Group offers a broad spectrum of products and services through six operating businesses: UnitedHealthcare, Ovations, AmeriChoice, OptumHealth, Ingenix and Prescription Solutions. Through its family of businesses, UnitedHealth Group serves more than 70 million individuals nationwide. Visit www.unitedhealthgroup.com for more information.

the *sick care* model of health delivery to an emphasis on *wellcare* (or healthcare), the health reform initiatives in the 21st century will be nothing more than a political fantasy and a windfall for the healthcare providers and insurance industries.

For the sake of this argument, let us assume that for every future dollar generated from sick care in the US, healthcare providers (the full range of organizations and professionals) would reinvest at least 30 cents toward improving health maintenance, prevention, and wellness initiatives with the goal of improving the community's health status. Under the universal healthcare model, *uncompensated care* would virtually disappear, and it would be possible to redirect existing government subsidies for indigent care (i.e., Disproportionate Share payments and tax abatement for non-profits) to increase payments to providers who are committed to the *well care* model. If the annual national healthcare budget in ten years were to settle in at about 20% of the GDP, or about $3.2 trillion, then a 30% commitment to prevention and wellness through public and private initiatives would amount to over $960 billion. Such a substantial investment in the nation's wellbeing is far greater than today's negligible budget of approximately *three percent* for prevention and public health services (Timmreck, 2003).

By redirecting approximately 30% of the total healthcare budget to health care, I believe that Americans could reap huge financial rewards during the next twenty-year horizon, containing the estimated total cost of healthcare in the US to about $4.8 trillion by 2080. This figure is almost half of the projected $8.5 trillion healthcare budget projected by the Congressional Budget Office (CBO) that economists based on the present spending trend. These savings could be accomplished by investing approximately $10 more per person in preventive health and wellness measures; researchers have demonstrated that for every $10 spent on primary care, prevention, wellness, and health maintenance, there is a corresponding *sevenfold* decrease in the amount of sick care dollars required by the population over a twenty-year timeline (see Chapter 8). This ROI certainly merits serious consideration.

The research reviewed for this book suggests that a *rational* public-private partnership that ensures basic healthcare services to all citizens (universal healthcare system) and uses a *fair* method for allocating limited health resources. This should reinforce the concept that healthcare is part of a *limited* human right. The "moral imperative" that President Obama spoke about during his speech to the joint session of the US Congress and the American people on September 9, 2009 pertained to the urgent need for enacting a sound healthcare policy that covers all Americans:

- A fair and equitable system of basic universal health services.
- A defined package of affordable healthcare benefits packet that promotes healthier lifestyles and accounts for medical needs.
- A reasonable and accountable methodology for allocating limited healthcare resources on the basis of their impact on prevention, wellness, and primary care, along with proven and cost-effective curative interventions.

- Better public and personal responsibility that becomes the cornerstone of a new moral attitude for improving the health status of Americans while maximizing life opportunity goals and productivity throughout society.

13.2 -- Relevance of this Book to Current Healthcare Reform Efforts

There is a loud clamor in support of major healthcare reform across America; it is expressed in newspapers, magazines, professional journals, Congressional hearings, associations, churches, town halls, etc. How to best accomplish reform is the trillion-dollar question. There is a different sense of urgency throughout the nation at this time as compared to the popular sentiment in 1993, when the Clinton Administration tried to advance a proposition for fundamentally changing the structure of the US healthcare system. Why did the previous efforts led by former First Lady Hillary Rodham-Clinton fail miserably in light of the well-staged rebellion by special interest groups? *AARP's* article in April 2009 explains how today's circumstances are vastly different than back in the 1990s:

> *The landscape has changed. What was a concern in 1993 has reached critical urgency in 2009. Senator Sheldon Whitehouse, D-R.I., told [President] Obama at a White House 'health care summit' of lawmakers and industry leaders last month, 'We're past the Harry and Louise moment [classic symbols of the anti-reform movement in 1993]. We're at the Thelma and Louise moment,' he said, referring to the popular 1991 movie. 'And we're heading for the cliff.' (AARP Bulletin, April 2009, p. 3)*

The metaphorical *cliff* that Senator Whitehouse alluded to was the fact that the current employer-sponsored, market-driven health system in the US has nearly tripled the overall annual cost of healthcare expenditures from $913 billion to $2.4 trillion during a 15-year period (1994 to 2009). The projected budget for healthcare expenditures in 2014 is expected to grow to over $4 trillion. The number of uninsured has escalated from close to 37 million in 1993 to approximately 47 million in 2008, according to the US Census Bureau. Add to the astonishing figures another 30 million *underinsured* Americans who are struggling to pay off thousands of dollars in debts that are owed even after the insurance companies have paid their share to providers for the care provided to insured patients. This scenario hardly seems like progress.

The *Urban Institute* released its report on the status of uninsured Americans in the first quarter of 2009. They analyzed the historical trend of uninsured individuals in the United States and judged that the number will probably reach between 57 and 66 million individuals by the year 2019, unless Congress takes drastic steps to reform the healthcare system.

The problems associated with the employer-sponsored health insurance system have become even more evident because of the worldwide economic recession, and the fact that the US unemployment rate topped 10% in 2009. It is difficult to imagine how policymakers can ignore the impending meltdown of the US *sick care* system that could rival the collapse of the banking industry last year. The 2009-2010 Congressional battleground over healthcare reform is split along ideological party lines that represent "irreconcilable" differences between *fiscal conservatism* and *foundational moral* philosophies. The contemporary healthcare reform debate, fueled primarily by *economic concerns* is bound to generate dramatically different solutions than a focus on *moral* reasons for dealing with the healthcare crisis. In the end, Congress will have to come to grips with the fact that healthcare cannot continue to be treated as an employer-sponsored, market-driven commodity that excludes millions of Americans from the system because of unreasonably high premiums with private for-profit health insurance companies. Congressional leaders have the unique opportunity to collaborate on behalf of the constituents they represent to forge a historical paradigm shift in the way Americans receive and pay for healthcare, as long as they act swiftly. A prolonged debate over healthcare reform legislation will undoubtedly thwart the momentum for approval, as it did in 1993.

"The conventional wisdom in politics and healthcare is that it's different this time," states Neil McLaughlin (2009, May 18, p. 21), managing editor of *Modern Healthcare*. His editorial continues: "the divisions and obstructionism that erupted among industry players in the 1990s won't recur, and all groups realize it's in their best interest to overhaul the dysfunctional US healthcare 'system.'" Time will tell! In the next section, two contrasting political positions are represented by political leaders Tom Daschle and Mitt Romney.

13.3 -- The Politics of Healthcare Reform
THE DEMOCRATIC POSITION

Former US Senate majority leader (D-SD) Tom Daschle and co-author of *Critical: What We Can Do about the Health Care Crisis* (2008) was President Obama's nominee for US Health and Human Services Secretary in November 2008. He was chosen to become the new Administration's point-person to help engineer the overhaul of the US healthcare system because of his intimate knowledge of the Congressional political process. Daschle withdrew his nomination in early 2009 when he became the subject of taxation scrutiny during Congressional hearings.[82] Nevertheless, he remains an influential force among Congressional leaders and key policymakers who are busy crafting alternative legislative healthcare reform proposals.

Daschle lays out in the May 11-18, 2009 issue of *Newsweek* the predominant Democratic agenda to achieve universal healthcare in the United States. Daschle explains that the proposal to establish a new "public health-insurance plan" to cover persons caught in the health insurance gap would help stimulate competition among private (and more expensive) market-driven

---

[82] Tom Daschle withdrew his nomination for HHS Secretary during the Senate confirmation process in early 2009 amidst allegations that he failed to pay necessary taxes on certain earned income and perks in previous years.

health plans. He believes that a public health plan would result in broader coverage alternatives and lower health insurance premium rates for all Americans. Essentially, the myths perpetrated by the health insurance industry and opponents of healthcare reform saying the public option would ultimately lead to a *single-payer* government-run health insurance system proved to be a smoke screen to derail Democratic reform initiatives in Congress. The Democratic plan, according to Daschle, advocates a substantial increase in the amount of funding for preventive health services and public health initiatives designed to attack the *root cause* of escalating acute and chronic sick care costs that negatively impact the US economy. Daschle notes:

> *Nevertheless, we must realize that reforming the health-care system is, first and foremost, for the American people – not the companies that profit from it…with health reform, Americans are likely going to have some kind of choice. Allow a public health-insurance plan or accept the fact that you are in for far more regulation as we construct a new system without it. With real competition, potentially far less regulation is warranted. (p. 38)*

Daschle (2008) suggests in *Critical* that an essential ingredient for transforming the American healthcare system consists of the establishment of a newly created *Federal Health Board* charged with the responsibility of establishing the reformed system's structural framework and filling in most of the operational details of the legislation approved by Congress. Daschle's proposal for a Federal Health Board was patterned after the *Health Services Commission* created by Oregon's Basic Health Services Act of 1989. This Act establishes a process for determining evidenced-based clinical value and cost-effectiveness of various treatment protocols (pp. 169-180). The OHP has been operating since 1994 as a "rational" mechanism for allocating limited Medicaid funding according to public values and priorities. Daschle asserts that the proposed Federal Health Board could be a key factor that finally unlocks the door to high-quality, high-value health care, helping to establish a scientific and participatory basis for implementing a rational health-care distribution process.

DEMOCRATS EASE IMPACT OF HEALTH BILL

> *WASHINGTON – Fearing a backlash, Democrats [on the Senate Finance Committee] worked Thursday to smooth the impact of sweeping health care legislation on working-class families as they pushed President Barack Obama's top domestic priority toward a crucial Senate advance. The most far-reaching overhaul in decades aims to protect millions who have unreliable coverage or none at all, and to curb insurance company abuse…Supporters said the overhaul's cost was in the range that Obama has set, about $900 billion over a decade, and would not raise federal deficits. Gradually, health care has grown to*

Mark G. Tozzio, M-IHHS, FACHE

dwarf all other issues in Congress, and is causing supporters and opponents to spend more than $1 million a day on television advertising to sway the outcome.

By Associate Press, October 2, 2009

The Republican Position

The Republican viewpoint was represented by former Governor Mitt Romney from Massachusetts. Massachusetts enacted a universal health plan for the state's uninsured and mandated coverage for all residents during Romney's gubernatorial term. Romney outlines the fundamental position of the Republicans' health reform plan as such: Republicans are adamant that less government interference is better for the country. "Republicans believe health care can be best guided by consumers, physicians and markets; Democrats believe government would do better," asserts Romney. Republicans would rather maintain the status quo because reform would increase healthcare costs and raise taxes. He fails to explain how Republicans reconcile their status quo stance with the overwhelming discontent voiced by Americans with high costs associate with the employer-sponsored, market-driven healthcare insurance system. Other concerns involve the growing number of uninsured, which has skyrocketed since the early 1990s. Even Republicans agree that the rise in national healthcare costs is unsustainable beyond 2016. The Republican formula, in Romney's words, is simple:

1. Get everyone insured. Help low-income households retain or purchase private insurance with a tax credits, vouchers, or co-insurance. Let's use the tens of billions we now give to hospitals to help offset the cost of free care and instead help people buy and keep their own private insurance...No more "free riders."
2. Make health insurance affordable and portable. Eliminate the tax discrimination against consumers who purchase insurance on their own.
3. Give people an incentive to be concerned about the cost of healthcare and how good the treatment system actually is compared to the rest of the world.
4. Provide citizens with information about the cost and quality of providers and the effectiveness of alternative treatments.
5. Reform Medicare and Medicaid, applying market competition principles to lower cost and improve patient care.
6. Control health reform at the state level...let the states serve as "the laboratories of democracy."

The problem with the Republican plan is that the historical record has demonstrated that normal market forces have not worked effectively for controlling the rising costs of provider services and private health insurance premiums. Health insurance executives and Wall Street have dictated lower reimbursement for medical providers and physicians and have charged high prices to consumers in order to maintain healthy margins. It is a common practice of the insurance industry to deny coverage for preexisting conditions and exclude higher-risk patients from plans. This "discriminatory" practice generally conflicts with the unwritten moral contract with society to ensure reasonable access to necessary healthcare services, regardless of one's lot in life.

The United States has experimented with the market-based model for delivering healthcare for nearly a century; the consensus is that the healthcare system is failing to meet expectations and is on the brink of financial collapse. Romney's argument that "the answer is unleashing markets – not government," has a poor historical track record during the past 50 years, as the cost of healthcare has skyrocketed and the uninsured and underinsured population has climbed to almost 70 million Americans.

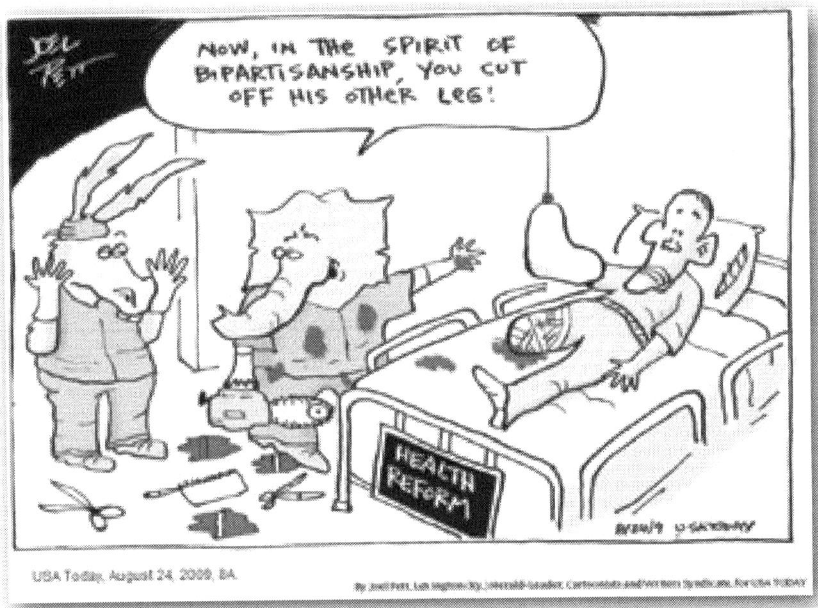

Illustration 1 – Congressional Bipartisanship and Healthcare Reform – The Battle Ground

THE MORAL POSITION

A quote from Len M. Nichols' (2006) essay *Outline of the New American Vision for a 21st Century Health Care System* seems apropos for wrapping up this section and reiterating why healthcare in the United States should be considered a fundamental pillar of a healthier and productive society:

> *There are 10,000 technical issues involved with health system reform, but one fundamental moral question: who shall be allowed to sit at our health care table of plenty? Many*

scriptural traditions and much humanistic philosophy admonish all communities to feed the hungry. Food was once the only indispensable commodity, the only thing one human being could give to another to guarantee and sustain life, the reason for communities in the first place. Health care has long since joined food as a unique gift, necessary to sustain and enrich lives stricken with certain kinds of illness. Too many uninsured Americans forgo treatment because of cost concerns, and don't see a doctor until it is too late in the disease progression – when treatments are most expensive or no longer effective and so they sometimes die needlessly. For us to deny health insurance – or access to effective health care – because of cost is tantamount to denying food to the starving poor. Few ethical teachers would approve. We can do far, far better than that. (New America Foundation, 2009, May 28)

If we are serious about instituting equitable healthcare reform legislation, it is not enough to just throw more money at the *sick care* system (as has been the case with the focus on employer-based, market-driven healthcare for decades). A case in point, the greatest positive impact on improving human health status over the past two hundred years or so related to enhanced, *clean potable water* and *hand-washing practices* – not necessarily expensive technological advances (Garrett, 2000).

> *Health care is a human right, not a commodity. Everyone in the United States has the human right to health care…This means that benefits and contributions should be shared fairly to create a system that works for everyone… [and] that the US government has a responsibility to ensure that care comes first.*
>
> BY AMNESTY INTERNATIONAL USA, MARCH 30, 2009

According to Nichols, a paradigm shift for the US healthcare system emphasizing personal and shared responsibility for wellness, prevention, and public health would be the best way to achieve long-term improvement in health status and help control rising healthcare costs. The moralist's position on healthcare reform is that basic universal healthcare reform is the (*human*) *right* thing to do.

Fourteen

Epilogue

14.1 -- Advice for Policymakers

Retired Professor of Health and Economics, Scott MacStravic, is regarded as one of the great healthcare policy leaders and futurists during the 1980s. He recently shared his thoughts regarding a viable course of action for healthcare reform in the United States:

> *As for healthcare reform, it is a vast challenge that will require disruptive changes in how every stakeholder in the 'system' behaves - particularly consumers, but also payers, providers, governments, etc. There is no simple answer despite those who favor 'solutions' such as consumer driven health plans (CDHPs) or even a single-payer system. It's a rat's nest. (MacStravic, 2007, personal communication)*

Japan's experience with a burgeoning aging population provides insight into the likely scenario that the United States will soon confront. The Japanese average life expectancy is the longest in the world – over 80 years (the United States is 77). Their per capita healthcare spending is approximately $2,500, compared to approximately $7,500 in the United States, yet the US ranks much lower on the health status list of developed nations. Over the past 40 years, healthcare expenditures in Japan grew from 4.4% of their GDP to 8.1% (Garret, 2000, pp.824-830). In order to cope with the country's escalating healthcare costs, the Japanese government began charging a special tax on individuals over 40 in order to fund home-based alternatives to institutionalization. They also encouraged healthier lifestyles for the younger population (wide-spread prevention and wellness programs) to curtail acute and chronic care inpatient utilization in later years of life. The Japanese experience is an important model for American policymakers to study.

Americans are increasingly demanding equal access to affordable healthcare services. This is only part of the solution - it also requires personal responsibility for taking better care of our bodies and promoting healthier lifestyles. It makes little sense, for example, to subsidize growing tobacco and permit cigarette sales while at the same time spend billions of dollars on treating preventable cancer diseases. Health promotion has to become the top priority for healthcare reform initiatives (Timmreck, 2003).

To achieve major shifts in personal and public responsibility for health improvement, change will either be (1) planned and orderly or (2) forced and chaotic. The impending impact on our healthcare system of the Baby Boom generation and continuing rise in the number of uninsured and underinsured individuals will strain providers and financial resources beyond reason. Transitioning to a balanced and progressive healthcare system in the US will take at least 10 years to accomplish, assuming that major healthcare reform legislation is adopted by 2010. The longer we delay healthcare reform and revamping the health insurance system in the United States, the greater the chances will be that the system will collapse because of the immense financial burden.

Larry McAndrews, President and CEO of the National Association of Children's Hospitals and Related Institutions (NACHRI) recently discussed his thoughts about the upward spiraling of healthcare costs in the United States:

In some sense, cost increases [referring to comments by economist Uwe Reinhardt in the same article concerning the relationship between increasing costs of healthcare and rise in US per capita income] in health care are perverse examples of Maslow's hierarchy of needs; as we have more discretionary income we are willing to expend more and more for marginal increases in health status, particularly when someone else is paying. (Children's Hospitals Today, 2009, Spring, p. 3)

President Obama appealed to members of Congress to pursue a bi-partisan solution for reforming the nation's healthcare system before it causes the havoc with the US economy. He reminded members of Congress that healthcare reform has been a key legislative priority in Washington, DC since 1943 when Congressman John Dingell, Sr. introduced the first healthcare reform bill. President Obama continued: "Our collective *failure* to meet this challenge, year after year, decade after decade, has led us to a breaking point." The President rebuked opponents of a Democratic-backed healthcare reform bill for spreading false rumors about the consequences of a government takeover of the health system:

Well the time for bickering is over. The time for games has passed. Now is the season for action. Now is when we must bring the best ideas of both parties together, and show the American people that we can still do what we were sent here to do. Now is the time to deliver on healthcare.

As President Obama fleshed his vision of healthcare reform, he alluded to a letter written to him by Senator Ted Kennedy (D-Mass) in May 2009 just prior to his death from brain cancer:

> *In it, he [Senator Ted Kennedy] spoke about what a happy time his last months were, thanks to the love and support of family and friends, his wife, Vicki, and his children, who are here tonight. And he expressed confidence that this would be the year that health care reform – 'that great unfinished business of our society,' he called it – would finally pass. He repeated the truth that health care is decisive for our future prosperity, but he also reminded me that 'it concerns more than material things.' 'What we face,' he wrote, 'is above all a moral issue; at stake are not just the details of policy, but fundamental principles of social justice and the character of our country.'*

During the final days of his life, Senator Ted Kennedy continued to fight fervently for a bi-partisan bill to reform the US healthcare system, one that would create a universal healthcare system for all American families. Senator Ted Kennedy served as Chairman of the influential Senate Finance Committee charged with the task of forging a saleable healthcare reform policy in Congress until his death on August 26, 2009 at age 77. The Senate Finance Committee passed the draft reform bill on September 2, 2009 and forwarded the document for review by the entire Senate body.

> *Healthcare reform must move our system from a volume to a value-driven care; doing nothing is not an option for Americans [paraphrased].*
>
> BY SENATOR BLANCHE LINCOLN, (D-AR), SENATE FINANCE COMMITTEE
> HEARING ON HEALTHCARE REFORM, OCTOBER 13, 2009.

The transition toward universal access to basic healthcare services and perhaps even a tiered medical system in the United States seems inevitable, as the demand for health resources continues to outstrip ordinary funding capabilities. As Americans grapple with the painful realities of the national economic crash in 2008, there is little room for error on the part of legislators and policymakers charged with the responsibility of implementing a strategic turnaround that should stimulate economic revitalization and simultaneously protect the health and wellbeing of Americans in all walks of life.

14.2 -- Advice for Providers

Why should society be so concerned with personal and community health status? A common presumption (backed by scientific evidence and common sense) is that healthier individuals are more productive citizens, and they contribute positively to society as a whole. A *healthier* society, in which members are free to maximize the "good life" and build a productive and prosperous community, is a widely-held philosophical goal around the world (Daniels, 1985). Amos Hawley, considered the father of the discipline of Human Ecology, preached that a critical aspect of successful human existence is humanity's commitment to *coexist* with several dimensions of our ecosystem. The science of Human Ecology is based on an *interdisciplinary* approach to societal progress (Hawley, 1950). Hawley postulated that a "healthy and integrated community" was able to more fully enjoy the biological, social, educational, scientific, technological, religious, cultural, political, environmental, and economic aspects of our world.

The presumption that good health and wellbeing are foundational aspects of human ecological existence is a central message of this book. *Universal access to basic healthcare should be a limited human right for all* because it enables individuals and society to reach their peak performance and productivity. Optimal health status is a complex matter. The health status of a population is based on numerous controllable and uncontrollable factors including those that are (1) externally imposed on individuals, (2) created by individuals themselves (self-inflicted or indirectly), and (3) caused by ecological circumstances beyond the individual's control.

Good health is both a *personal obligation* and a *moral communal responsibility* in order to promote the "greater good." The moral standards we choose to abide by make humanity "superior" to other life forms on this planet, along with our propensity to protect human life and mitigate suffering of the less fortunate in society. How does this philosophy of life make healthcare a human entitlement, a *right* for everyone, and at what cost to society? Should each individual have a moral obligation to contribute to the overall wellbeing of the community-at-large and help ensure that the basic necessities of life are available in a reasonable and equitable manner? These crucial concerns frame the moral, social, political, and economic basis for determining what are *reasonable* and *equitable* standards pertaining to the attainment of general health and wellbeing. This brings us to the pivotal question for policymakers: What are the appropriate criteria for ascertaining *basic* healthcare that maximizes communal wellbeing and productivity in America?

It is essential for healthcare providers to work collaboratively to explore creative means for offering the best possible health services and programs to all communities in this country without losing sight of the fact that medicine is a "special calling," first and foremost. Second, healthcare is a huge business enterprise that must run efficiently and with sufficient profitability to sustain this special calling. This is the essence of the moral imperative that urges Americans to regard health and healthcare as *foundational* elements of our society.

14.3 --Advice for Consumers

Individuals are personally responsible for making rational and responsible choices about their own healthcare future and for practicing healthier life-styles. While there are many circumstances beyond the individual's control that impact health status, Daniels (1983) cautions that we can do a lot of ordinary things to influence our health – "by avoiding smoking, excess alcohol, and certain foods, and by getting adequate exercise and rest" (Daniels, 1983, p. 35). Add to the list of prohibitions the deliberate and harmful acts of aggression toward each other, as in the case of suicide, homicide, reckless driving, assault in the commission of a crime, terrorism, etc. If we accept that healthcare should be a limited human right for all and employ distributive justice principles to ensure that basic health resources are available to maximize individuals' opportunity for personal achievement, how then do we reconcile compassionate care for those who disregard their own bodies and jeopardize the welfare of others? Is it really fair for society to devote equal amounts of limited health resources to individuals who suffer from the ravages of lung cancer because they chose to exercise their freedom to smoke cigarettes and abuse their body?

What about situations where environmental pollution by manufacturers is the cause of cancer and other maladies? Should society allocate equal amounts of health resources to care for individuals in both these types of circumstances? My point is that making healthcare decisions on the basis of merit, severity of illness, ability to recover and become a productive member of society, cost-effectiveness of treatment, profitability of services, and other considerations are all moral and ethical judgments. It seems evident that if we all share in the economic burden to offer basic healthcare resources, then we also have a mutual obligation to take care of our physical and mental wellbeing and avoid voluntarily causing injury to ourselves as much as possible. This is the reason that healthcare is a two-way street for individuals and providers of care.

Mark Lisa, Chief Executive Officer of Tenet Health System's Doctors Hospital in Manteca, California, echoes the sentiment of conservative politicians that claim solving our healthcare woes is not simply a matter of dumping more money and resources into the system. The long-term (and lasting) solution for America's healthcare system, Lisa emphasizes, "needs to be a wholesale and complete change in the personal health philosophy of every American…we want 100% freedom to do what we want to our bodies, but accept zero percent responsibility when it comes to the prevention or cure of what we allowed to happen because of that freedom." Lisa offers these commonsensical suggestions for promoting healthier life-styles:

- Ban the cultivation, sale and use of tobacco – in lieu of that move then we should tax smokers at a higher rate to offset the costs of their (government-funded) chronic care.
- Mandate every school child to have two hours of exercise a day – as part of school curriculum.
- Instead of requiring employers to offer health insurance as a benefit, mandate that all employers make their employees exercise vigorously for an hour a day.
- People that don't wear seatbelts [or motorcycle helmets] should lose the privilege of driving for a least six months: it's cheaper than hospital care or a funeral.

- All restaurants should provide nutritional information to all customers.
- Alcohol should contain nutritional information, be heavily taxed, or banned. (*ModernHealthcare.com*, 2009, May 23)

Each of these suggestions has the potential for significantly reducing voluntary injury to our bodies. They can also reduce unnecessary healthcare expenditures. Unfortunately, these suggestions are regarded by many as infringements by Big-brother on personal freedom and *civil liberties*. The truth about defending the *freedom* of a cyclist to ride a motorcycle without protective headgear (to cite one glaring example of a voluntary health preventive measure) is that it makes *no* sense from a personal or societal perspective when the person crashes and suffers from permanent traumatic brain injury (TBI). Voluntary assaults on our personal wellbeing cost billions of healthcare dollars each year, not to mention the associated pain and suffering to oneself and loved ones (Gutmann, 1983, pp. 43-67). Each of us has the moral obligation to society to care for our bodies in a logical and responsible manner without bringing about the need for additional laws and regulations to protect us.

14.4 -- Next Steps for Reforming the US Healthcare System

Every American should learn more about healthier behaviors and life-styles through public health initiatives and education, and become actively engaged in personal awareness and monitoring of health status. Americans are demanding that the private and public sectors allocate more resources to enhance preventive services, wellness programs, and primary care, and that everyone have reasonable access to affordable and basic healthcare services, regardless of socioeconomic circumstances.

This is the *moral imperative* that President Obama has alluded to on several occasions. There is no moral or ethical justification for anyone or any group to stand in the way of healthcare reform just because the proposed legislation is not perfected, or that it does not fully address each and every concern. Certainly, profiting from the business of sick care is no reason to preserve the status quo. Collectively, we must constantly strive to perfect social initiatives that contribute to healthier life-styles, and be willing to shed the status quo, so that our actions constantly produce the *greatest good* for all Americans.

This is…

Why Healthcare in the United States *Should* be a Limited Human Right for All.

Postscript - March 23, 2010

Obama Signs Historic Health Care Bill: 'It Is the Law of the Land'

The $938 Billion Bill, Facing Fire from Republicans, Brings Significant Changes to American Health Care
BY HUMA KHAN, ABC News

After more than a year of negotiations, debate and political drama, President Obama today signed the historic health care bill that could reshape care for millions of Americans while setting up a divisive battle with Republicans that's expected to spill into the November elections and beyond.

"After a century of striving, after a year of debate, after a historic vote, health care reform is no longer an unmet promise," Obama said at an event after the signing ceremony at the Department of Interior. "It is the law of the land."

The president took a direct stab at critics of health care overhaul, saying they are "still making a lot of noise" about what the new law means. "I heard one of the Republican leaders say this was going to be Armageddon. Well, two months from now, six months from now, you can check it out. We'll look around and we'll see," Obama said to applause.

The president signed the health care bill into law at the White House this morning. He was joined by Americans whose stories have touched the president, and Democrats who voted for the health care bill.

"Today, after almost a century of trying, today, after over a year of debate, today, after all the votes have been tallied, health insurance reform becomes law in the United States of America," Obama said to a standing ovation.

"It's easy to succumb to the sense of cynicism about what's possible in this country. But today, we are affirming that essential truth, a truth every generation is called to rediscover for itself: That we are not a nation that scales back its aspirations. We are not a nation that falls prey to doubt or mistrust," the president added. "We are a nation that faces its challenges and accepts its responsibilities."

The attendees chanted "Fired up, ready to go" -- Obama's campaign slogan -- as the president and Vice President Joe Biden arrived at the East Room. "Ladies and gentleman, to state the obvious, this is a historic day," Biden said to a cheering crowd before the president took the podium.

As Biden finished his remarks and shook Obama's hand, he was heard on the microphone whispering, "This is a big f-ing deal." White House Press Secretary Robert Gibbs tweeted soon afterward, "And yes Mr. Vice President, you're right..."

Postscript - June 28, 2012

Supreme Court Upholds Health Care Law, 5-4, in Victory for Obama
http://www.nytimes.com/
by ADAM LIPTAK

June 28, 2012

WASHINGTON — The Supreme Court on Thursday upheld President Obama's health care overhaul law, saying its requirement that most Americans obtain insurance or pay a penalty was authorized by Congress's power to levy taxes. The vote was 5 to 4, with Chief Justice John G. Roberts Jr. joining the court's four more liberal members.

The decision was a victory for Mr. Obama and Congressional Democrats, affirming the central legislative achievement of Mr. Obama's presidency.

"The Affordable Care Act's requirement that certain individuals pay a financial penalty for not obtaining health insurance may reasonably be characterized as a tax," Chief Justice Roberts wrote in the majority opinion. "Because the Constitution permits such a tax, it is not our role to forbid it, or to pass upon its wisdom or fairness."

At the same time, the court rejected the argument that the administration had pressed most vigorously in support of the law, that its individual mandate was justified by Congress's power to regulate interstate commerce. The vote was again 5 to 4, but in this instance Chief Justice Roberts and the court's four more conservative members were in agreement.

The court also substantially limited the law's expansion of Medicaid, the joint federal-state program that provides health care to poor and disabled people. Seven justices agreed that Congress had exceeded its constitutional authority by coercing states into participating in the expansion by threatening them with the loss of existing federal payments.

Justice Anthony M. Kennedy, who had been thought to be the administration's best hope to provide a fifth vote to uphold the law, joined three more conservative members in an unusual jointly written dissent that said the court should have struck down the entire law. The majority's approach, he said from the bench, "amounts to a vast judicial overreaching."

The court's ruling was the most significant federalism decision since the New Deal and the most closely watched case since Bush v. Gore in 2000. It was a crucial milestone for the law, the Patient Protection and Affordable Care Act of 2010, allowing almost all — and perhaps, in the end, all — of its far-reaching changes to roll forward.

Mr. Obama welcomed the court's decision on the health care law, which has inspired fierce protests, legal challenges and vows of repeal since it was passed. "Whatever the politics, today's decision was a victory for people all over this country whose lives are more secure because of this law," he said at the White House.

Republicans, though, used the occasion to attack it again.

"Obamacare was bad policy yesterday; it's bad policy today," Mitt Romney, the presumptive Republican presidential nominee, said in remarks near the Capitol. "Obamacare was bad law yesterday; it's bad law today." He, like Congressional Republicans, renewed his pledge to undo the law.

The historic decision, coming after three days of lively oral arguments in March and in the midst of a presidential campaign, drew intense attention across the nation. Outside the court, more than 1,000 people gathered — packing the sidewalk, playing music, chanting slogans — and a loud cheer went up as word spread that the law had been largely upheld. Chants of "Yes we can!" rang out, but the ruling also provoked disappointment among Tea Party supporters.

In Loudoun County, Va., Angela Laws, 58, the owner of a cleaning service, said she and her fiancé were relieved at the news. "We laughed, and we shouted with joy and hugged each other," she said, explaining that she had been unable to get insurance because of her diabetes and back problems until a provision in the health care law went into effect.

After months of uncertainty about the law's fate, the court's ruling provides some clarity — and perhaps an alert — to states, insurers, employers and consumers about what they are required to do by 2014, when much of the law comes into force.

The Obama administration had argued that the mandate was necessary because it allowed other provisions of the law to function: those overhauling the way insurance is sold and those preventing sick people from being denied or charged extra for insurance. The mandate's supporters had said it was necessary to ensure that not only sick people but also healthy individuals would sign up for coverage, keeping insurance premiums more affordable.

Conservatives took comfort from two parts of the decision: the new limits it placed on federal regulation of commerce and on the conditions the federal government may impose on money it gives the states.

Five justices accepted the argument that had been at the heart of the challenges brought by 26 states and other plaintiffs: that the federal government is not permitted to force individuals not engaged in commercial activities to buy services they do not want. That was a stunning victory for a theory pressed by a small band of conservative and libertarian lawyers. Most members of the legal academy view the theory as misguided, if not frivolous.

"To an economist, perhaps, there is no difference between activity and inactivity; both have measurable economic effects on commerce," Chief Justice Roberts wrote. "But the distinction between doing something and doing nothing would not have been lost on the framers, who were practical statesmen, not metaphysical philosophers."

Justice Ruth Bader Ginsburg, in an opinion joined by Justices Stephen G. Breyer, Sonia Sotomayor and Elena Kagan, dissented on this point, calling the view "stunningly retrogressive." She wondered why Chief Justice Roberts had seen fit to address it at all in light of his vote to uphold the mandate under the tax power.

Akhil Reed Amar, a Yale law professor and a champion of the health care law, said that it was "important to look at the dark cloud behind the silver lining."

Why The United States Healthcare System Should Be A Limited Human Right For All

"Federal power has more restrictions on it," he said, referring to the new limits on regulating commerce. "Going forward, there may even be laws on the books that have to be re-examined."

The restrictions placed on the Medicaid expansion may also have significant ripple effects. A splintered group of justices effectively revised the law to allow states to choose between participating in the expansion while receiving additional payments or forgoing the expansion and retaining the existing payments. The law had called for an all-or-nothing choice.

The expansion had been designed to provide coverage to 17 million Americans. While some states have indicated that they will participate in the expansion, others may be resistant, leaving more people outside the safety net than the Obama administration had intended.

Although the decision did not turn on it, the back-and-forth between Justice Ginsburg's opinion for the four liberals and the joint opinion by the four conservatives — Justice Kennedy and Justices Antonin Scalia, Clarence Thomas and Samuel A. Alito Jr. — revisited the by-now-familiar arguments. Broccoli made a dozen appearances.

"Although an individual might buy a car or a crown of broccoli one day, there is no certainty she will ever do so," Justice Ginsburg wrote. "And if she eventually wants a car or has a craving for broccoli, she will be obliged to pay at the counter before receiving the vehicle or nourishment. She will get no free ride or food, at the expense of another consumer forced to pay an inflated price."

The conservative dissenters responded that "one day the failure of some of the public to purchase American cars may endanger the existence of domestic automobile manufacturers; or the failure of some to eat broccoli may be found to deprive them of a newly discovered cancer-fighting chemical which only that food contains, producing health care costs that are a burden on the rest of us."

All of the justices agreed that their review of the health care law was not barred by the Anti-Injunction Act, which allows suits over some sorts of taxes only after they become due. That could have delayed the health care challenge to 2015. The conservative dissenters said that the majority could not have it both ways by calling the mandate a tax for some purposes but not others.

"That carries verbal wizardry too far, deep into the forbidden land of sophists," they said.

As a general matter, Chief Justice Roberts wrote that the decision in the case, National Federation of Independent Business v. Sebelius, No. 11-393, offered no endorsement of the law's wisdom.

Some decisions, the chief justice said, "are entrusted to our nation's elected leaders, who can be thrown out of office if the people disagree with them."

Justice Ginsburg, speaking to a crowded courtroom that sat rapt for the better part of an hour, drew a different conclusion.

"In the end," she said, "the Affordable Care Act survives largely unscathed."

Reporting was contributed by John H. Cushman Jr., Robert Pear, John Schwartz, Ethan Bronner and Sabrina Tavernise.

Supreme Court Ruling, see http://www.supremecourt.gov/opinions/11pdf/11-393c3a2.pdf

References for Section One

Abelson, Reed. (2009, August 25). Policy experts call fear of medical rationing unfounded. *The New York Times*. Retrieved August 26, 2009, from http://www.nytimes.com/2009/08/25/us/25georgiaside.html?_r=1&reed Abelson&st=cs…

Adler, Nancy, Boyce, Thomas, Chesney, Margaret, Cohen, Sheldon, Folkman, Susan, Kahn, Robert & Syme, S. Leonard. (1999). Socioeconomic status and health: The challenge of the gradient. In Mann, Jonathan M., Gruskin, Sofia, Grodin, Michael A., & Annas, George (Eds.). *Health and human rights: A reader* (pp.181-201). New York: Routledge.

Altman, Stuart H., Reinhardt, Uwe E., & Shields, Alexandra E. (Eds.). (1998). *The future US healthcare system: Who will care for the poor and uninsured?* Chicago: Health Administration Press.

American Hospital Association. (2009). *TrendWatch Chart Book 2009*. Retrieved April 27, 2009, from http://www.aha.org/aha/trendwatch/chartbook/2009/*chart3-1.pdf*

American Hospital Association. (2009). *TrendWatch Chart Book 2009*. Retrieved April 27, 2009, from http://www.aha.org/aha/trendwatch/chartbook/2009/*chart7-1.pdf*

American Hospital Association. (2009). *TrendWatch Chart Book 2009*. Retrieved April 27, 2009, from http://www.aha.org/aha/trendwatch/chartbook/2009/*chart1-29.pdf*

American Association of Retired Persons. (2008, June). Health Care '08. *AARP Bulletin*.

American Association of Retired Persons. (2009, April). We're at the Thelma and Louise moment. *AARP Bulletin*, 3.

Amiel, Yoram & Cowell, Frank A. (1999). *Thinking about inequality*. New York: Cambridge University Press.

Avorn, Jerry. (1983). Needs, Wants, Demands, and Interests. In Bayer, Ronald, Caplan, Arthur, & Daniels, Norman (Eds.), *In search of equity: Health needs and the healthcare system* (Chapter 7). New York: Plenum Press

Ayres, Stephen. (1992). Rationality, not rationing, in health care. In Strosberg, et al. (Eds.), *Rationing America's medical care – The Oregon plan and beyond* (pp. 132-143). Washington, DC: The Brookings Institution.

Baumrin, Bernard. (2002). Why there is no right to health care. In Rhodes, Rosamond, Battin, Margaret P., and Silvers, Anita. (Eds.). (2002). *Medicine and social justice* (pp. 79-82). New York: Oxford University Press.

Bayer, Ronald, Caplan, Arthur, & Daniels, Norman. (Eds.). (1983). *In search of equity: Health needs and the healthcare system.* New York: Plenum Press

Beehner, Lionel (2009, September 24). A world in pursuit of quantifiable happiness. *USA Today,* 11A.

Berg, Bruce L. (2007, 6th ed.). Qualitative research methods for social sciences. New York: Pearson Education, Inc.

Book, Robert A. (2009, April 3). Single payer: Why government-run health care will harm both patients and doctors. *The Heritage Foundation,* Webmemo #2381.

Brannigan, Michael. (1993). Oregon's Experiment. *Health Care Analysis,* Vol. 1, 15-32.

Brannigan, Michael & Boss, Judith A. (2001). *Healthcare ethics in a diverse society.* Mountain View, CA: Mayfield Publishing Company.

Bryan, Willie V. (2007, 2nd ed.). *Multicultural aspects of disabilities: A guide to understanding and assisting minorities in the rehabilitation process.* Springfield, IL: Charles C. Thomas Publisher, Ltd.

Cantor, David. (2002). *Reinventing Hippocrates.* Burlington, Vermont: Ashgate Publishing Company.

Carlson, Joe. (2009, April 27). Some hefty paydays. *Modern Healthcare,* 24-29.

Cassel, Christine & Harris, Jeffrey. (2009, May 11). Help us help ourselves: Reform should aim to boost medical professionalism for physicians. *Modern Healthcare,* 21.

Centers for Disease Control and Prevention. (2008). *Health Insurance Coverage: Early Release of Estimates from the National Health Interview Survey, January – March 2008.* Retrieved May 29, 2009, from http://www.cdc.gov/nchs/data/nhis/ earlyrelease/insur200809.htm.

Ciulla, Joanne B. (2003). *The ethics of leadership.* Belmont, California: Wadsworth/Thompson Learning.

Coffman, Donna, MD. (2004, January/February). Is Health Care a Right or a Commodity? *Unique Opportunities – The Physician's Resource*. Retrieved May 14, 2009, from http://www.uoworks.com

Commonwealth Fund. (2008a, July). *Commission's 2008 report: Why not the best?* Retrieved on March 15, 2009, from http://www.commonwealthfund.org/~/media/Files/Publications/Fund%20Report/2008/Jul/Why%20Not%20the%20Best%20%20Results%20from%20the%20National%20Scorecard%20on%20U%20S%20%20Health%20System%20Performance%20%202008/Scorecard_Chartpack_2008%20pdf.pdf.

Commonwealth Fund. (2008b, July). *National scorecard on US health system performance, 2008 chart pack* [companion to the *Commission's 2008 report: Why not the best?* Results from a national scorecard on US health system performance, 2008]. Retrieved March 25, 2009, from http://www.commonwealthfund.org.

Congressional Budget Office. (2009, January). *The Budget and Economic Outlook: Fiscal Years 2009 to 2019*, Budget Analysis Division (Publication No. 3187).

Cooter, Robert & Gordley, James. (1995). Cultural justification of unearned income. In Cowan, Robin, & Rizzo, Mario J. (1995). *Profits and morality* (pp. 150-175). Chicago: The University of Chicago Press.

Cowan, Robin, & Rizzo, Mario J. (1995). *Profits and morality* (pp. 150-175). Chicago: The University of Chicago Press.

Daniels, Norman. (1983). Health care needs and distributive justice. In Bayer, Ronald, et al. (Ed.), *In Search of Equity* (Chapter 1). New York: Plenum Press.

Daniels, Norman. (1985). *Just Health Care*. Cambridge: Cambridge University Press.

Daniels, Norman. (1988). *Am I My Parent's Keeper?* New York: Oxford University Press.

Daniels, Norman, Editor. (1989, 2nd Ed.). *Reading Rawls: Critical studies on Rawls' 'A Theory of Justice.'* Stanford, California: Stanford University Press.

Daniels, Norman, & Sabin, James E. (2008, 2nd Ed.). *Setting limits fairly: Learning to share resources for health*. New York: Oxford University Press.

Daniels, Norman. (2009). Just health: Replies and further thoughts. *Journal of Medical Ethics*, Vol. 35, 36-41.

Daschle, Tom, Greenberger, Scott S., & Lambrew, Jeanne M. (2008). *Critical: What we can do about the health care crisis.* New York: St. Martin's Press, Inc.

Daschle, Tom, & Romney, Mitt. (2009, May 11 / 18). Obama's health-care conundrum: DC is likely to get tangled up over a 'public plan' option. Two opposing viewpoints. *Newsweek,* 38-39.

DiPrete, Bob & Coffman, Darren. (2007, March). A brief history of health services prioritization in Oregon. *Health Services Commission Web Site.* Retrieved August 31, 2009, from http://www.oregon.gov/OHPPR/HSC/docs/PrioritizationHistory.pdf

Dobias, Matthew. (2007, April 30). Sensitive trigger: After the latest report from Medicare trustees, providers issue more calls for reform as they fear even harsher cuts to come. *Modern Healthcare,* 6-7.

Dunham, William. (2009, March 12). Obama's public health insurance idea draws fire. *Reuters News.* Retrieved April 4, 2009, from http://www.reuters.com/ article/politics News/idUSTRE52B4BK20090312

Dychtwald, Ken & Flower, Joe. (1989). *Age wave: the challenges and opportunities of an aging America.* New York: St. Martin's Press.

Dychtwald, Ken. (1999). *Age Power.* New York: Penguin Putnam, Inc.

Econometrica, Inc. (2007, March). Structural factors affecting the health insurance coverage of workers at small firms. *Small Business Research Summary,* SBA, No. 295, Contract SBAHQ-05-M-436. Retrieved March 23, 2009, from http://www.sba.gov/advo.

Emanuel, Ezekiel J. (2008). *Healthcare, guaranteed: A simple, secure solution for America.* New York: Public Affairs.

Englehardt, Tristram H. Jr. (2000). Bioethics at the end of the millennium: Fashioning healthcarecare policy in the absence of a moral consensus. In Wear, Stephen, Bono, James J., Logue, Gerald & McEvoy, Adrianne (Eds.). *Ethical issues in health care on the frontiers of the twenty-first century* (pp. 1-16). Great Britain: Kluwer Academic Publishers.

Engstroem, Timothy H., & Robison, Wade L. (Eds.). (2007). *Health care reform: Ethics and politics.* Rochester: University of Rochester Press.

Fisher, Elliot, MD. (Ed.). (2009). *Dartmouth Atlas of Health Care*. Retrieved September 20, 2009, from http://www.dartmouthatlas.org/; also http://money.cnn.com/ 2009/06/15/ news/economy/health_care_costs.moneymag/index.htm.

Fisk, Milton. (2000). *Toward a healthy society: The morality and politics of American health care reform*. Lawrence, Kansas: University Press of Kansas.

Futrelle, David. (2009, July 16). Too much money for too much medicine. *Money Magazine*, pp.82-86.

Galloro, Vince, Vesely, Rebecca & Zigmond, Jessica. (2009, August 3). The big pay (scale) back. *Modern Healthcare*, 6-12.

Gardner, Howard. (1999). *Intelligence Reframed: Multiple intelligences for the 21st century*. New York: Basic Books.

Garrett, Laurie. (2000). *Betrayal of trust: The collapse of global public health*. New York: Hyperion.

Gawande, Atul, MD. (2009, June 1). The Cost Conundrum: What a Texas Town Can Teach us About Health Care [Electronic version]. *The New Yorker*. Retrieved July 11, 2009, from **http://www.newyorker.com/reporting/2009/06/01/** 090601fa_fact_gawande.

Gawande, Atul, MD. (2009, June 23). Atul Gawande: The Cost Conundrum Redux, *The New Yorker* - News Desk, p. x.

Goldberg, Bruce, MD. (2009, June 12). A historic accomplishment in health care. *DHS Director's Message on the Web*. Retrieved September 22, 2009, from http://www.dhs.state.or.us/tools/news/dir_msg/2009/2009-0612.html.

Gould, Elise, with assistance from Garr, Emily. (2009, October 9). Most states suffer large declines in employer-sponsored health coverage. Economic Policy Institute. Retrieved October 13, 2008, from http://www.epi.org/ economic_snapshots/entry/webfeatures_snapshots_20081009/

Hannibal, Karl & Lawrence, Robert. (1999). The health professional as human rights promoter: Ten years of physicians for human rights (USA). In Mann, Jonathan M., Gruskin, Sofia, Grodin, Michael A., & Annas, George (Eds.). *Health and human rights: A reader* (pp. 404-416). New York: Routledge.

Have, Henk A.M.J. (1993). The Netherlands: Choosing core health services in the Netherlands. *Health Care Analysis*, Vol. 1. (Have is a Professor with the Department of Ethics, Philosophy and History of Medicine, Catholic University of Nijmegen, The Netherlands).

Hawley, Amos H. (1950). *Human ecology: A theory of community structures.* New York: The Ronald Press Company.

Hayry, Matti. (2007, 2nd ed.). Utilitarianism and Bioethics. In Ashcroft, Richard, Dawson, Angus, Draper, Heather, & McMillian (Eds.). *Principles of health care ethics* (pp. 57-64). Somerset, NJ: John Wiley & Sons Ltd.

Herman, Barbara. (2001, Summer). The scope of moral requirement. Philosophy and Public Affairs, Vol. 30, No. 3, 227-256.

Himmelstein, David U., MD, Thorne, Deborah, Warren, Elizabeth, JD, Woolhandler & Steffie, MD. (2009, August). Medical bankruptcy in the United States, 2007: Results of a national study. *The American Journal of Medicine*, Vol. 122, Issue 8, 741-746.

Holahan, John, Bowen, Garrett, Headen, Irene, & Lucas, Aaron. (2009). *Health reform: The cost of failure.* Washington, DC: Urban Institute (funded by the Robert Wood Johnson Foundation).

Institute of Medicine. (1982). *Health and behavior: Frontiers of research in the biobehavioral sciences.* Washington, DC: National Academy Press.

Institute of Medicine. (2001). *Health and behavior: The interplay of biological, behavioral, and societal influences.* Washington, DC: National Academy Press.

Institute of Medicine. (2002). *Care without coverage: Too little, too late.* Washington: National Academy Press.

Johansson, Ingvar, & Lynoe, Niels. (2008). *Medicine & philosophy: A twenty-first century introduction.* Piscataway, New Jersey: Transaction Books

Johnson, Glen. (2007, August 24). Romney: Mass. health plan be copied. *Yahoo!News.* Retrieved August 24, 2007, from http://news.yahoo.com/s/ap/20070824/ ap_on_el_pr/romney_ health_care&printer...

Kant, Immanuel, translated by Ellington, James W. (1993). *Grounding for the Metaphysics of Morals*. Indianapolis, Indiana: Hackett Publishing Company, Inc.

Knowlton, David. (2009, August 24). Grow better carrots: Improve incentives, prevention to find money to cover the uninsured. *Modern Healthcare*, 26.

Konner, Melvin. (1993). *Medicine at the crossroads: The crisis in health care*. New York: Pantheon Books.

Kuhn, Thomas (1996). *The structure of scientific revolutions* (3rd ed.). Chicago: University of Chicago Press.

Lalonde, Marc. (1981). *A new perspective on the health of Canadians*. Government of Canada, National Health and Welfare Ministry / Supply and Services [Cat. No. H31-1374].

Levi, Jeffrey, Segal, Laura M. & Juliano, Chrissie. (2008). *The Trust for America's Health Report*. Retrieved August 21, 2009, from http://healthyamericans.org/reports/prevention08/Prevention08.pdf.

Lisa, Mark. (2009, May 23). Personal accountability needs to be a priority. *ModernHealthcare.com*. Retrieved June 23, 2009, from http://www.modernhealthcare.com/apps/pbcs.dll/article?AID=/20090323/REG/303239950&AssignSessionID=373359975306137

Lundberg, George D. & Stacy, James. (2002, Revised Edition). *Severed trust: Why American medicine hasn't been fixed*. New York: Basic Books, Perseus Books Group.

Mahar, Maggie. (2006). *Money-driven medicine: The real reason health care costs so much*. New York: HarperCollins Publishers.

May, David. (2009, September 28). Editorial. Doing a number on the uninsured: Whatever the figure, it's too high and cries out for some solutions. *Modern Healthcare*, 18.

McLaughlin, Neil. (2009, May 18). Editorial. *Modern Healthcare*, 21.

Mann, Jonathan M., Gruskin, Sofia, Grodin, Michael A., & Annas, George. (1999). Health and human rights. In Mann, Jonathan M., Gruskin, Sofia, Grodin, Michael A., & Annas, George (Eds.). *Health and human rights: A reader* (pp. 7-28). New York: Routledge.

Marcum, James A. (2008). *An introductory philosophy of medicine: Humanizing modern medicine.* New York: Springer Science+Business Media B.V.

Marks, Stephen (1999). Common strategies for health and human rights: From theory to practice. In Mann, Jonathan M., Gruskin, Sofia, Grodin, Michael A., & Annas, George (Eds.). *Health and human rights: A reader* (pp. 396-403). New York: Routledge.

McAndrews, L. A. (2009, Spring). Dateline: August 2012 – the election of the President of the United States. *Children's Hospitals Today*, Vol. 17, 3.

McCain, John. (2008, October 9). Access to quality and affordable health care for every American. *New England Journal of Medicine*, Vol. 359, No. 15, 1537-1541.

Mill, John Stuart, with an introduction by Berlin, Isaiah. (1992), On *liberty and utilitarianism*. New York: Alfred A. Knopf, Inc., Everyman's Library Series.

Mill, John Stuart, with an introduction by Davis, Scott. (2005, rev. ed.). *Utilitarianism*. New York: Barnes & Noble, Inc.

Modern Healthcare Survey Results. (2009, June 15). Healthcare - A random poll conducted by Greenberg Quinian Rosner Research between May 7 and 12, 2009. *Modern Healthcare*, 9.

Mokdad, Ali, Marks, James, Stroup, Donna, & Gerberding, Julie. (2004, March 19). Actual causes of death in the US, 2000. *JAMA*, Vol. 291, No. 10, 1238-1245.

National Institute of Health. (2009). Hippocratic Oath. *NIH Historical Records.* Retrieved August 20, 2009, from http://www.nlm.nih.gov/hmd/greek/greek_oath.html.

National Center for Health Statistics. (2008). Uninsured population in the US – early release of information. *National Health Insurance Survey.* Retrieved May 29, 2009, from http://www.cdc.gov/nchs/data/nhis/earlyrelease/insur200809.htm.

Nichols, Len M. (2006). *Outline of the new America vision for a 21st century health care system.* Washington, DC: New America Foundation. Retrieved May 28, 2009, from http://www.newamerica.net/files/archive/Doc_File_2855_1.pdf

Obama, President Barack. (2009, July 29). What Health Insurance Reform Means for You. *The White House.* Retrieved July 29, 2009, from http://www.info.whitehouse.gov.

Obama, President Barack. (2009, July 1). President's public address on healthcare at Northern Virginia Community College, Annandale, Virginia. *CNN Television*.

Obama, President Barack. (2009, September 9). President's address to the joint members of Congress at the US Capitol concerning the need to overhaul health care in the United States, Washington, DC. *Transcript released by the White House*.

Office for Oregon Health Policy and Research. (2009, February). *Trends in Oregon's health care market and the Oregon Health Plan: Report to the 75th Legislative Assembly*. Retrieved June 8, 2009, from http://www.oregon.gov/ OHPPR/RSCH/docs/Trends/ Trends_in_Oregons_Health_Care3.pdf

Oregon Health Policy and Research. (2009, June). Gearing up for health reform. *OHPPR Official Web Site*. Retrieved September 22, 2009, from http://www.oregon.gov/OHPPR/index.shtml.

Oregon Health Fund Board. (2009, June 20). The essential benefit package – recommendations of the Oregon Health Fund Board's Benefits Committee. *OHPPR Official Web Site*. Retrieved September 24, 2009, from http://www.oregon.gov/OHPPR/index.shtml.

Oregon Health Services Commission. (2005, April 12). *Report presented to the National Governor's Association describing the savings associated with the Oregon's Prioritized List of Health Services during the 2005-2007 period*. (Received summary information from Darren Coffman, Executive Director of the Health Services Commission, April, 15, 2009).

Page, Susan. (2009, August 10). Health care fight tricky to wage – Poll: Americans' goals all over map. *USA Today*, 1A.

Parsons, Patricia, and Parsons, Arthur. (1995). *Hippocrates now! Is your doctor ethical?* Toronto, Canada: University of Toronto Press.

Porter, Michael. (2004, November 15). Solving the health care conundrum. *Working Knowledge – Harvard Business School*. Retrieved May 15, 2009, from http://hbswk.hbs.edu/cgi-bin/print?id=4486.

Posner, Richard A., Judge. (2007, April 29). Health care reform: A presidential fantasy. *LTVN Expert Analysis/Editorial Opinion & Commentary*. Retrieved May 31, 2007, from http://www.legalnews.tv/commentary/health_care_reform…200704

Rachels, James. (2003, 4th ed.). *The elements of moral philosophy*. New York: McGraw-Hill.

Rawls, John. (1971). *A theory of justice*. Cambridge, Massachusetts: Harvard University Press.

Rawls, John. (1999, rev. ed.). *A theory of justice*. Cambridge, Massachusetts: The Belknap Press of Harvard University Press.

Rawls, John; Edited by Kelly, Erin. (2001). *Justice as fairness: A restatement*. Cambridge, Massachusetts: The Belknap Press of Harvard University Press.

Reid, T.R. (2009, September 21). No country for sick men: To judge the content of a nation's character, look no further than its health-care system. *Newsweek*, 42-45.

Relman, Arnold S. (2009, July 2). The health reform we need & are not getting. *The New York Review of Books*, Vol. 56, No. 11. Retrieved August 5, 2009, from http://www.nybooks.com/articles/22798.

Satcher, David M., MD. (2006). Securing the right to healthcare and well-being. In Smiley, Tavis (Ed.), *The covenant with Black America*. Chicago: Third World Press.

SCORE Counselors to America's Small Business, Retrieved March 25, 2009, from http://score.org/small_buz_stats.html

Seiber, Eric E., and Florence, Curtis S. (2008, March). Changes in family health insurance coverage for small and large firm workers and dependents: Evidence from 1995 to 2005. *Small Business Research Summary*, SBA, No. 321, Contract SBAHQ-06-M-0513, Retrieved March 23, 2009, from http://www.sba.gov/advo.

Scruton, Roger. (1994). *Modern philosophy: An introduction and survey*. New York: Penguin Books.

Scruton, Roger. (2001, rev. ed.). *Kant: A very short introduction*. New York: Oxford University Press.

Schramme, T. (2009). On Norman Daniels' interpretation of the moral significance of healthcare. *Journal of Medical Ethics*, Vol. 35, 17-20.

Seedhouse, David. (1993). Putting the horse first: The practical value of philosophical analysis. *Health Care Analysis*, Vol. 1, 1-3.

Sen, A.K. (1989, 2nd ed.). Rawls versus Bentham: An axiomatic examination of the pure distribution problem. In Daniels, Norman (Ed.), *Reading Rawls: Critical Studies on Rawls' 'A Theory of Justice* (p. 289). Stanford, California: Stanford University Press.

Senate Finance Committee. (2009, April 29). *Transforming the health delivery system: Proposals to improve patient care and reduce health care costs.* Washington, DC: US Congressional Printing Office.

Simmons, Janice. (2009, September 24). Making the jump to value. *HealthLeaders Media.* Retrieved September 25, 2009, from http://webmail.aol.com /28200/aol/en-us/mail/PrintMessage.aspx

Simmons, Janice. (2009, October 1). Senate Finance gives ok to raise limits on employee healthy behavior rewards. *HealthLeaders Media.* Retrieved October 1, 2009, from http://www.healthleadersmedia.com/print/content/239865/topic/WS_HLM2_LED/Senate

Simmons, Janice. (2009, October 13). Can Senate Finance bill bend the cost curve? *HealthLeaders Media.* Retrieved October 14, 2009, from http://www.healthleadersmedia.com/print/content/240319/topic/WS_HLM2_LED/Can -Senate-…

Stanford Encyclopedia of Philosophy. Retrieved September 2, 2009, from http://plato.stanford.edu/about.html.

Stanton, Mark W. (2004, September). Employer-sponsored health insurance: Trends in cost and access. *DHHS Agency for Healthcare Research and Quality.* Retrieved October 16, 2009, from http://www.ahrq.gov.

Starr, Paul. (1982). *The Social Transformation of American Medicine: The rise of a sovereign profession and the making of a vast industry.* New York: Basic Books, Inc.

Strosberg, Martin, Wiener, Joshua, Baker, Robert, & Fein, I. Alan. (1992). *Rationing America's Medical Care: The Oregon Plan and Beyond.* Washington, DC: The Brookings Inst.

Smiley, Tavis. (Ed.). (2006a). *The covenant with Black America.* Chicago: Third World Press

Smiley, Tavis. (Ed.). (2006b). *The covenant in action.* Carlsbad, California: Smiley Books

Smiley, Tavis and Robinson, Stephanie. (2009, unabridged audio CD). *Accountable: Making America as good as its promise.* New York: Simon & Schuster Audio Division

Tozzio, Mark, with assistance from Bryan, Willie V. (2008, June 25). Understanding cultural diversity and the interplay with health status of the population in Southeast District of Columbia. *Unpublished White Paper.* United Medical Center, Washington, DC.

Trust for America's Health. (2009a, July). *F as in fat 2009: How obesity policies are failing America.* Retrieved July 2, 2009, from http://healthyamericans.org/ reports/obesity2009/

Trust for America's Health. (2009b). *Blueprint for healthier America.* Retrieved July 5, 2009, from http://healthyamericans.org/report/55/blueprint-for-healthier-america.

US Census Bureau. (2008, August) *Income, Poverty, and Health Insurance Coverage in the United States: 2007* (Current Population Reports, P60-265). Retrieved June 20, 2009, from http://www.census.gov/ prod/2008pubs/p60-235.pdf

US Department of Health and Human Services. (2001, with subsequent updates). *Healthy People 2010.* Rockville, Maryland: Office of Disease Prevention and Health Promotion. Retrieved March 15, 2009, from http://www.healthypeople.gov/Publications/

USA Today. (2009, August 18). In family medicine, you get to be part of your patient's life story (p. 2A). Retrieved August 18, 2009, from http://ee.usatoday.com/Subscribers/.

Vladeck, Bruce. (2003). Universal health insurance in the United States: Reflections on the past, the present, and the future. *American Journal of Public Health,* Vol. 93, No. 1, 16–19. Retrieved August 7, 2009, from http://www.pubmedcentral.nih.gov/articlerender.fcgi?artid=1447684.

Weil, Andrew. (1995, updated in 2004). *Natural health, natural medicine: The complete guide to wellness and self-care for optimum health.* New York: Houghton Mifflin Company.

Will, George F. (2009, June 21). Arguments for public health option don't hold water. *Houston Chronicle,* B 10.

You said: Would the USA be better off with a single-payer, government-run healthcare insurer? (2007, August 17, p. 22). *Medical Economics.* Retrieved August 25, 2009, from http://www.memag.com.

Zwart, Hub. (1993). Rationing in the Netherlands: The liberal and the communitarian perspective. *Health Care Analysis,* Vol. 1. (Zwart is a Professor of Philosophy with the Centre for Ethics, Catholic University of Nijmegen, The Netherlands).

Exhibit A – Community Forum on Healthcare Reform

Nexus Health Systems, LTD
General Staff Discussion on Healthcare Reform
December 22, 2008, 12:00 to 1:00 PM
Facilitator: Mark Tozzio, FACHE

Summary of Discussion
Our group consisted of 14 healthcare workers at the corporate business level that were both consumers and providers of health care. Our company takes care of (1) seriously ill children, (2) traumatic brain injury patients recovering over a period of 3 to 18 months, and (3) LTAC patients. This diversified group had many personal and family encounters with hospital and medical care instances – their comments listed below were reflective of local and personal experiences.

The group reviewed and discussed the sample questions provided in the Obama-Biden Participant's Guide relating to healthcare reform:

1. Briefly, from your own experience, what do you perceive is the biggest problem in the health system?
   See below
2. How do you choose a doctor or hospital? What are your sources of information? How should public policy promote quality health care providers?
   The insurance companies dictate where to go. There are not reliable sources of information about quality of providers – a national web site that is prepared by the government could be helpful.
3. Have you or your family members ever experienced difficulty paying medical bills? What do you think policy makers can do to address this problem?
   The cost of employer-based insurance is escalating. Many participants described situations of people they knew that we destroyed financially because of healthcare bills, even though they paid a lot for insurance. An affordable government sponsored plan could compete with price and services offered along side of the traditional private plans.
4. In addition to employer-based coverage, would you like the option to purchase a private plan through an insurance-exchange or a public plan like Medicare?
   YES (unanimous)
5. Do you know how much you or your employer pays for health insurance? What should an employer's role be in a reformed health care system?

The employer is at the mercy of the area insurance company charges – they should be the main source of coverage but be able to buy coverage through a government subsidized program if they wanted to.
6. Below are examples of the types of preventive services Americans should receive. Have you gotten the prevention you should have? If not, how can public policy help?
Much more funding should be channeled to prevention programs instead of "sick care" system consuming all of the money. It should not be the program of last resort – prevention should be available to all citizens.
7. How can public policy promote healthier lifestyles?
TV campaigns like the ones that were used in the election process (paid with federal dollars) would be very effective. Education in the schools is going to reach the youth and change adult habits in the long run – anti-smoking campaigns have worked well.

The group discussed at length two main questions posed by the facilitator:

1. What is most seriously wrong about the American health system from a personal standpoint?
    - We are paying more for less healthcare services
    - The present system offers a piece meal approach to care
    - The processes are inefficient compared to the technology and resources that should be available in this country
    - Getting care is very time consuming – needs to be streamlined
    - Lack of technology to maximize care – information technology is not available to make processes quick and efficient
    - Must make careful assumption based on good and reliable information to back up statements
    - Uninsured must have adequate care – this is a human right, not a privilege for those who can pay for regular insurance
    - Universal care = bad care (HMOs don't offer adequate care to the masses)
    - There is run away cost in our health system
    - Care for the poor is seriously lacking
    - Too much greed in our system makes it detrimental to the average "Joe"
    - There needs to be more patient education involved in medical care
    - Physicians need to take more time to explain problems and issues that affect health
    - Capitalistic market-based model of health care in the US is not "good" system
    - Preventive care must be a central part of the American health care system – our current "sick care" system is too expensive and inefficient

Why The United States Healthcare System Should Be A Limited Human Right For All

2. What ideas do you have that would significantly improve the current system?
   - A single payer nationalized care system is NOT the answer – maintain a private sector insurance system
   - Changes must be staged or incremental – don't wipe out the current system overnight
   - Government, insurers and employers must partner together to incorporate healthy behaviors and preventive care approaches in everyday activities (Japanese have a great system to follow)
   - Set a reasonable maximum profit level for hospitals and providers of care that allows for replacement of equipment and facilities but does not result in excessive profit-making – perhaps 6% to 8% would be appropriate range (not like the for-profits that make 15% to 35%)
   - Focus on helping people in the GAP (between poor and rich that are covered) and the underinsured – working poor
   - Illegal immigrants are taxing our healthcare system in the border states – we need a humanistic policy for dealing with these individuals that fall outside of our traditional system (some members said that we should not pay for illegal's' care and others said that we must pay – difficult situation to address)

The group reviewed and discussed the survey questions provided in the Obama-Biden Participant's Guide relating to healthcare reform:

1. What do you perceive is the biggest problem in the health system?
   Exhibit A – Community Forum on Healthcare Reform

   (5 votes)   a. Cost of health insurance
   (4 votes)   b. Cost of health care services
   (3 votes)   c. Difficulty finding health insurance due to a pre-existing condition
   (2 votes)   d. Lack of emphasis on prevention
   (1 vote)   e. Quality of health care

2. What do you think is the best way for policy makers to develop a plan to address the health system problems?

   (10 votes) a. Community meetings like these
               b. Traditional town hall meetings
   (2 votes)   c. Surveys that solicit ideas on reform
   (1 vote)   d. A White House Health Care Summit
   (1 vote)   e. Congressional hearings on C-SPAN

3. After this discussion, what additional input and information would best help you to continue to participate in this great debate?

   (3 votes)   a. More background information on problems in the health system
   (8 votes)   *b. More information on solutions for health reform*
   (3 votes)   c. More stories on how the system affects real people
   (1 vote)   d. More opportunities to discuss the issues

The group appreciated the opportunity to input at the grass roots level…but will the government and politicians really pay attention to the consumer public? This is an excellent forum and the special effort to reach out to the public is a great start for the Obama-Biden-Daschle team. Thanks!!!!!!!!!

Supplemental Bibliography for Section One

AARP Bulletin. (2006, Winter). Per capita spending on health care in the United States. Retrieved August 28, 2007, from http://www.aarp.org/bulletin/medicare/issues

AARP Bulletin. (2007, September). The number of people without health insurance is increasing. Retrieved September 27, 2007, from http://www.aarp.org/bulletin/

American Hospital Association. (2007, July 25). Health for life. *AHA.org*, Retrieved September 24, 2007, from http://www.aha.org.

Alexander, John M. (2008). Capabilities and social justice: The political philosophy of Amartya Sen and Martha Nussbaun. Burlington, VT: Ashgate Publishing Company.

American Hospital Association Policy Forum. (2005, May). *Trends Affecting Hospitals and Health Systems: TrendWatch Chartbook 2005* (Chapter 1). Archived at http://ahapolicyforum.org/ahapolicyforum/trendwatch/chartbook2005.html

American Medical Student Association. (2007, May 31). The senior boom is coming: Are primary care physicians ready? *AMSA*, Retrieved May 31, 2007, from http://www.amsa.org/programs/gpit/seniors.cfm

Andersen, Hanne, Barker, Peter and Chen, Xiang (1996). Kuhn's mature philosophy of science and cognitive psychology. *Philosophical Psychology, 09515089, 9,12p*. Retrieved February 20, 2007, from http://web.ebscohost.com.ezproxy1.lib.ou.edu/ host/detail?vid=7&hid.

Appleby, Julie. (2007, July 2). Country is watching Massachusetts insurance plan. *USA Today*, A1.

Archer, Kim. (2007, April 4). Better habits mean longer life, health official says. *Tulsa World*. Tulsa, Oklahoma, A9.

Associated Press. (2006, May 9). US gets poor grades for newborns' survival: Nation ranks near bottom among modern nations, better only than Latvia. *MSNBC*. Retrieved May 20, 2008, from http://www.msnbc.msn.com/id/12699453/.

Bacon, Perry, Jr. (2007, September 18). Clinton presents plan for universal coverage. *washingtonpost.com*, Retrieved September 18, 2007, from http://washingon post.com/wp-dyn/content/article/2007/09/17/AR2007091701026…

Baird, Macaran, MD. (2002). Comments on the commissioned report – Health and behavior: The interplay of biological, behavioral, and societal influences. *Families, Systems & Health*, Vol. 20, No. 1, 1-6.

Bello, Marisol. (2008, February 28). Goals for black America not met. *USA Today*, 1A.

Bennis, Warren, Goleman, Daniel, and O'Toole, James. (2008). *Transparency: How leaders create a culture of candor.* New York: Jossey-Bass.

Bobadilla, Jose Luis, Costello, Christine A., and Mitchell, Faith (1997). *Premature death in the new independent states.* OU Netlibrary (Chapters 1, 2, 5, 7, 9, and 12). Retrieved July 7, 2008, from http://books.nap.edu/openbook/0309057345/gifmid/220.gif

Biggerstaff Jr., Ray P. and Syre, Thomas R. (1991, winter). The Dynamics of Hospital Leadership. *Hospital Topics,* Vol. 69 (1), 36-40. Retrieved October 9, 2006 from Academic Search Elite database [EBSCOhost].

Buchanan, Joy. (2008, February 14). Medicine meets a culture gap – simple awareness can be bridge between patient and doctor. *USA Today*, 9A.

Cain, Brad. (2007, May). Coverage crisis. *HealthLeaders*, pp. 27-32.

Centers for Disease Control and Prevention. (2008). Various articles - (1) AIDS – Rumors, myths, and hoaxes. (2) Why is injecting drugs a risk for HIV? (3) Can I get HIV from anal sex? (4) Can I get HIV from vaginal sex? (5) Can I get HIV from kissing? (6) Which body fluids transmit HIV? (7) Are lesbians or other women who have sex with women at risk for HIV? *Centers for Disease Control and Prevention*, US Department of Health and Human Services. Retrieved June 24, 2008, from http://www.cdc.gov/hiv/resources/qa/...

Centers for Disease Control and Prevention. (2008). AIDS 101 Quiz. *Centers for Disease Control and Prevention*, US Department of Health and Human Services. Retrieved June 20, 2008, form http://www.hivatwork.org. delivery?vid=13&hid

Ciulla, Joanne B. (1995). Leadership ethics: Mapping the territory. *Business Ethics Quarterly*, Vol. 5, Issue 1, 5-28.

Ciulla, Joanne B. (1998, June 10). Want to choose good leaders? Consider their ethical records. *Access Work News.* Retrieved January 27, 2008), from http://infoweb.newsbank.com/iw-search/we/InfoWeb

Ciulla, Joanne B., Editor (2004). *Ethics, the heart of leadership*. Westport, CT: Praeger Publisher.

Cohen, Jon (1999). The march of paradigms. *Science, 283*, 5410, p1998, 2p, 2graphs. Retrieved February 20, 2007, from http://web.ebscohost.com.ezproxy1.lib.ou.edu/ehost/delivery?vid=13&hid

Cohen, R. A., Martinez, M. E., Free, H. L. (2008, September). *Health insurance coverage: early release of estimates from the National Health Interview Survey, January – March 2008*. Washington, DC: US Center for Disease Control and Prevention, Center for Health Statistics - National Health Insurance Survey. Retrieved May 29, 2009, from http://www.cdc.gov/nchs/data/nhis/early release/insur20080p.htm.

Colwill, Jack M. and Cultice, James M. (2003). The future supply of family physicians: Implications for rural America. *Health Affairs* (The Policy Journal of the Health Sphere), Vol. 22, No. 1, 190-198.

Covey, Stephen R. with Merrill, Rebecca. (2006). *The Speed of Trust*. New York: Simon & Schuster, Inc.

Cowell, Frank A. (1995). *Measuring inequality*. New York, NY: Prentice Hall/Harvester Wheatsheaf.

Dawkins, Richard (1989). *The selfish gene*. (2nd ed.). Oxford: Oxford University Press.

Dunn, John. (1990). Reconceiving the content and character of modern political community. In Dunn, John (Ed). *Interpreting political responsibility*. Oxford: Polity Press.

Dye, Carson F. and Garman, Andrew N. (2006). *Exceptional leadership: 16 critical competencies for healthcare executives*. Chicago, IL: Health Administration Press.

Eckersley, Richard, Dixon, Jane, and Douglas, Bob. (2001). *The social origins of health and well-being*. New York: Cambridge University Press.

Editorial. (1996, March 16). Uninsured in the USA, and still waiting. *Lancet, 347*, 9003. Retrieved July 19, 2007, from http://web.ebscohost.com.ezproxy1. lib.ou.edu/ehost/detail?...

Edwards, John. (2007, July 23). One for all: My plan is the only true universal coverage initiative in this campaign. *Modern Healthcare*, p. 22.

El Nasser, Haya. (2008, February 12). US growth spurt seen by 2050. *USA Today*, 3A.

Epstein, Helen. (2008, New Ed.). *The invisible cure: Why we are losing the fight against AIDS in Africa*. New York: Picador – Farrar, Straus and Giroux.

Evans, Daryl Paul. (1984, January). Reviewed work(s): The social transformation of American medicine. *Contemporary Sociology*, 13, 1, 11-13. Retrieved July 19, 2007, from http://links.jstor.org/sici?sici=0094-3061%28198401%2913%...

Evans, Abigail Rian. (1999). *Redeeming marketplace medicine: A theology of health care*. Cleveland, Ohio: The Pilgrim Press.

Farmer, Paul. (2003). *Pathologies of power: Health, human rights, and the new war on the poor*. Berkeley: University of California Press.

Farrelly, Colin P. (2007). *Justice, democracy and reasonable agreement*. New York: Palgrave MacMillan.

Gardner, Howard. (1995). *Leading Minds: An Anatomy of Leadership*. New York: Basic Books.

Garman, Andrew N., Butler, Peter and Brinkmeyer, Lauren. (2006, November/December). Leadership. *Journal of Healthcare Management*, Volume 51, Number 6, 360-364. Chicago: ACHE Press.

Glatthorn, Allan A. and Joyner, Randy L. (2005). *Writing the winning thesis*. Thousand Oaks, California: Corwin Press.

Globalization and Health (2007, August 11). The maladies of affluence. *The Economist*, Vol. 384, No. 8541, 49-50.

Goleman, Daniel. (1998). *Working with Emotional Intelligence*. New York: Bantam Books.

Goldstein, Myrna Chandler and Goldstein, Mark A. (2001). *Controversies in the practice of medicine*. Westport, Connecticut: Greenwood Press.

Graham, Judith. (2007, August 21). Screening for staph are now the law: State first to apply mandatory testing. *Chicagotribune.com*, Retrieved August 21, 2007, from http://www.chicagotribune.com/news/local/chicago/chi-mrsaaug21,0,3659820.story

Grazier, Kyle L. (2006). Interview with Larry Sanders, FACHE, chairman and chief executive officer, Columbus Regional Healthcare System. *Journal of Healthcare Management,* Vol. 51 (4), 212-213.

Griffith, John R. and White, Kenneth R. with Cahill, Patricia. (2003). *Thinking Forward: Six strategies for highly successful organizations.* Chicago: Health Administration Press.

Gross, David (1998, June 27). How will America stay healthy? *Lancet,* 351, 9120. Retrieved July 19, 2007, from http://web.ebscohost.com.ezproxy1.lib.ou.edu/ehost/detail?...

Hackler, Chris. (1993). Health care reform in the United States. *Health Care Analysis,* Vol. 1, 5-13.

Haeser, Jamie L. and Preston, Paul. (2005, January/February). Communication Strategies for Getting the Results You Want. *Healthcare Executive,* 16-20.

Hall, Robert T. (2000). *An introduction to healthcare organizational ethics.* New York: Oxford University Press.

Harris, Dean M. (2007, 3rd ed.). *Contemporary issues in healthcare law and ethics.* Chicago: AUPHA/HAPC.

Helman, Cecil G. (2007, 5th ed.). *Culture, Health and Illness.* United Kingdom: Hoddler Arnold.

Hollingsworth, Rogers. (1983, September). Review: Causes and consequences of the American medical system. *Reviews in American History,* 11, 3, 326-332. Retrieved July 19, 2007, from http://links.jstor.org/sici?sici=0048-7511%28198309%...

Jimenez, Ramon and Lewis, Valerae. (2007). *Culturally competent care guidebook.* American Academy of Orthopedic Surgeons, Rosemont, IL. [Free for the asking, www.aaos.org]

Jonas, Steven (1984, March). Editorial - The social transformation of American medicine. *Quarterly Review of Biology,* 59, 1, 105. Retrieved July 19, 2007, from http://www.jstor.org.ezproxy1.lib.ou.edu/view/00335770/dm994743/99p1106m/

Judson, Karen. (2001). *Medical ethics: Life and death issues.* Berkeley Heights, New Jersey: Enslow Publishers, Inc.

Jung, K and Smeeding T. (1999). Abstract - Income inequality and population health among 18 developed countries: The evidence from Luxemburg income study. *Association for Health Services Research*, Vol. 16, pp. 389-90. Retrieved on June 8, 2008, from http://gateway.nlm.nih.gov/MeetingAbstracts/ma?f=10219478.html.

Kant, Immanuel, edited and translated by Zweig, Arnulf. (1986). *Philosophical correspondence*. Chicago: The University of Chicago Press.

Kelley, Robert. (2009, October 26). Press release: Waste in the US healthcare system pegged at $700 billion. Thomson Reuters. Retrieved October 27, 2009, from http://thomsponrueters.com/content/press_room/tsh/wates_US_healthcare_system.

Khaliq, Amir A., Walston, Stephen L. and Thompson, David M. (2005, spring) [University of Oklahoma, College of Public Health]. The Impact of Hospital CEO Turnover In US Hospitals – Final Report. Prepared for the American College of Healthcare Executives (ACHE), archived at http://www.ache.org/PUBS/Research /pdf/ hospital_ceo_turnover_06.pdf

Klein, Jo-Ellyn Sakowitz. (1998, November). The Stark laws: Conquering physician conflicts of interest? *Georgetown Law Journal*, Washington, DC. Retrieved November 24, 2008, from http://findarticles.com/p/articles/mi_qa3805/ is_199811/ ai_n8819444/print?tag=art Body;c...

Kobayashi, Karen M. (2003). Do intersections of diversity matter? An exploration of the relationship between identity markers and health for mid- to later-life Canadians. *Canadian Ethnic Studies*, (Calgary), Vol. 35, Issue 3, 85.

Kouzes, James M. and Posner, Barry Z. (2006). *A Leader's Legacy*. San Francisco: Jossey-Bass.

Kozlowski, Kim, et al. (2004, December 19). Suburbs' black babies die at higher rates: The disparity is especially glaring in Oakland County, where death is four times more likely. *The Detroit News*. Retrieved May 20, 2008, from http://detnews.com/2004/specialreport/ 0412/20/A01-36533.htm.

Kucinich, Dennis. (2007, September 3). Get rid of the for-profits. *Modern Healthcare*, p. 40.

Levine, Susan. (2008, January 31, B01). District lacking in access to care: 1 in5 has no medical provider, Rand Report says. *Washingtonpost.com*. Retrieved February 1, 2008, from http://www.washingtonpost.com/wp-dyn/content/article/2008/01/30/ AR2008013001228_pf...

Lewis, O. (1975). *Five families; Mexican case studies in the culture of poverty.* New York: Basic Books.

Lewis, Shawn D., et al. (2004, December 20). Michigan steps up effort to curb baby deaths: Experts say a focus on why black infants are more likely to die will help find answers. *The Detroit News.* Retrieved May 20, 2008, from http://detnews.com/2004/specialreport/0412/20/A01-37563.htm.

Locke, Don C. (1998, 2nd Edition). *Increasing multicultural understanding.* Thousand Oaks, California: Sage Publications.

Lofland, John, Lofland, Lyn, Anderson, Leon, and Snow, David. (2006). *Analyzing social settings.* Belmont, CA: Wadsworth.

Lollar, Donald J. and Crews, John E. (January 2003). Redefining the role of public health in disability. *Annual Review of Public Health*, Vol. 24, 195-208. Retrieved February 4, 2008, from http://arjournals.annualreviews.org.ezproxy1.lib.ou.edu/doi/full/10.1146...

Lorentzen, Amy. (2007, September 2). Edwards backs mandatory preventive care. *Yahoo!News*, Retrieved September 19, 2007, from http://news,yahoo.com/s/ap/20070903/ap_on_el_pr/edwards&printer...

McAdams, Lisa. (2006, May 1). Russia readies radical health care reform. *News VOA.com.* Retrieved July19, 2008, from http://www.voanews.com/english/archive/2006-05/2006-05-01-voa31.cfm?renderfoprint=...

McAdoo, Harriette Pipes. (1999, 2nd Ed.). *Family ethnicity: Strength in diversity.* Thousand Oaks, California: SAGE Publications, Inc.

Mechanic, David. (1966, Winter). The sociology of medicine: Viewpoints and perspectives. *Journal of Health and Human Behavior*, Vol. 7, No. 4, 237-248.

MedlinePlus. (2008). AIDS. *National Library of Medicine*, US Gov. (7 pages). Retrieved June 24, 2008, from http://www.nlm.nih.gov/medlineplus/aids.html.

MedlinePlus. (2008, December 22). By the numbers: An annual resource guide filled with the numbers, rankings and financial figures that shape healthcare –. *Modern Healthcare*, Supplement 2008-2009 Edition.

Mill, John Stuart. (2005, rev. ed.). *Utilitarianism*. New York: Barnes & Noble, Inc.

Morris, Tom. (1999). *Philosophy for dummies*. New York: Wiley Publishing.

Munro, Barbara H. (1997). *Statistical methods for health care research*. New York: Lippincott-Raven Publishers.

National Center for Health Statistics. (2007). Fast stats A to Z - Deaths / Mortality. *Centers for Disease Control*. Retrieved August 30, 2007, from http://www.cdc.gov/nchs/fastats/deaths.htm

Nelson, William A. (2005, July/August). An Organizational Ethics Decision-Making Process. *Healthcare Executive*, 8-14.

Nichols, Len M. (2007). *A sustainable health system for all Americans,* Washington, DC: New America Foundation.

Nightingale, Carl H. (2008, February). Before race mattered: Geographies of the color line in Colonial Madras and New York. *American Historical Review*, pp.48-71.

Obama, Barack. (2007, July 29). My cure for an ailing system. *Modern Healthcare*, p. 22.

Pear, Robert. (2008, January 23). At house party on health care, the diagnosis is it's broken. *Nytimes.com*. Retrieved on December 23, 2008, from http://www.nytimes.com/2008/12/23/health/23health.html?_r=1&em=&page wanted=print.

Peterson, Alan. (2003). Review - Betrayal of trust: The collapse of global public health. *Sociology of Health & Illness*, Vol. 25, 7, pp. 889-890.

Pollmar, Ph.D., Terry, Brandt, Jr., MD, Ph.D., Edward and Baird, MD, MS, Macaran (2002, March-April). Summary of an Institute of Medicine report - Health and behavior: The interplay of biological, behavioral, and societal influences. *American Journal of Health Promotion*, Vol. 16. No. 4, 206-219.

Polsby, Nelson (1989). Social science and scientific change: A note on Thomas S. Kuhn's contribution [Electronic version]. *Political Science, 1, 199-210*

Porter, Michael E. and Teisberg, Elizabeth O. (2006). *Redefining health care: Creating value-based competition on results.* Boston, Massachusetts: Harvard Business School Press.

Rashford, Marleise. (2007, January-March). A universal healthcare system: Is it right for the United States? [Electronic version]. *Nursing Forum, 42, 1, 3-11.*

Reid, T.R. ((2009). *The healing of America: A global quest for better, cheaper, and fairer health care.* New York: Penguin Press.

Rescher, Nicholas. (2000). *Kant and the reach of reason: Studies in Kant's theory of rational systemization.* Cambridge, Massachusetts: Cambridge University Press.

Reynolds, Issable. (2007, September 18). Aging Japan struggles to rein in health costs. *Yahoo!News,* Retrieved September 19, 2007, from http://news,yahoo.com/s/nm/20070919/lf_nm/japan_ageing_health_dc

Rhodes, Rosamond, Battin, Margaret P., and Silvers, Anita. (Eds.). (2002). *Medicine and social justice.* New York: Oxford University Press.

Richardson, Bill, Governor. (2007, August 27). Coverage for all, at the right price. *Modern Healthcare,* p. 44.

Roberts, Laura Weiss, Johnson, Mark E., Brems, Christiane, and Warner, Teddy. (2007, Fall). Ethical disparities: Challenges encountered by multidisciplinary providers in fulfilling ethical standards in the care of rural and minority people. *The Journal of Rural Health,* Vol. 23, Supplemental Issue, 89-97.

Robinson, Mary, Novelli, William, Pearson, Clarence, and Norris, Laurie. (2007). Global health and global aging. New York: Jossey-Bass.

Rost, Joseph C. (1995). Leadership: A discussion about ethics. *Business Ethics Quarterly,* Vol. 5, Issue 1, 129-142.

Ryan, Maura A. (2006, October). The politics of risk: A human rights paradigm for children's environmental health research. Environment Health Perspectives, Vol. 114 [full version available free]. Retrieved May 20, 2008, from http://www.ehponline.org/docs/2006/9002/abstract.html.

Sanders, Cindy. (2008, June). Tennessee Institute for Public Health releases county health rankings. *Nashville Medical News*, p. 1 and 20.

Scruton, Roger. (2005, rev. ed.). *Philosophy: Principles and problems*. New York: Continuum.

Semmes, Clovis E. (1996). *Racism, health, and post-industrialism: A theory of African-American health*. Westport, Connecticut: Praeger Publishers.

Shope, Robert E. (2001, January 12). Things fall apart. *Science's Compass*. Vol. 291, p. 258.

Small, Mario Luis. (2007, June). Racial differences in networks: Do neighborhood conditions matter? *Social Science Quarterly*, Vol. 88, No. 2, pp. 320-343.

Tozzio, Mark. (2008, March 27). Presentation to the board of directors of Greater Southeast Community Hospital – Market Assessment, *Unpublished Paper, HPPD, Inc.*

Tozzio, Mark. (2004, January - February). Critical nature of the J-1 Visa Waiver Program for foreign medical graduates, [selected as an ACHE Best Case Report for the Year (2002)], *Journal of Healthcare Management*, volume 49, No.1, pp. 61-69.

Tozzio, Mark. (2007, July 23). Critique - The future US healthcare system: Who will care for the poor and uninsured? By Altman, S.H., Reinhardt, U.E., and Shields, A. E. (Ed.), 1998. *Unpublished Paper.*

Tozzio, Mark. (2007, July 30). Critique – The social transformation of American medicine. By Paul Starr, 1982. *Unpublished Paper.*

Tozzio, Mark. (2008, March 27). Presentation to the board of directors of Greater Southeast Community Hospital – Healthcare market assessment, *Unpublished Paper, HPPD, Inc.*

Ubel, Peter A. (2000). *Pricing life – Why it's time for health care rationing*. Cambridge, Massachusetts: The MIT Press.

Wagner, Natalie. (2006, April 17). Health care cost comparison of the United States and Canada. *OLR Research Report* (2006-R-0289). Retrieved November 30, 2008, from http://www.caga.ct.gov/2006/rpt/2006-R-0289.htm.

Weil, Andrew. (2004). *Health and healing: The philosophy of integrative medicine and optimum health*. New York: Houghton Mifflin Company.

Wilkinson, Richard G. (1997, June 14). Commentary: Income inequality summarizes the health burden of individual relative deprivation. *BMJ*, 314, 1724. Retrieved June 8, 2008, from http://www.bmj.com/cgi/content/full/314/7096/1727.

World Health Organization. (2008). *Primary health care now more than ever.* The World Health Organization Report 2008. Retrieved November 29, 2008, from https://www. who.int/whr/2008/whr08_en.pdf

SECTION TWO (2010 – 2017)

WHY THE UNITED STATES HEALTHCARE SYSTEM *SHOULD* BE A LIMITED HUMAN RIGHT FOR ALL

MARK G. TOZZIO, M-IHHS, FACHE

SECTION TWO (2010-2017)

Foreword for Section Two (2010-2017)

Since the signing of the Affordable Care Act (ACA) into law by President Barack Obama March 23, 2010, a lot of changes have occurred in the United States healthcare system. Most are positive and some need fixing badly. On the whole, there seems to be a change in attitude among health leaders and providers at all levels – most have come to accept the principle goals of ObamaCare: "The right care for every patient, every time." The push to improve healthcare quality and outcomes using measurable targets and integrated health information systems has resulted in better care and more cost effective delivery to a broader segment of Americans.

Universal Health Insurance Coverage has added some 25 million persons through the individual / employer mandates and Marketplaces in all states. Medicaid eligibility has expanded family coverage for lower income families. New incentive-based payment options are rewarding providers for meeting and exceeding CMS and commercial insurers' quality targets and controlling the rapid rise in the cost of healthcare – in 2016 it reached $3.2 trillion, or about 18% of the national Gross Domestic Product (GDP). Section 2 (2010-2017) documents key aspects of the impact of the ACA on quality and cost indicators in the United States. In the *e-book* version, there are many "live" URL links in the footnotes that provide additional valuable information to those who are interested.

A new Republican Administration has vowed to ***"repeal and replace"*** the ACA. Section Two expands on the findings of Section One (2009). Mark's offers recommendations as to how regulators might alternatively ***"revise and enhance"*** on the progress made over the ACA implementation period. The conclusions in Section Two reaffirm Mark's original conviction that: "A healthier population significantly increases the chances of being a highly productive nation, from an economic standpoint. If one accepts this foundational premise, isn't there a significant advantage for United States to vigorously pursue having a healthier population?"

Mark's **current** book provides readers with factual information about progress made in the health delivery system since 2010. He also identifies ways to enhance the law rather than *"throw the baby out with the bath water,"* and strengthen the weaker links of the ACA. You will

Mark G. Tozzio, M-IHHS, FACHE

appreciate the new material included in Section Two from his interdisciplinary point of view — then formulate your own ideas and opinions regarding the next steps the nation should embark on from 2017 and beyond.

David Woodrum, FACHE

Table of Contents for Section Two (2010-2017)

	Foreword for Section Two (2010-2017)	255
	Table of Contents for Section Two (2010-2017)	257
	List of Graphs and Tables	259
	List of Figures	261
	Acknowledgements for Section Two (2010-2017)	263
One	Universal Healthcare Becomes a Reality	267
	1.1 -- President Barack Obama Signs PPACA into Law	267
	1.2 -- The ACA is Really About Insurance Reform	269
	1.3 -- Americans both Love and Loathe the ACA	277
	1.4 -- Legal Challenges to the ACA Reach the US Supreme Court	282
Two	Health Insurance Reform	290
	2.1 – Key Milestones of the ACA: 2010 to 2016	290
	2.2 -- Healthcare Industry Embraces ACA Changes	298
	2.3 -- Transitioning from Volume to Value-Based Care	302
	2.4 -- ACOs, Bundled Payments, Systems Consolidations, Population Health Management - Today's Collaborative Care Movement	308
Three	Weathering of the Political Storm	320
	3.1 -- The "Unprecedented" Presidential Election of 2016	320
	3.2 -- The Proverbial Monetary Coin of America's Healthcare System Has Two Distinct Sides to the Argument	326
	3.3 -- Do Politics Trump Logic?	337
Four	Going Forward in a New Post-ObamaCare Era	342
	4.1 -- Revisiting Why the United States Healthcare System Should be a Limited Human Right for All in 2017 and Beyond	342
	4.2 -- Conclusions and Recommendations	345

Appendix A (2017) 353
Appendix B (2017) 355
Appendix C (2017) 359
Supplemental Resources for Section Two (2010-2017). 367

List of Graphs and Tables

GRAPHS

Graph 1 – Types of Networks on Marketplaces 271
Graph 2 – Percent Approval and Disapproval of the 2010 ACA 279
Graph 3 – Quarterly Uninsured Rate Estimates for Non-Elderly Wellbeing Index 294
Graph 4 – Quarterly Uninsured Rate Estimates for Non-Elderly by Race and Ethnicity 295
Graph 5 – Marketplace Enrollment by Income - Expansion v Non-Expansion States. 295
Graph 6 – Medicaid Enrollment Through ACA Expansion 296
Graph 7 – Aggregate Hospital Margins: 1994-2014 301
Graph 8 a, b, c, and d - ACO Activity from 2011 to 2016 317
Graph 9 – Ratio of Primary Working-Age Americans to Those 65 and Older 336
Graph 10 – Larry Sobal's "Value" Tipping Point 348

TABLES

Table 1 – ACA Essential Health Benefits Categories 270
Table 2 – ACA's Most Popular Provisions 273
Table 3 – Evaluation of Major Elements of ACA Since 2013 275
Table 4 – Profitability of For-Profit Insurance Companies: 9 Months in 2010 300
Table 5 – CMS Parts A and B Shared Risk Arrangement Levels 314
Table 6 – 2017 Push in the US Congress to Address Changes to PPACA 333
Table 7 – Tozzio's [original] Prescription for Healthcare Reform: 2009 346
Table 8 – Tozzio's Updated Prescription for Healthcare Reform: 2017 349
Table 9 – Trend of US Healthcare Expenditures: 2006 to 2014 351

List of Figures

FIGURES

Figure 1 – Percent of Individuals in US Without Insurance 274
Figure 2 – Political Party Support of ACA Elements 281
Figure 3 – Summary of Supreme Court Ruling on NFIB v Sebelius 283
Figure 4 – Summary of Supreme Court Ruling on King v Burwell. 284
Figure 5 – Map of America's Health Rankings Composite Measures: 2012-2015 288
Figure 6 – CMS ACA Benefits Wheel 293
Figure 7 – CMS ACA Core Strategies and Goals: 2013-2017. 304
Figure 8 – Progression of Payment Arrangement Risk Models. 309

Acknowledgements for Section Two (2010-2017)

I am deeply appreciative of the time and counsel from my colleagues David Woodrum, Rich Miller, Edwin Hanson, Joseph Philipp, and Dr. Delroy Jefferson during the preparation of Section 2 of my book about healthcare reform in the United States. Their contributions have made the topics discussed more relevant and focused; and insured that I provided interesting and objective information to the readers of **Why the United States Healthcare System Should Be A Limited Human Right For All – Sections One and Two 2009-2017.**

However, the comments and contents this book are my responsibility alone, and do not reflect the beliefs, opinions, or comments of reviewers or editors referenced in these Acknowledgements.

Once again I am grateful to my wife Darlina for her patience and love, and the support of our daughter Aungela Spurlock and her family, during the latest update of my book. I also acknowledge the special contributions of Carolla Kosel to this project. Carolla helped with the technical edits to the text prior to its publication – it is definitely a better book because of her excellent writing skills and talent.

I could not have succeeded in this endeavor without the dedication of these and many other individuals.

Thanks again to all!

Mark Tozzio

Why the United States Healthcare System *Should* Be A Limited Human Right for All
Section Two (2010-2017)

One

UNIVERSAL HEALTHCARE BECOMES A REALITY

1.1 -- President Barack Obama Signs PPACA into Law

"Today, after almost a century of trying, today, after over a year of debate, today, after all the votes have been tallied, health insurance reform becomes law in the United States of America," Obama said to a standing ovation...

"It's easy to succumb to the sense of cynicism about what's possible in this country. But today, we are affirming that essential truth, a truth every generation is called to rediscover for itself: That we are not a nation that scales back its aspirations. We are not a nation that falls prey to doubt or mistrust," the president added. "We are a nation that faces its challenges and accepts its responsibilities..."

As Biden finished his remarks and shook Obama's hand, he was heard on the microphone whispering, "This is a big f-ing deal." White House Press Secretary Robert Gibbs tweeted soon afterward, "And yes Mr. Vice President, you're right..."

HUMA KHAN, MARCH 23, 2010, ABC NEWS.

Since my original "thesis" published in November 2009, **Why The United States Healthcare System Should Be A Limited Human Right For All**,[83] The *Patient Protection and Accountable Care Act*, also called *ObamaCare*, became a reality in the United States on March

---

[83] Mark Tozzio, (November 2009), *Why the United States Healthcare System Should Be A Limited Human Right for All*, Printed by *CreateSpace*, An Amazon.com Company (paperback and e-book versions).

23, 2010. This accomplishment ushered in **Universal Health Insurance Coverage** after 50 years of political wrangling at the local, state and federal levels of government. Although the *Patient Protection and Affordable Care Act of 2010* (P.L. 111-148 approved by the 111th Congress of the United States, commonly known as PPACA or ACA for short, https://www.gpo.gov/fdsys/pkg/PLAW-111publ148/pdf/PLAW-111publ148.pdf) is far from perfect, this historical law promised to radically change the health insurance approach from fee-for-service to outcomes-based payment incentives and dramatically improve access to healthcare services. The ACA's complexity is outlined in nearly 2,000 pages of legislation which generated 33,000 pages of regulations approximately 8 months after the ACA was signed into law. [See *https://**www.healthcare.gov*** for details on the implementation of this legislation].

ObamaCare is one of the most controversial federal law of all time to say the least. The US Congressional House of Representatives passed the Senate version of the ACA bill by a slim margin of 219-212 on March 21, 2010 – 178 Republicans and 34 Democrats voting against the legislation. President Obama signed the ACA into law on March 23rd. Since that momentous day, the GOP (Republican Party) introduced federal legislation to *repeal all or part* of the ACA at least *63 times* through "Groundhog Day," February 2016, with the President blocking the move.[84]

Enrollment in the ACA *Marketplace* health insurance plans (originally called *Exchanges*) began its turbulent process early October 2013. The **Healthcare.gov** ACA website experienced serious operational challenges with the online systems that managed the insurance information and sign-up mechanism of millions of Americans in the federal and state subsidized private insurance plans that were qualified by the US Health and Human Services Department (HHS). By the end of the second enrollment period of 2014, *Healthcare.gov* performed more effectively and the numbers of subscribers reached approximately 8 million individuals according to the *Kaiser Family Foundation* reducing the uninsured population.[85]

Nationally, the sentiment over *ObamaCare* has remained about half of Americans favoring the ACA, and the other half against. The mandate for universal health insurance coverage for all Americans through traditional commercial insurance plans, and the so called federal / state *Marketplace Exchanges* programs, and government programs such as Medicaid and Medicare has expanded coverage to about 25 million citizens during the past six years of implementation (who previously could not afford health insurance).[86] The journey toward universal health insurance coverage has been a struggle, however, the lower income families and "working poor" have gained access to *limited* healthcare services through individual health insurance tax credit to subsidize insurance premiums. The proposed "government option" (either expanding Medicare to Americans under 65 years old or creating a government-sponsored health plan

---

[84] See https://thinkprogress.org/gop-lawmakers-vote-to-repeal-obamacare-again-on-groundhog-day-6f0c931a8549#.8vbd199kd
[85] See http://kff.org/health-reform/issue-brief/assessing-aca-marketplace-enrollment
[86] See http://kff.org/health-reform/poll-finding/kaiser-health-policy-news-index-december-2014/

similar to Medicare, Medicare or government employee coverage for individuals of all ages) was not made part of the 2010 healthcare reform legislation.

While the overall cost of healthcare in the United States has steadily to climbed, reaching $3.2 trillion in 2016 (up from $2.5 trillion in 2009, close to 18% of the Gross Domestic Product), the rate of annual growth of healthcare spending has declined from and average of more than 10% to under 6.5%, the lowest rate since the early 1960s. Healthcare providers have come to embrace parts of the ACA, particularly provisions that reduce the uninsured patient population – resulting in a reduction in "bad debt and uncompensated care" across the country's health systems. In my opinion, the ACA has finally moved Americans closer to accepting the concept that "the United States Healthcare System Should be a *Limited* Human Right for All."[87]

With the election of Donald Trump November 8, 2016 as the 45th President of the United States, the fate of *universal healthcare* insurance coverage[1] is once again up in the air. Trump has promised to "repeal and replace" *ObamaCare* with a *Republican version* of health insurance legislation within the first 100 days of his new Republican administration. This political initiative reopens the long-standing argument: **Is healthcare a right or a privilege in America?** Section Two re-examines this crucial and ethical subject.

1.2 -- The ACA is Really About Insurance Reform

Most Americans believe that the main intent of enacting the ACA was about reforming the health delivery systems, incenting value-based high-quality care, and promoting universal healthcare for all. *This is not necessarily true.* The ACA is *really* about **health insurance reform** and regulation of commercial health insurance companies that dominate health coverage for millions of Americans. Health insurance coverage *conditions of participation* and ever-increasing premiums have prevented nearly **52 million individuals** (excluding those under 65 years of age and the most impoverished) from accessing the health systems' resources in the richest country in the world.[88] This is why the legislation is titled: **Affordable Care Act of 2010**. The ACA did not strongly address quality and cost initiatives, however HHS did have the latitude to develop these types of strategic goals in the guidelines that followed over the next six years of implementation.

ACA Marketplaces were designed to attract qualified health insurance plans offering (1) "essential health benefits (EHB)," (2) competitive premium prices for different levels of coverage – *Bronze, Silver, Gold, and Platinum* (the "**Metals**" plans), (3) non-discriminatory enrollment guidelines (including **no** preexisting illnesses exclusions), (4) broader choice, and (5) federal tax-credit subsidies based on family income / size ranges (only available through the Marketplace). EHBs are categorized as follows:[89]

---

[87] Mark Tozzio, 2009, *Why the United States Healthcare System Should Be A Limited Human Right For All,* Printed by *CreateSpace*, An Amazon.com Company (paperback and e-book versions).
[88] https://obamawhitehouse.archives.gov/blog/2010/09/16/affordable-care-act-helps-america-s-uninsured
[89] http://www.healthpocket.com

Table 1 – ACA Essential Health Benefits Categories

ACA Essential Health Benefit Categories for Marketplace Insurance Plans

Category	Principal Attributes
Ambulatory Coverage	Primary care visit, specialty visit, outpatient facility, and physician follow-ups
Emergency Care Coverage	Emergency room, emergency transport, and urgent care
Hospitalization Coverage	Hospitalization, home care, hospital facility, and hospital physician
Maternity Care Coverage	Prenatal care and outpatient services
Mental Health Coverage	In and outpatient mental health services
Substance Abuse Coverage	In and outpatient substance abuse services
Prescription Drug Coverage	Generic drugs, brand name drugs, non-preferred brand drugs, and specialty drugs
Pediatric Coverage	Children's dental check-up and children eye care
Preventative Coverage	Preventive care services Lab, Diagnostic, Imaging Services
Optional Benefits	Can be offered for additional cost

Note: In 2014, less than 2% of existing health plans in the commercial insurance market were found to offer all of the EHBs; on average, 76% of health plans qualified by the ACA Marketplaces provided EHBs.[90]

In many cases, plans with lower insurance premiums and higher deductibles means less choice of provide networks. In the August 19, 2013 issue of *Modern Healthcare*, M. P. McQueen wrote about "tight networks" prevalent with Marketplace insurance plans. He states: "Insurers including Aetna and Health Net say narrower networks [of providers], made up of hospitals and physicians selected using cost and patient-outcomes criteria, are necessary to keep their exchange plan premiums affordable while still meeting the requirements of the Patient Protection and Affordable Care Act."[91]

---

[90] Healthpocket Infostat, March 7, 2013, see https://www.healthpocket.com/healthcare-research/infostat/few-existing-health-plans-meet-new-aca-essential-health-benefit-standards#.WIUVg5L21mA
[91] *Modern Healthcare*, August 19, 2013, p. 8.

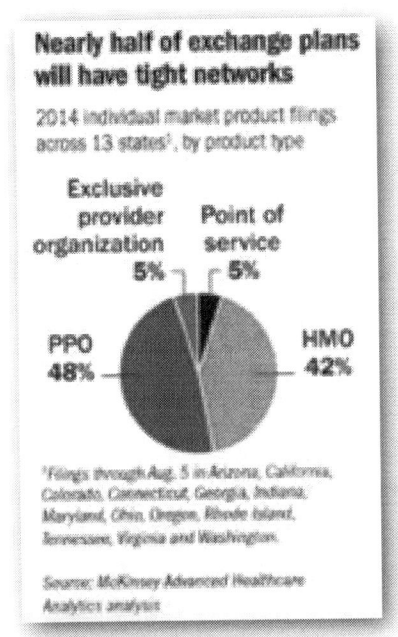

Graph 1 – Types of Networks on Marketplaces

In order for the ACA program to work economically, **all** Americans have to participate in the health insurance pool, regardless of health status and age (thus, universal coverage requirement). For healthy young individuals this *coverage mandate* is a contentious imposition. However, if the entire population (healthy, chronically ill, sick, disabled, and aging cohorts) consume limited healthcare resources without expanding the revenue base of health insurers, the ACA requirements will result in an unfair economic burden for insurance companies and will drive up premiums sky high for enrollees.

The major elements of the ACA intended to improve consumer benefits according **Healthcare.gov**, encompass the following summary:[92]

Improving Quality and Lowering Health Care Costs through Insurance Reform
o   Free preventive care services
o   Prescription discounts for seniors
o   Protection against health care fraud
o   Small Business Tax Credits

New Consumer Protections
o   Pre-existing conditions
o   Consumer assistance

---

[92] Adapted from information published by HHS, see https://www.hhs.gov/healthcare/facts-and-features/key-features-of-aca/benefits-of-the-affordable-care-act-for-americans/index.html

Access to Health Care
- Creation of Health Insurance Marketplaces (run by states, federal government or combination)
- Sliding scale for individual / family Income Tax Credits to help defray the cost of insurance premiums (only those purchasing health insurance on Marketplaces are eligible)

Benefits for Women
- Providing expanded insurance options
- Covering preventive services
- Lowering costs
- Insurers can no longer charge higher insurance premiums to women than their male counterparts for similar benefits

Young Adult Coverage
- Coverage available to children up to age 26 on parents' insurance policies

Strengthening Medicare Protection
- Yearly wellness visits
- Many free preventive services for some seniors with Medicare

Expanding Medicaid Coverage
- Funding to states for expansion of low income families

Holding Insurance Companies Accountable
- Insurers must justify any premium increase of 10% or more before the rates can take effect
- Enforcing a minimum medical loss ratio (MLR) requiring 80 to 85% investment of health premiums for healthcare to subscribers

In a national poll administered by the *Kaiser Family Foundation* in March 2013, the top four most favorable (popular) benefits flowing from the implementation of the ACA were: (1) tax credits for small businesses and individual / family subscribers, (2) drug / medicine cost assistance, (3) Marketplaces to buy insurance, and (4) extension of dependent coverage to age 26.[93] The chart below details the percentage of persons surveyed that were *in favor* of benefits offered by the ACA, and those who were actually *aware* of the new benefits.

---

[93] Kaiser Family Foundation Health Tracking Pool, conducted March 5-10, 2013, see http://ObamaCarefacts.com/benefitsofObamaCare/

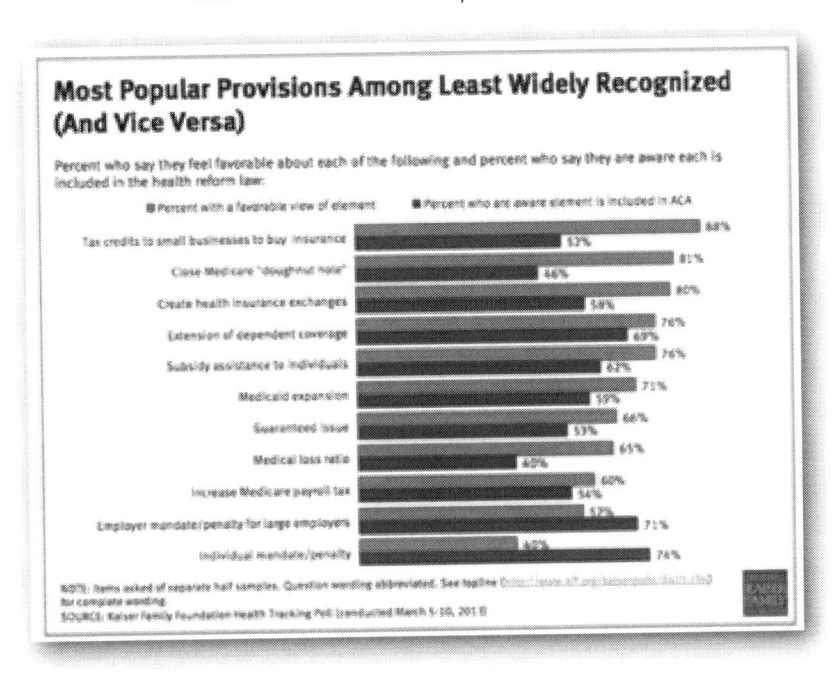

Table 2 – ACA's Most Popular Provisions

As noted, Congress chose to subsidize the purchase of health insurance through Marketplaces via a sliding scale Federal Income Tax Credit system managed by the IRS. The credits are awarded to Marketplace subscribers with family incomes up to 400% of the federal poverty level (FFPL). Families with incomes above 400% can purchase health insurance through the Marketplaces but do not receive federal assistance with the premiums. Consumer education was a high priority for the Obama Administration to explain and promote the benefits of ACA's Marketplaces. Eligibility for state *Medicaid* coverage was extended from 100% to 133% of the FFPL to significantly reduce the number of lower income uninsured. In 2013, eligibility criteria for federal tax assistance to pay health insurance premiums purchased through the Marketplaces ranged from an annual family income of $11,490 (family with one person) to $110,280 (family with 5 or more persons). Data from Health and Human Services [Department] "show only 52% [of subscribers] knew they were eligible for aid."[94]

The IRS manages tax subsidies paid directly to approved commercial companies insuring Marketplace subscribers during the calendar year using multiple federal data sources and projected income figures furnished by subscribers. The agency reconciles the total amount paid on behalf of subscribers at the end of the tax year. Guides were published by HHS to help subscribers evaluate the "Best Value" of insurers offered on the Marketplaces. Persons / families that do not purchase *any* health insurance coverage are subject to an annual income tax penalty or fine determined by the ACA's individual mandate guidelines.

---

[94] Jayne O'Donnell, October 15, 2016, "About 2.5 million miss out on ObamaCare tax credits," *USA Today*, p. 3A.

The *Journal of American Medical Association* (JAMA) reported in August 2016 that ObamaCare substantially impacted access to health insurance since it was signed into law March 2010. The chart below shows that the uninsured rate in the United States dropped from 16.0% (49 million) in 2010 to an all time low of 9.1% (29 million) in 2015 of Americans.[95]

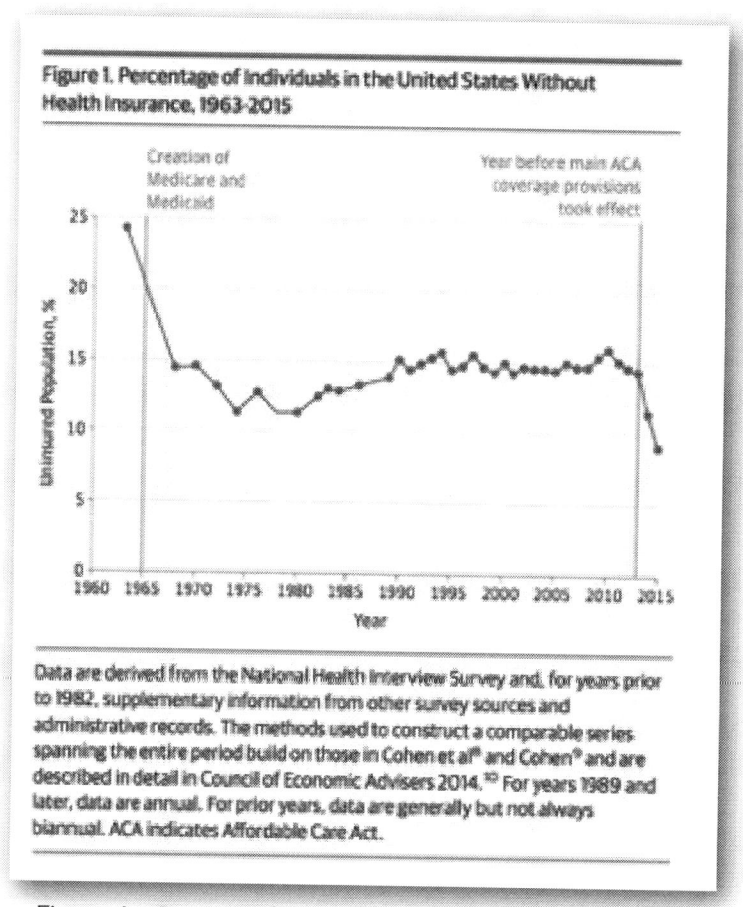

Figure 1 – Percent of Individuals in US Without Insurance

As discussed in Chapter 3.3 below, financial incentives to create alternative healthcare payment methodologies by CMS and commercial insurers were also stimulated by the ACA. This approach fostered a connection between providers' better quality of care, cost containment, and more affordable services with the health insurance reform legislation. The formation of *Accountable Care Organizations*, *Population Health Management* programs, *shared savings arrangements, etc.* between providers and payers has lead to enhanced efforts regarding care

---

95 Barack Obama, JD, ACA Special Report, **JAMA**, August 2, 2016, Volume 316, Number 5, page 526, see http://jama-network.com/journals/jama/fullarticle/2533698

and quality systems for the ultimate benefit of consumers. It is fair to say that by 2016, providers in the United States widely *embraced* the transition from insurance payments based on volume to a "value-based" reimbursement system thanks to the ACA.

Before moving to Section 1.3, I want to share with you a *scorecard* I developed to measure the effectiveness of major ACA elements in the initiatives since 2013. This is *my perception* and I encourage readers to offer your own evaluation of these key elements of the ACA in the third column of the tool present below:

Table 3 – Evaluation of Major Elements of ACA Since 2013

Evaluation of Major Elements of the ACA Initiatives Since 2013

Key Elements	Percent Success – 0>100 (Tozzio's Score)
Incenting value-based high-quality care	40% - CMS and some large insurance companies have promoted ACOs, Bundled Payments, etc.
Promoting universal healthcare	**50% - Still 20 million uninsured in US**
Marketplaces were designed to attract qualified health insurance plans	25% - Insurers are dropping out of Marketplaces; some states have only one plan to choose from
Essential health benefits (EHB)	**40% - Compared to 2 percent of insurers offering these types of benefits prior to the ACA**
Competitive premium prices	30% - Affordable policy deductibles and co-insurances are way too high
Non-discriminatory enrollment guidelines	**80% - Pre-existing and lifetime limits of coverage are enforced**
Broader coverage choices	35% - Cost of "Metals" going up too much for Platinum and Gold options
Federal tax-credit subsidies	**85% - Since affirmation by the Supreme Court, subsidies are secure and beneficial to subscribers**
Alternatives for "tight networks" to deal with price control	40% - Cheaper plans have very limited choice of providers

All Americans have to participate in the health insurance pool	**90% - Most Americans are reluctantly buying insurance instead of paying fines**
Improving Quality and Lowering Health Care Costs	*25% - The ACA is insurance reform at this point; limited incentives for meaningful value-based reimbursement*
New Consumer Protections	**70% - CMS is going after violators**
Access to Health Care	*80% - Access has improved, yet the cost remains a serious problem*
Benefits for Women	**75% - Women has more leverage to demand specialized care**
Parental policy coverage available to children up to age 26	*95% - This is a major attraction to young adults that typically do not buy health insurance*
Many new free preventive services	**90% - Critical to improve health status and reduce unnecessary utilization**
Expanding Medicaid Coverage	*70% - Great for the states that are participating – several Republican Governors have refused to take federal money to expand coverage*
Holding Insurance Companies Accountable	**40% - Accountable and collaborative care arrangements are spreading and moving away from pure fee-for-service reimbursement**
Enforcing a minimum medical loss ratio (MLR)	*75% - Various large insurance companies have been forced to refund subscribers (more prevalent in early years of ACA)*
IRS manages tax subsidies	**95% - Complicated but working well for Marketplace subscribers**
ObamaCare substantially impacted access to health insurance	*95% - Huge changes in insurance company practices compared to pre-ACA (EHB and discrimination)*

Financial incentives to create alternative healthcare payment methodologies by CMS	**65% - Providers are embracing value-based compensation and taking advantage of EHR system subsidized by the ACA in early years**
Other (a) Public Option Insurance for <65 population	0% - As system run by the government similar to the Federal Employees Benefit Program and Medicare should be adapted for < 65 Marketplace subscribers as viable option to private for-profit insurers
Other (b) Healthcare as Human Right	**40% - The debate is still alive and well especially with the new Republican-lead Administration**
Other (c) COOP non-profit insurers with federal loan guarantees (CMS / CCIO)	20% - This was a disaster thanks to the budget cuts and Sequestration by Congress (could have been a valid non-profit insurer option of Marketplaces to stimulate competition and lower policy prices)

1.3 -- Americans both Love and Loathe the ACA

"More Americans negative than positive about ACA."

Art Swift, Gallup, September 8, 2016.

The nation is divided on the merits of the ACA for years before President Barack Obama signed the legislation into law in 2010.[96] Perhaps supporters knew that it was imperative to *fast track* the implementation of the ACA's incremental transformation steps in order for Americans to *experience* its benefits early on. Accessing and navigating the Marketplace health plans was a disaster on the first *open enrollment period* in October 2013. The government website – **Healthcare.gov** – crashed at the start of enrollment causing embarrassment to HHS officials and the President. Although the problems were eventually resolved, public perception was seriously damaged and the confidence

---

[96] The debate about whether health insurances is a human right or privilege has been raging for nearly a half century… with universal health coverage and subsidized coverage being the "party line" focus of these discussions.

of subscribers dwindled to a record low. This rocky launch, or the *failure to launch* ObamaCare successfully, gave opponents (particularly Republican politicians at all levels) plenty of fodder to assert that the government healthcare reform program was a total failure and should be scrapped.

However, the second enrollment period in 2014 went much smoother, and by the end of 2015 enrollment close to 17.7 million Americans had secured "affordable" ACA healthcare insurance through the individual-market policies.[97] Many of these individuals had previously been part of the growing uninsured / uninsured population in the US who gained *essential health benefits (US Federal Register, Vol 78, No. 37, published February 25, 2013)*[98] required of all insurers participating in the online Marketplace shopping sites.[99] [100] According to testimony by Edmund Haislmaier before the US House of Representatives' Committee on the Budget, January 24, 2017, [CMS] reported "that subsidized enrollees accounted for about 45 percent of the total individual market, with about 10 million people enrolled in unsubsidized individual-market coverage."[101] Haislmaier concluded his remarks by stating:

In general, enrollment data indicate that the implementation of the ACA appears to have had three effects on health insurance coverage: (1) a substantial increase in individual-market enrollment; (2) an offsetting decline in fully insured employer-group plan enrollment; and (3) a significant increase in Medicaid enrollment in states that adopted the ACA Medicaid expansion.

In an article authored by Elizabeth Fender,[102] December 13, 2016, in *The Daily Signal,* discussed the historical perception of Americans regarding the ACA during 2013 to 2016 saying: "Gallup's tracking, for instance, shows that since the law took effect in 2013, a majority of Americans have consistently disapproved of it, ranging from a low of 48 percent in July 2015 – just after the Supreme Court's ruling upholding the law's federal subsidies – to a high of 56 percent."[103] The Gallup Poll Fender referring to included 1,015 randomized respondents between the ages of 18 and 64 surveyed during the term of 2012 to 2016 – it asked the American public: "Do you

---

97 Testimony before the Committee on Budget, US House of Representatives by Edmund F. Haislmaier, Senior Research Fellow, Health Policy Studies Center for Health Policy Studies, "The Real Changes in Health Insurance Enrollment Under the Affordable Care Act," January 24, 2017, see http://www.heritage.org/research/reports/2017/01/the-real-changes-in-health-insurance-enrollment-under-the-affordable-care-act
98 https://www.gpo.gov/fdsys/pkg/FR-2013-02-25/pdf/2013-04084.pdf
99 https://www.cms.gov/CCIIO/Resources/Fact-Sheets-and-FAQs/ehb-2-20-2013.html
100 http://healthaffairs.org/blog/2015/02/22/implementing-health-reform-2016-benefit-and-payment-final-rule-consumer-provisions/
101 Also see note 14 above; qualified enrollees received premium subsidies in the form of Tax Credits paid to insurers to make the cost of health insurance affordable based on family income criteria.
102 Elizabeth Fender is Market Research Associate for *The Heritage Foundation.*
103 See http://dailysignal.com/2016/12/13/ObamaCare-may-soon-be-over-heres-what-americans-have-thought-of-the-law-since-2010/

generally approve of disapprove of the 2010 Affordable Care act, signed into law by President Obama that restructured the US healthcare system?" The results of this important Gallup Poll are graphically depicted below:[104]

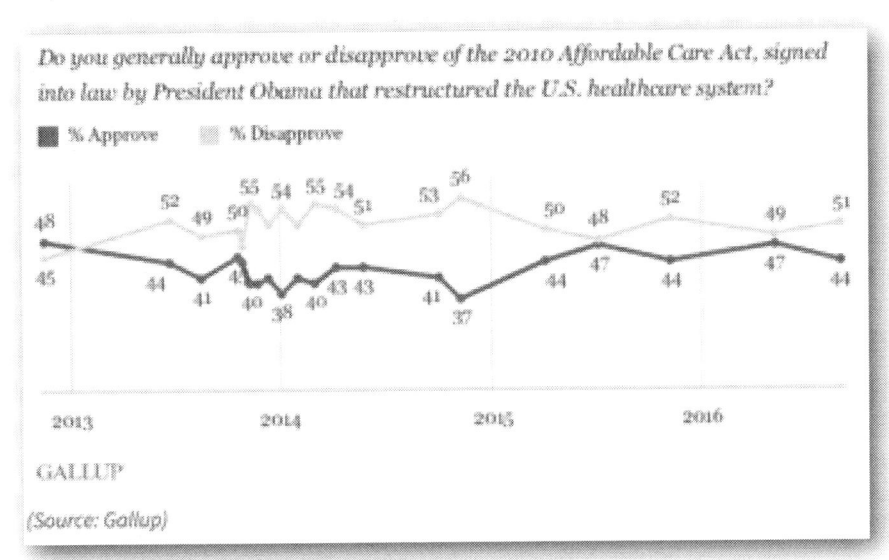

Graph 2 – Percent Approval and Disapproval of the 2010 ACA

This Gallup Poll indicates that "the American public hasn't embraced the healthcare law and still holds serious reservations about it... Americans have remained at least slightly more negative than positive about the law for three years."[105] Several other reputable national polls affirmed Gallup's findings. Another question posed by the Gallup Poll asked the perception of Americans how they felt about "the ACA's ability to improve their family's healthcare situation" in the short and long run[106] –

- 18 percent say the law has helped their families
- 29 percent say it hurt them
- Long-term, most Americans say the law will hurt or not make much difference

---

104 GALLUP NEWS SERVICE AFFORDABLE CARE ACT APPROVAL Results are based on telephone interviews with a random sample of – 1,015 -- national adults, aged 18+, living in all 50 states and the District of Columbia, conducted August 30-31, 2016. For results based on the total sample of National Adults, the margin of error is ±4 percentage points at the 95% confidence level. Interviews are conducted with respondents on landline telephones and cellular phones, with interviews conducted in Spanish for respondents who are primarily Spanish-speaking. Samples are weighted to correct for unequal selection probability, non-response, and double coverage of landline and cell users in the two sampling frames. They are also weighted to match the national demographics of gender, age, race, Hispanic ethnicity, education, region, population density, and phone status. In addition to sampling error, question wording and practical difficulties in conducting surveys can introduce error or bias into the findings of public opinion polls. See http://www.gallup.com/poll/195383/americans-negative-positive-aca.aspx?version=print
105 http://www.gallup.com/poll/195383/americans-negative-positive-aca.aspx?version=print
106 ibid.

I have first hand experience with health insurance plans on the ACA Marketplace. As an independent consultant, the continual rise in commercial health insurance premiums caused my wife and me to seek coverage on the Oklahoma Marketplace in 2014.[107] The enrollment process was filled with confusion, errors, bad information, and frustration. We finally decided on the *Gold Plan* with Blue Cross of Oklahoma offered through the Marketplace. For us, the ACA provided a **monthly** Federal Tax Credit subsidy of $1,185.00 to help pay for the premium (my wife and I) of $1,588.95, leaving a monthly balance for us to pay of $403.95. The plan had reasonable health insurance coverage, however, with a *narrow network* of providers. The annual deductible was $3,700.00, and there was a co-pay of $25.00 for primary care visits and 100% co-pay for specialists' care until the deductible was satisfied. We were definitely satisfied with the alternative ACA insurance cost *after* the federal subsidy compared to our experience with commercial market rates (before the enactment of the universal health program) of $1,643.27 per month for a small 2-person consulting business.[108]

Researching the most cited reasons behind the public's discontent with ObamaCare, here are the culprits:

1. Intense negative publicity (and sometimes falsehoods about the ACA)[109] perpetrated by opposition politicians has strongly influenced American sentiment about the law
2. Since the ACA's insurers are predominantly private for-profit insurance companies, premiums rose steadily from year-to-year to offset higher costs to comply with the EHBs (although to overall average increase from 2013 to 2016 was lower than previous years in the United States)
3. Failure of the Federal Government to provide the promised "risk corridor" protection to insurance companies (non-profit COOPs were decimated by this move).
4. Too narrow of provider networks limiting consumer choice
5. Escalating out-of-pocket costs and unrealistic annual family deductibles
6. Lack of a *Public Insurance Option* similar to the coverage for government employees or Medicare to compete with private for-profit plans
7. The cost of national healthcare in America continued to grow from $2.3 trillion in 2013 to $3.2 trillion in 2016
8. Strong opposition to the "individual mandate" to secure health insurance coverage and associated tax penalties for non-compliant healthy / younger population participating in the ACA.[110]

---

107 See *Section One* of this book, Chapter 9.3, page 118 – *Joe the Consultant*. The monthly rate in 2009 was $1,643.27; it rose to $2,400.00 per month by 2013.
108 Mark Tozzio, personal health insurance cost information in 2016.
109 David Hunke, President and Publisher, "Nonsense about 'death panels' spring back to life," *USA Today*, January 7, 2011, p. 8A.
110 The 2010 PPACA law requires that all Americans shall have health insurance coverage or pay an income tax penalty with their annual federal tax obligation. **No one is obligated to buy health insurance under ObamaCare**. Also see

9. Diminishing number of insurers offering plans on the Marketplaces (some states in the 2016 open enrollment period reported only **one option** to choose from).

As is the case with many complex new federal laws, this list points to several important opportunities for enhancing healthcare legislation to address these concerns and problems instead of simply subscribing to the "repeal and replacement" the ACA.

What are the most admired features of the ACA? A national poll conducted by the *Kaiser Family Foundation* and published March 2014 sheds light on this question:[111]

Percent who say they have a FAVORABLE opinion of each provision of the law	Total Public	Democrat	Independent	Republican
Extension of dependent coverage	80%	87%	76%	76%
Close Medicare "doughnut hole"	79	89	75	73
Subsidy assistance to individuals	77	89	74	65
Eliminate out-of-pocket costs for preventive services	77	81	76	75
Medicaid expansion	74	89	69	62
Guaranteed issue	70	74	70	69
Medical loss ratio	67	68	64	54
Increase Medicare payroll tax on upper income	56	77	54	33
Individual mandate/penalty	35	56	31	16

FIGURE 12: Many Elements Of ACA Continue To Be Popular Across Parties

Figure 2 – Political Party Support of ACA Elements

Clearly there are redeeming attributes of the ACA that have improved healthcare coverage in the United States since the implementation of universal coverage in 2013. The most popular benefits are:

1. Federal Tax Credit subsidy assistance to individuals and families with income up to 400 percent of the FFPL[112]
2. Extension of dependent coverage on parents' health insurance policy up to the age of 26
3. Expanded coverage of the poor under states Medicaid programs facilitated by Federal assistance to participating states (from 100 to 133 percent of the FFPL)
4. Guaranteed issue of insurance regardless of preexisting illnesses and employment status (portability of insurance between jobs)
5. Elimination of the life-time insurance coverage limitation of coverage

---

discussion about the US Supreme Court's decision of June 28, 2012.
111 See http://kff.org/health-reform/poll-finding/kaiser-health-tracking-poll-march-2014/
112 Federal Family Poverty Limit; according to HHS, in 2012 a family of four could earn up to $92,200 annually and still qualify for a subsidy computed on a sliding scale.

6. Free preventive care services
7. Addition of EHB[113] for all plans offered on the Marketplace

The election of President Donald Trump November 8, 2016 seems to have sealed the fate of ObamaCare in 2017. In spite of the political rhetoric, ACA subscribers are wondering if the new Trump Administration and Republican-lead Congress can actually devise and approve a better and brighter solution for universal health coverage which is affordable to *all* Americans in the near term without reversing progress made by the ACA since 2013?

1.4 -- Legal Challenges to the ACA Reach the US Supreme Court

The Centers for Medicare and Medicaid (CMS) reported that the national healthcare spending reached $2.34 trillion and projected the tab would reach $4.5 trillion by 2019.[114] Most healthcare policy experts, health system executives, providers of care, politicians, and the American public generally agree that the historical health expenditure trend is not sustainable in the near future. They also support major reform of the volume-based payment system for the good of the nation's economic solvency -- that is where the agreement ends.

Several legal challenges to the implementation of the ACA followed the law's enactment on March 23, 2010. Two specific suits threatened the viability of the ACA and made their way to the *United States Supreme Court* and were decided June 28, 2012 and June 25, 2015. These two core arguments against the ACA deserve our special attention:

- The first challenge reviewed by the highest court in America known as the 2012 NFIB v Sebelius[115] *(no. 11-392)* ruled in favor in part, and reversed in part, of the ACA -- https://www.supremecourt.gov/opinions/11pdf/11-393c3a2.pdf
- The second was known as the 2015 King vs Burwell[116] *(no. 14-114)* ruled in favor of the ACA / Obama Administration's contention --https://www.supremecourt.gov/opinions/14pdf/14-114_qol1.pdf

The premise of the suit in **NFIB v Sebelius** was summarized in the June 28, 2012 Supreme Court ruling –

---

113 Essential Health Benefits (EHB).
114 CMS, Office of the Actuary, 2010.
115 National Federation of Independent Business et al. versus Kathleen Sebelius, Secretary of Health and Human Services et al.
116 David King et al., Petitioners, versus Sylvia Burwell, Secretary of Health and Human Services et al.

Figure 3 – Summary of Supreme Court Ruling on NFIB v Sebelius

In 2010, Congress enacted the Patient Protection and Affordable Care Act in order to increase the number of Americans covered by health insurance and decrease the cost of health care. One key provision is the individual mandate, which requires most Americans to maintain "minimum essential" health insurance coverage. 26 U. S. C. §5000A. For individuals who are not exempt, and who do not receive health insurance through an employer or government program, the means of satisfying the requirement is to purchase insurance from a private company. Beginning in 2014, those who do not comply with the mandate must make a "[s]hared responsibility payment" to the Federal Government. §5000A(b)(1). The Act provides that this "penalty" will be paid to the Internal Revenue Service with an individual's taxes, and "shall be assessed and collected in the same manner" as tax penalties. §§5000A(c), (g)(1).

Another key provision of the Act is the Medicaid expansion. The current Medicaid program offers federal funding to States to assist pregnant women, children, needy families, the blind, the elderly, and the disabled in obtaining medical care. 42 U. S. C. §1396d(a). The Affordable Care Act expands the scope of the Medicaid program and increases the number of individuals the States must cover. For example, the Act requires state programs to provide Medicaid coverage by 2014 to adults with incomes up to 133 percent of the federal poverty level, whereas many States now cover adults with children only if their income is considerably lower, and do not cover childless adults at all. §1396a(a)(10)(A)(i)(VIII). The Act increases federal funding to cover the States' costs in expanding Medicaid coverage. §1396d(y)(1). But if a State does not comply with the Act's new coverage requirements, it may lose not only the federal funding for those requirements, but all of its federal Medicaid funds. §1396c. Twenty-six States, several individuals, and the National Federation of Independent Business brought suit in Federal District Court, challenging the constitutionality of the individual mandate and the Medicaid expansion. The Court of Appeals for the Eleventh Circuit upheld the Medicaid expansion as a valid exercise of Congress's spending power, but concluded that Congress lacked authority to enact the individual mandate. Finding the mandate severable from the Act's other provisions, the Eleventh Circuit left the rest of the Act intact.

In layman's language, the first US Supreme Court suit was about: (1) the ACA requirement for the *individual mandate*, and (2) the expansion of Medicaid at the state level. The individual mandate imposed a universal health insurance coverage on all Americans OR pay a graduated income tax penalty in lieu of participation. As for the Medicaid expansion provision of the ACA, states unwilling to adopt the 133 percent FFPL for eligibility would not only loose future federal funds for covering the cost of additional participants, but also have ALL federal assistance for the state Medicaid program withheld.

On November 14, 2011, the Supreme Court of the United States issued a "writ of certiorari"[117] to the United States Appeals Court for the Eleventh Circuit in order to consolidate two similar law suits: **NFIB v Sebelius** and **Florida v United States Department of Health and Human Services** into a single review. The Court heard oral arguments March 26–28, 2012 and decided the consolidated case on June 28, 2012. In a stunning 5-4 ruling[118] in favor of upholding the ACA, Supreme Court Chief Justice John Roberts delivered the court's affirmative decision with the following caveats:

- ✓ *ObamaCare individual mandate was actually deemed a tax (penalty) rather than a mandate, thus determined in keeping with the US Constitution under the Commerce Clause (granting Congress the power to impose a tax on citizens).*
- ✓ *Declared that the Administration could not withhold Medicaid funds to states electing not to expand coverage to poor families with incomes up to 133 percent of FFPL.*

The majority of Republican-lead states did not expand their Medicaid programs' eligibility criteria affecting an estimated 7 percent of the poorest Americans.[119] This landmark decision by the Supreme Court breathed life back into the ACA enrollment process that was under threat of a "claw back" action by the IRS for persons enrolling and receiving tax credit subsidies. It also cleared the way for a major HHS advertising campaign across the nation to enlist Americans in ObamaCare starting with the Marketplaces' open enrollment period October 2013.

The syllabus of the suit in **King v Burwell** is included in the Supreme Court's decision on June 25, 2015 is presented below –

Figure 4 – Summary of Supreme Court Ruling on King v Burwell

The Patient Protection and Affordable Care Act grew out of a long history of failed health insurance reform. In the 1990s, several States sought to expand access to coverage by imposing a pair of insurance market regulations—a "guaranteed issue" requirement,

---

[117] For definition of writ of certiorari at http://www.nolo.com/dictionary: "Latin for 'to be fully informed.' In cases in which there is not appeal as a matter of right, certiorari is a writ (order) by the appeals court to a lower court to send all the documents in a case so that the appeals court can review the decision. Certiorari is most commonly used by the United States Supreme Court, which grants certiorari when at least four Justices believe that the case involves a sufficiently significant federal issue."

[118] Voting in favor of the majority decision were Justices John Roberts, Ruth Bader Ginsburg, Stephen Breyer, Sonya Sotomayor, and Elena Kagan; voting against were Justices Antonin Scalia, Clarence Thomas, Anthony Kennedy, and Samuel Alito.

[119] see http://ObamaCarefacts.com/supreme-court-ObamaCare

which bars insurers from denying coverage to any person because of his health, and a "community rating" requirement, which bars insurers from charging a person higher premiums for the same reason. The reforms achieved the goal of expanding access to coverage, but they also encouraged people to wait until they got sick to buy insurance. The result was an economic "death spiral": premiums rose, the number of people buying insurance declined, and insurers left the market entirely. In 2006, however, Massachusetts discovered a way to make the guaranteed issue and community rating requirements work—by requiring individuals to buy insurance and by providing tax credits to certain individuals to make insurance more affordable.

The combination of these three reforms—insurance market regulations, a coverage mandate, and tax credits—enabled Massachusetts to drastically reduce its uninsured rate. The Affordable Care Act adopts a version of the three key reforms that made the Massachusetts system successful. First, the Act adopts the guaranteed issue and community rating requirements. 42 U. S. C. §§300gg, 300gg–1. Second, the Act generally requires individuals to maintain health insurance coverage or make a payment to the IRS, unless the cost of buying insurance would exceed eight percent of that individual's income. 26 U. S. C. §5000A. And third, the Act seeks to make insurance more affordable by giving refundable tax credits to individuals with household incomes between 100 per cent and 400 percent of the federal poverty line. §36B.

In addition to those three reforms, the Act requires the creation of an "Exchange" in each State—basically, a marketplace that allows people to compare and purchase insurance plans. The Act gives each State the opportunity to establish its own Exchange, but provides that the Federal Government will establish "such Exchange" if the State does not. 42 U. S. C. §§18031, 18041. Relatedly, the Act provides that tax credits "shall be allowed" for any "applicable taxpayer," 26 U. S. C. §36B(a), but only if the taxpayer has enrolled in an insurance plan through "an Exchange established by the State under [42 U. S. C. §18031]," §§36B(b)–(c). An IRS regulation interprets that language as making tax credits available on "an Exchange," 26 CFR §1.36B–2, "regardless of whether the Exchange is established and operated by a State . . . or by HHS," 45 CFR §155.20. Petitioners are four individuals who live in Virginia, which has a Federal Exchange. They do not wish to purchase health insurance. In their view, Virginia's Exchange does not qualify as "an Exchange established by the State under [42 U. S. C. §18031]," so they should not receive any tax credits. That would make the cost of buying insurance more than eight percent of petitioners' income, exempting them from the Act's coverage requirement. As a result of the IRS Rule, however, petitioners would receive tax credits. That would make the cost of buying insurance less than eight percent of their income, which would subject them to the Act's coverage requirement. Petitioners challenged the IRS Rule in Federal District Court. The District Court dismissed the suit, holding *that the Act unambiguously made tax credits available to individuals enrolled through a Federal Exchange. The Court of Appeals for the Fourth Circuit affirmed. The Fourth Circuit viewed the Act as ambiguous, and deferred to the IRS's interpretation under Chevron U. S. A. Inc. v. Natural Resources Defense Council, Inc., 467 U. S. 837.*

The second critical challenge to the ACA dealt with the eligibility of Marketplace subscribers receiving taxes credit subsidies paid directly to insurance companies by the IRS for residents in states that **did not** implement their own "state run exchanges" (original name for Marketplaces). In this instance (some 26 states and possibly 8 million people), the federal government instituted and managed national Marketplaces operated by HHS. Non-participating states claimed that the ACA language limited tax credits to individuals / families securing health insurance on Exchanges established by the *states*. The argument the Supreme Court worked with is that:

> *… the Act requires the creation of an "Exchange" in each State—basically, a marketplace that allows people to compare and purchase insurance plans. The Act gives each State the opportunity to establish its own Exchange, but provides that the Federal Government will establish "such Exchange" if the State does not. 42 U. S. C. §§18031, 18041. Relatedly, the Act provides that tax credits "shall be allowed" for any "applicable taxpayer," 26 U. S. C. §36B(a), but only if the taxpayer has enrolled in an insurance plan through "an Exchange established by the State under [42 U. S. C. §18031]," §§36B(b)–(c). An IRS regulation interprets that language as making tax credits available on "an Exchange," 26 CFR §1.36B–2, "regardless of whether the Exchange is established and operated by a State . . . or by HHS," 45 CFR §155.20.*

Legal scholars have argued that this dispute was a matter of *semantics*. The use of the word "**states**" in the healthcare law referred to the fact that *government sponsored Exchanges or Marketplaces* did not hinge on whether or not individual states created their own entities. The expectation of the Obama Administration was that most states *would* want to manage their own Marketplaces and receive federal assistance to do so, rather than defer to HHS to operate them completely. The strict interpretation of the word states became the crux of the legal dispute. Proponents of the ACA claimed it was merely a *red herring* by Republicans to bring down the legislation.[120]

The Obama Administration asserted that the narrow interpretation of the language in the ACA was politically motivated to defeat the program. Congressional representatives (the Democratic majority in the House and Senate) stated they intended for the law to apply equally

---

120 In logic and rhetoric, a *red herring* is an observation that draws attention away from the central issue in an argument or discussion; an informal logical fallacy. Also called a *decoy*. See http://grammar.about.com/od/rs/g/redherrterm.htm

to all Americans buying insurance coverage on Exchanges, regardless of who sponsors or operates them (i.e. no distinction between federal and state run Marketplaces).

On June 25, 2015, Supreme Court Chief Justice Roberts delivered the court's 6-3 decision[121] based on the following interpretation of the ACA verbiage:

- ✓ *Congress passed the Affordable Care Act to improve health insurance markets, not to destroy them,* Roberts wrote in the majority opinion. *"If at all possible, we must interpret the Act in a way that is consistent with the former, and avoids the latter.*
- ✓ *The context and structure of the Act compel us to depart from what would otherwise be the most natural reading of the pertinent statutory phrase,"* Roberts wrote.

Republicans vowed to continue the battle to "repeal and replace" ObamaCare in spite of these two Supreme Court's "liberal" rulings (2012 and 2015) in favor of the ACA.

In 2012, if the Supreme Court had interpreted the so called *individual mandate* as an obligation of Americans to buy health insurance instead of a tax levied against those who opt out of the universal health coverage requirement, this financial obligation (tax) could have been struck down as unconstitutional. The broad risk-sharing population including young healthy cohorts along with other healthcare consuming individuals and families spreads the cost over a larger premium-paying group required by the ACA. Without having *all* Americans share equally in the burden of healthcare insurance, the cost for unhealthy persons would be prohibitive. Unless everyone is part of universal health insurance coverage, it can't work without heavy government subsidy.

As for the favorable Supreme Court decision in 2015, it was felt that excluding 26 states and a population of approximately 6.5 million covered lives from the IRS tax credit assistance would cause the remaining participating state-run Marketplaces to collapse under high-cost low-revenue conditions.[122] Without nation-wide tax credit subsidies, participation in the ACA will disappear. The only way for universal health insurance to thrive is to significantly grow the membership and promote primary care and value-based incentives to control rising healthcare costs.

Ironically, Oklahoma's government officials have been leading opponents to the ACA since its enactment in 2010, even as the state ranked *45th worst* in health status in America at the time of the 2012 and 2015 Supreme Court decisions.[123] The south-central states

---

[121] Voting in favor of the majority decision were Justices John Roberts, Anthony Kennedy, Ruth Bader Ginsburg, Stephen Breyer, Sonya Sotomayor, and Elena Kagan; voting against were Justices Antonin Scalia, Clarence Thomas, and Samuel Alito.

[122] *Modern Healthcare*, "Beyond the Decision", June 29, 2015, pp. 7-18.

[123] *America's Health Rankings*, 2015, see http://cdnfiles.americashealthrankings.org/SiteFiles/Reports/2015AHR_Annual-v1.pdf

traditionally suffer from the highest rates of uninsured, high prevalence of obesity, high cardiovascular and related diseases, and limited access to primary care services. This map published by *America's Health Rankings* depicts states in our country from highest to lowest health status:

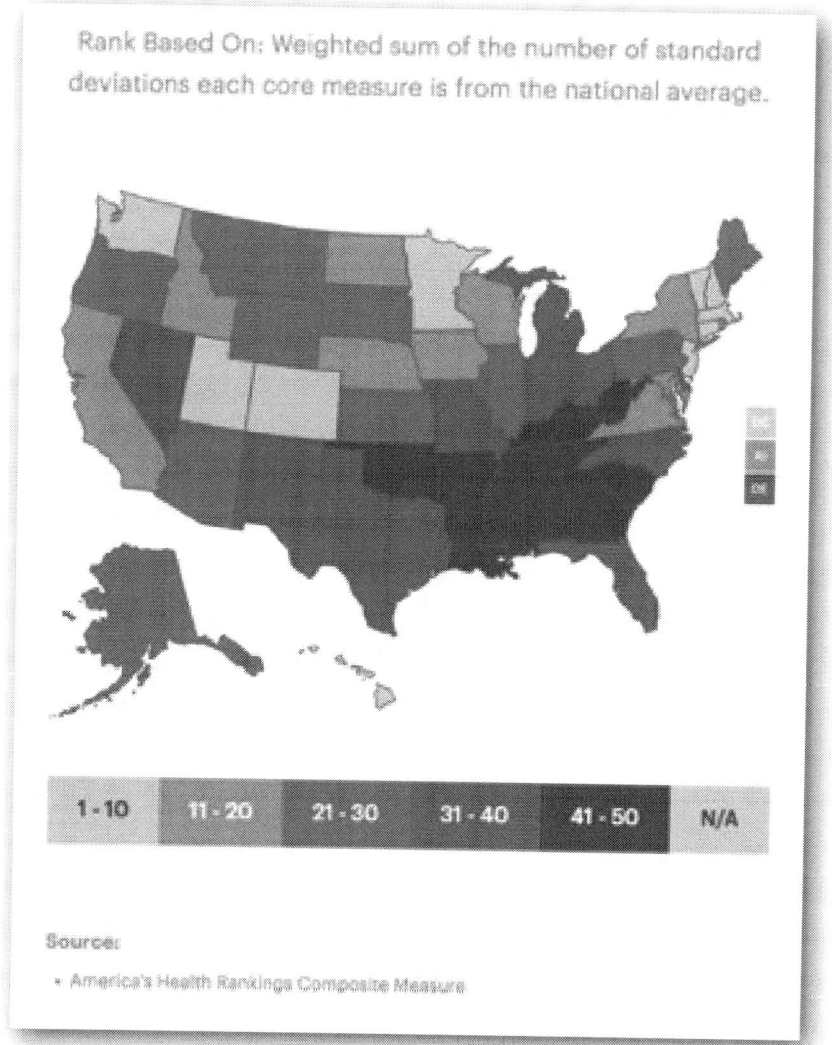

Figure 5 – Map of America's Health Rankings Composite Measures: 2012-2015

John Silva, CEO of *Morton Comprehensive Health Care* (non-profit Community Health Center) in Tulsa spoke to the *Tulsa World* newspaper on June 26, 2015 regarding the Supreme Court's decision to uphold ObamaCare: "I'm hoping now the state [Oklahoma] can stop these stupid challenges and work together with the community to make sure our poorest and most vulnerable residents have access to health-care coverage." Silva went on to say: "Anybody who thinks that this is a bad decision [by the *Supreme Court*] is not representing the needs of the people of this state."[124]

Silva's comments support the tenet that universal access to affordable health insurance coverage is a foundational precept of the ACA, and *healthcare should be a limited human right* for Oklahoman's.

---

[124] *Tulsa World*, Friday, June 26, 2015, pp. A1 and A6.

Two

Health Insurance Reform

2.1 – Key Milestones of the ACA: 2010 to 2016

"I am as confident as ever that looking back 20 years from now, the nation will be better off because of having the courage to pass this law [ACA] and persevere. As this progress with health care reform in the United States demonstrates, faith in responsibility, belief in opportunity, and the ability to unite around common values are what makes this nation great."

President Barack Obama, July 11, 2016, JAMA, Vol. 316 (5), p.530

The United States has a rich history when it comes to healthcare legislation and policy. There has been a careful balance for the government to provide necessary protection against sickness and pestilence for all citizens without excessive control and cost that impinges of freedom and rights of individuals. Beaufort Longest, Jr. presents a superb recap of Health Policymaking in the United States in his book published in 2006.[125] He shares his definitions of health early in his book (pp. 1-2):

Health is a universally important aspect of human life... Good health is also an integral part of thriving modern societies, a cornerstone of well performing economics, and a shared principle [of all] democracies... The way in which health is defined by any nation is important because it reflects the nation's values regarding health the resources it is

---

[125] Beaufort B. Longest, Jr., 2006, *Health Policymaking in the United States*, 4th Ed., Health Administration Press, Chicago, Il.

prepared to devote to the pursuit of health, and how far the nation would be willing to go in aiding or supporting the pursuit of health among its citizens.

My interpretation of Longest's statement is that it reinforces the belief that a state of good health is a *human right* that enriches countries that provide universal healthcare to all citizens. This has been the impetus for establishing and refining laws pertaining to health benefits in our nation starting with the passage of federal legislation by the *Fifth Congress* of the United States compelling "employers of merchant seamen to fund arrangements for their healthcare through the Marine Hospital Service" way back in July 16, 1798.[126]

Another transformational healthcare milestone transpired with the passage of the **Social Security Amendments of 1965** set forth in P.L.89-97 establishing the **Medicare** insurance program (Title XVIII) for those over 65 and **Medicaid**, Grants to the States for Medical Assistance Programs (Title XIX) to help care for the poor.[127] Today, Medicare and Medicaid expenditures represent approximately *35 percent* of the $3.2 trillion spent on health related services in United States.[128] Yet, nearly 50 million Americans remained uninsured or seriously underinsured when Barack Obama became the 44th President of the United States on January 20, 2009.

One of President Obama's central campaign promises was to help bring *universal health insurance coverage for all Americans* and "eliminate" the millions of uninsured and underinsured that were a shameful blemish on this great nation.[129] Several presidents preceding Barack Obama had tried to bring universal coverage to Americans, and failed. He was determined to fight for the legislation introduced in the Democratically controlled Congress. President Obama devoted a substantial part of his first year in the White House working toward the passage of the **Patient Protection and Affordable Care Act of 2010**.[130] The ACA was not designed to *replace* Medicare and Medicaid / CHIP programs, nor the private insurance coverage purchased **off** the Marketplaces or through employers.

From 2010 to 2013, when Marketplace enrollment began in November, it was a contentious period of healthcare reform fraught with ACA enrollment information overload, intense program education, implementation preparation, failed online processes, government and public confusion, opposition propaganda, and massive regulations promulgation by HHS and the IRS and state agencies.

---

126 Ibid., p. 379.
127 Ibid., p. 387.
128 Centers for Medicare and Medicaid statistics (CMS).
129 See discussion about calculating the national uninsured rate in the United States at https://aspe.hhs.gov/basic-report/understanding-estimates-uninsured-putting-differences-context
130 PPACA was signed into law on March 23, 2010.

When the ACA dust finally settled by the end of 2013, these were the major achievements pertaining to ObamaCare[131] [132] [133] that stand out:

- President Barack Obama nominated Kathleen Sebelius (D) as US Secretary of Health and Human Services Administration (HHS) serving in this Cabinet role from April 28, 2009 to June 9, 2014. Secretary Sebelius had served as 44th Governor of Kansas from 2003 to 2009, and prior to this post she was appointed as the 23rd Insurance Commissioner of Kansas from January 9, 1995 to January 13, 2003.[134] Sebelius' experience in the insurance industry was a key asset as head of the HHS.
- President Obama signed the PPACA into law on March 23, 2010 "expanding affordability, quality, and availability of private and public health insurance through consumer protections, regulations, subsidies, taxes, tax credit subsidies, insurance exchanges, and other reforms."[135]
- CMS / CCIIO established criteria for participation of *Qualified Health Plans* selling insurance on the Marketplaces including the EHB requirements.
- 16 states and Washington, DC embraced ObamaCare and created their own Marketplaces, while HHS established federal-state partnerships or government-run Marketplaces for the remaining 35 states and the District of Columbia.[136]
- CMS / CCIIO awarded start-up loans and funding for 23 non-profit health insurance entities called **Consumer Operated and Oriented Plans** (CO-OPs) totaling $2.4 billion under the provisions of the ACA (Section 1322 of the Act).[137] The new CO-OPs were intended to compete on the Marketplaces with established health insurers and help drive premium costs down and enhance consumer benefits. As of July 2016, 16 of the 23 CO-OPs had ceased operations primarily due to heavy losses and Congressional refusal to fund the "risk corridors" stipulated in the original government contracts.[138]

---

[131] Abstracted from http://obamacarefacts.com/obamacare-facts/
[132] Abstracted from https://www.hhs.gov/sites/default/files/fy-2016-hhs-agency-financial-report.pdf
[133] Abstracted from https://aspe.hhs.gov/pdf-report/health-insurance-coverage-and-affordable-care-act-2010-2016
[134] https://www.britannica.com/biography/Kathleen-Sebelius
[135] "What is ObamaCare?", see http://obamacarefacts.com/obamacare-facts/, page 1.
[136] See *Kaiser Family Foundation.org* at http://kff.org/health-reform/state-indicator/state-health-insurance-marketplace-types/?activeTab=map&currentTimeframe=0&selectedDistributions=marketplace-type&selectedRows=%7B%22nested%22:%7B%22all%22:%7B%7D%7D,%22wrapups%22:%7B%22united-states%22:%7B%7D%7D%7D
[137] CCIIO, see https://fas.org/sgp/crs/misc/R44414.pdf
[138] The term *risk corridor* refers to a guarantee by HHS to CO-OPs to limit loss thresholds after program reinsurance and risk adjustments are factored into margins during the three initial start-up years, see https://www.cms.gov/CCIIO/Resources/Files/Downloads/3rs-final-rule.pdf

- Created **Healthcare.gov** information / educational materials and enrollment online system for federal and state Marketplaces staffed by trained full-time program *Navigators* and assignment of traditional insurance brokers.[139] [140]

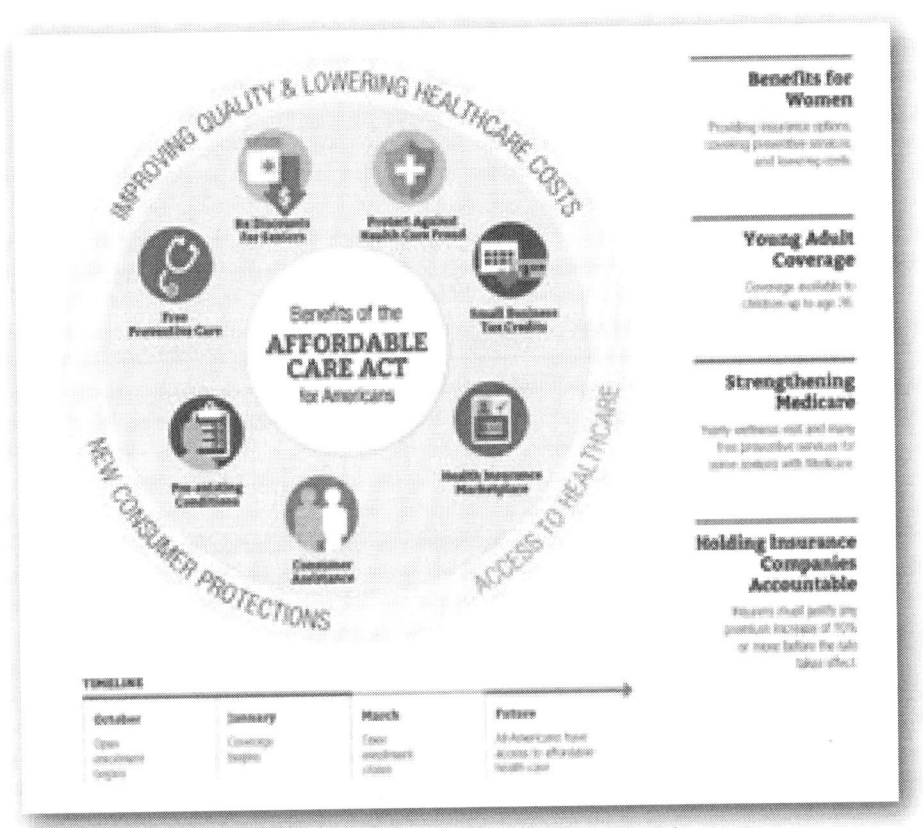

Figure 6 – CMS ACA Benefits Wheel

- Federal and state Marketplaces launched operations across America for open enrollment starting November 1, 2013 (in spite of big problems with the Healthcare.gov site).[141] [142]

What are the key participation factors and figures relating to implementation of ObamaCare during the operational phase from 2013 to 2016?[143]

---

139 *The Center for Consumer Information & Insurance Oversight*, see https://www.cms.gov/cciio/index.html
140 See "How Health Insurance Works," at http://obamacarefacts.com/obamacare-facts/
141 https://www.healthcare.gov/topics/
142 http://obamacarefacts.com/obamacare-glitch/
143 https://www.cms.gov/About-CMS/Agency-Information/CMS-Strategy/Downloads/CMS-Strategy.pdf

- The United States health uninsured rate for non-elderly adults (18-64 years old) fell *43 percent* (or a net decrease of close to 20 million adults including 2.3 million young adults remaining on their parents insurance plans until age 26) from 20.3% of the total population in 2013, to its historical low in decades of 11.5% in 2016.[144] [145] [146]

    NOTE: All graphs and statistics in this section were produced by ASPE Issue Brief, 2016, unless specifically referenced otherwise.[147]

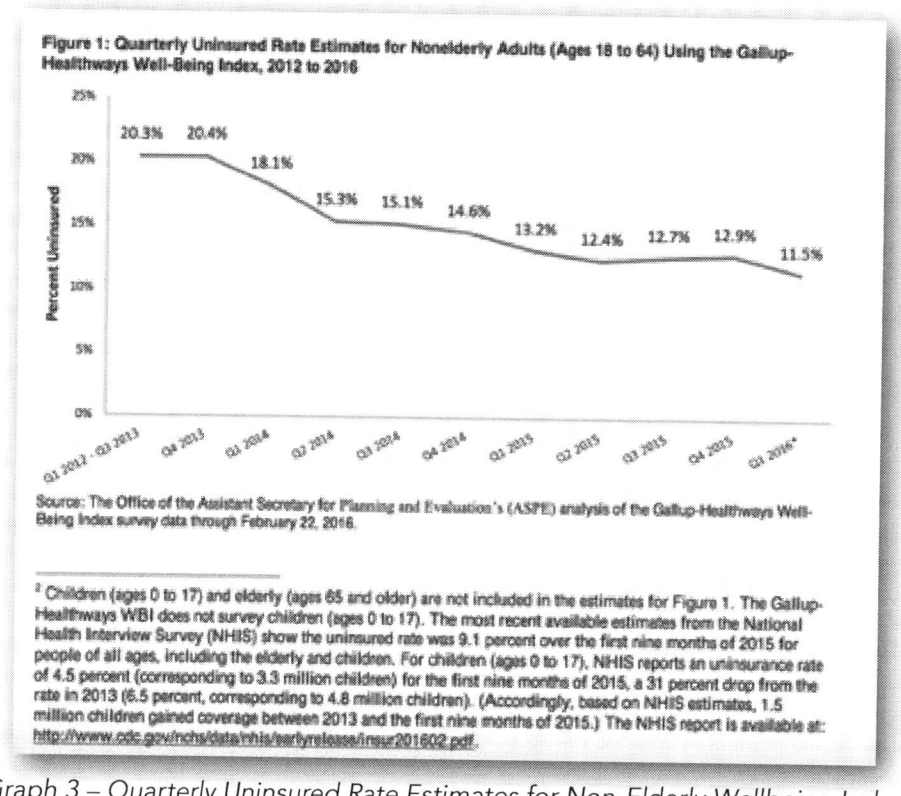

Graph 3 – Quarterly Uninsured Rate Estimates for Non-Elderly Wellbeing Index

- Uninsured rate for non-elderly adults by *largest racial categories* in the United States fell significantly for all groups between 2013 and 2016:

---

144 The 2016 rate of 11.5% is the lowest uninsured rate on record in several decades; see *KFF.org* report: "Key Facts About the Uninsured Population," at http://kff.org/uninsured/fact-sheet/key-facts-about-the-uninsured-population/
145 https://www.cdc.gov/nchs/data/nhis/earlyrelease/insur201605.pdf
146 http://www.gallup.com/poll/193556/uninsured-rate-remains-historical-low.aspx
147 https://aspe.hhs.gov/pdf-report/health-insurance-marketplace-summary-enrollment-report-initial-annual-open-enrollment-period

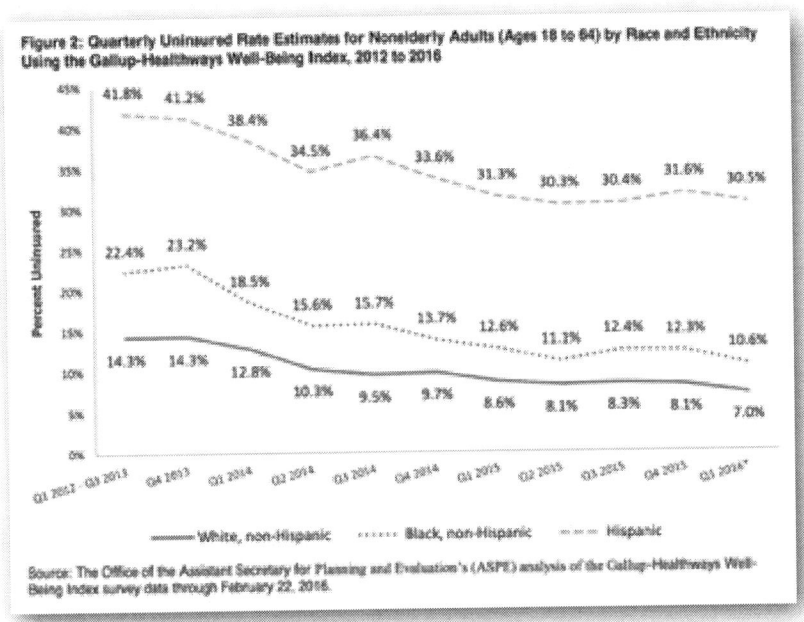

Why The United States Healthcare System Should Be A Limited Human Right For All

Graph 4 – Quarterly Uninsured Rate Estimates for Non-Elderly by Race and Ethnicity

- Uninsured rate for non-elderly adults in the United States by comparison of **major survey entities** between 2013 and 2016 is similar for six tracking agencies.
- Overall **enrollment trends** through US Marketplaces between 2013 and 2016 grew by 12.7 million overall.
- **Enrollment trends by *FFPL*** (percentage of the poverty limits) ranges through the Marketplaces were heaviest from >100% to <300% poverty level between 2013 and 2016.

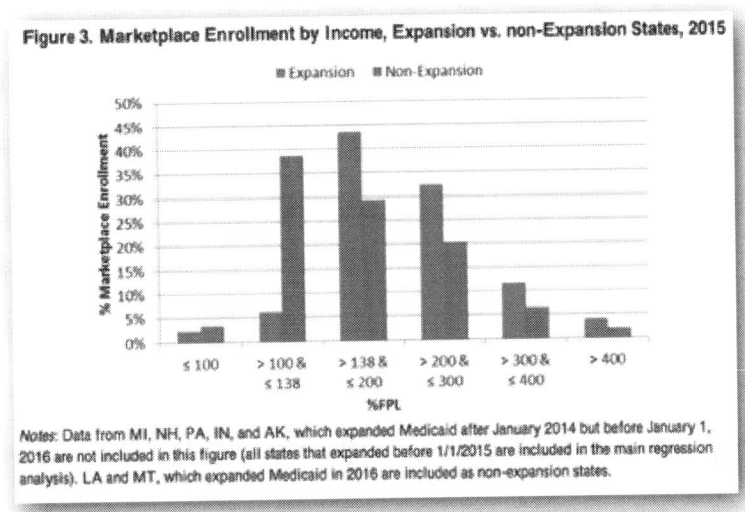

Graph 5 – Marketplace Enrollment by Income - Expansion v Non-Expansion States

- State Medicaid Program enrollment expansion related to the ACA reached 11.2 million *new* participants between February 2014 and January 2015:

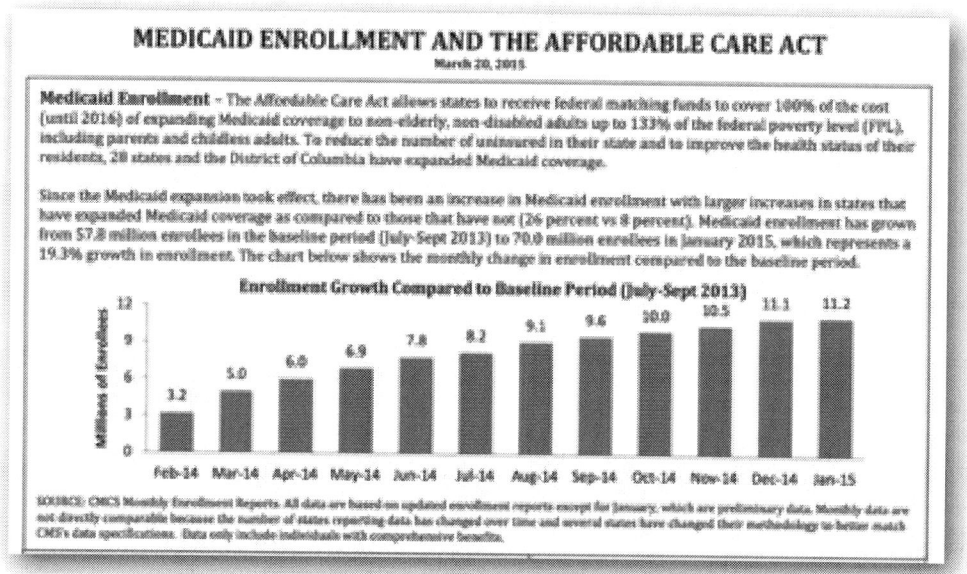

Graph 6 – Medicaid Enrollment Through ACA Expansion

- Young adults who sought health insurance coverage through the Marketplaces for the first time through 2016 amounted to 3.8 (ages 19 to 25). This number excludes young adults that remained / added to their parents' health insurance plans per the ACA expanded regulations. This group of healthier young adults is especially important to normalize the ACA and spread the healthcare costs across a broad sector of Americans.
- The percentage decline in the overall number of uninsured is similar by gender and race throughout the country.
- According to estimates by the HHS, healthcare annual spending growth from year-to-year grew at its slowest rate since 1960, and the healthcare price inflation also slowed to the lowest rate in 50 years.[148]
- ObamaCare extended *free* (insurers cannot charge extra premiums) preventive health services to over 47 million women.
- ObamaCare enabled about 54 million insurance subscribers to access coverage that might of previously excluded them because of *pre-existing conditions and high-risk conditions* (cancer, heart ailments, diabetes, etc.) prohibited in the new law.[149] Insurance

---

[148] See https://obamawhitehouse.archives.gov/sites/obamawhitehouse.archives.gov/files/achievements/theRecord_health.pdf

[149] See http://obamacarefacts.com/pre-existing-conditions/

companies are forbidden to terminate coverage of existing subscribers for any reason other than failure to pay monthly premiums or fraud.
- In 2010, an estimated 53.8% of working Americans received health insurance through their employers – the ACA *employer mandate* requires all business with more than 50 full time employees to offer coverage to at least 95% of workers or pay a "per-employee" contribution to the government by 2016.[150] Small employers (under 25 workers) can access the State Health Insurance Programs or *SHOP*[151] offered on the Marketplaces.
- After 2015, some states could add a premium surcharge to *smokers* after offering free smoking cessation incentives / programs to the public.
- **ObamaCare does not guarantee "affordable insurance"** to participants on Marketplaces – it does **limit premium cost** for the *Bronze Plan* to 8 percent of adjusted annual household family income and 9.5 percent for employee-only coverage.
- HHS estimates that as a result of the implementation of the ACA, the health system providers will experience a drop of approximately $50 billion each year in bad debt and charity care because of the employer and individual mandates and universal health insurance coverage. This figure could increase as the uninsured rate in the United States continues to drop as a result of ObamaCare.
- Obamacare eliminated the *lifetime benefits limitation* as well as the *annual coverage ceilings* imposed by most pre-2013 health plans operating in this nation.
- HHS estimated that some 86 million Americans paid co-pays and deductibles in 2011 for *free preventive health services* presently covered by insurers as a requirement of the ACA.

This list of major benefits resulting from ObamaCare are truly impressive and support the concepts behind universal healthcare insurance coverage in America. We have come a long way in providing better access to healthcare services in the rather short timeframe since the ACA legislation was signed into law in 2010. The data seems irrefutable -- The ACA has cut the number of uninsured and underinsured citizens in half, protected subscribers from abuses by insurers, significantly enhanced primary and preventive care services for millions, and slowed the pace of healthcare cost annual increases. This is not to say that improvements and refinements to the ACA are not necessary. It seems fitting to conclude this section with the words of President Barack Obama, a principal champion of the ACA legislation:[152]

---

150 See http://obamacarefacts.com/obamacare-employer-mandate/
151 See http://obamacarefacts.com/obamacare-small-business/
152 Barack Obama, JD, ACA Special Report, **JAMA**, August 2, 2016, Volume 316, Number 5, page 525, see http://jama-network.com/journals/jama/fullarticle/2533698

Mark G. Tozzio, M-IHHS, FACHE

Policy makers should build on the progress made by the Affordable Care Act by continuing to implement the Health Insurance Marketplaces and delivery system reform, increasing federal financial assistance for Marketplace enrollees, introducing a public plan option in areas lacking individual market competition, and taking actions to reduce prescription drug costs. Although partnership and special interest opposition remain, experience with the Affordable Care Act demonstrates that positive change is achievable on some of the nation's most complex challenges.

For the new Trump Administration and Republican-controlled Congress to pursue a strategy to **"repeal and replace"** ObamaCare at a time when the US health system is experiencing huge improvements over three short years of implementation seems *unfounded and risky*. If the values of our nation actually advocate that *healthcare is a limited human right for all Americans*, then why don't the policy makers work together to improve the current law rather than start healthcare reform from scratch, and turn back progress many years? Why not simply **"revise and enhance"** the ACA?

2.2 -- Healthcare Industry Embraces ACA Changes

GOP Obamacare replacement plan could prove "disastrous"

Republicans seem intent on pursuing a disastrous Obamacare replacement plan that couples catastrophic coverage with subsidized health savings accounts. Such high-deductible plans will make achieving good health much harder for patients. They will raise uncompensated-care costs and thus everyone's rates. And they will undermine the system's efforts at delivering better, more cost-effective care. Whether Republicans implement this alternative in three months or three years, the bottom line will be people paying more out of pocket. Preventive medicine and chronic disease management will get thrown under a bus filled with price-sensitive, ill-informed consumers left to their own devices to figure out what to buy in an overpriced and opaque healthcare marketplace.

Merrill Goozner, January 7, 2017, Modern Healthcare, Editorial.

For decades, healthcare providers have complained about the growing number of uninsured in the United States which translates into serious **bad debt and charity care** costs for hospitals, health systems, physicians and other providers of health services. In certain parts of the country that experience excessive poverty, unemployment, and under-employment, uncompensated care can reach as high as 15 percent of revenue. The average uncompensated care for all hospitals in the United States is between 6 to 8 percent of charges. On top of these losses, Medicare and Medicaid contracts reimburse provider services at their schedule of **"usual and customary"** rates that are typically near, or below, actual cost of delivering care. Commercial / private insurance companies pay for services on a **"discount from billed charges"** basis, or flat rates for different types of care. Community hospitals as a whole end up with *slim* operating margins between 2 to 4 percent of revenue after operating expenses. The old practice of shifting cost and losses to the commercial / private insurers has virtually ceased as insurers became more sophisticated and aggressive negotiators with providers.

An important feature of the ACA's reform is universal health insurance coverage – it helps spread insurers' risk over an expand number of covered lives (through the individual and business mandates). Advocates of a government sponsored **"single payer system"** coupled with universal health insurance similar to the Medicare system for the 65+ population believe this would be the most cost effective way to improve access and control healthcare cost in America. However, this approach would virtually eliminate commercial / private health insurers from the payment system. The single payer system is a politically suicidal strategy for a President and Congress to pursue because of the power and control that insurance companies exert in Washington, DC.

The political compromise reached by the US Congress during the 2009-2010 healthcare reform negotiations resulting in the *Accountable Care Act* (ACA) established *universal health insurance coverage* for non-seniors using the *existing* commercial / private insurance companies. These insurers are subject to strict controls designed to protect consumers from financial abuses. Nearly all commercial / private insurers in the United States operate as *for-profit* organizations, and accountable to their investors.

The ACA also created tough restrictions for insurance companies participating on the Marketplaces including the obligation to invest at least 85% (for larger insurance groups) of revenue from premiums back into the actual care of subscribers. Insurers of the individual and small business are allowed 80% for start-up insurance companies for a limited period to promote competitive prices for the *Metals on the exchanges*. This requirement is referred to as the **Medical Loss Ratio** (MLR), and is administered by HHS / CCIIO and state insurance regulators.[153] [154] According to the *Kaiser Family Foundation's* website:[155]

> Health insurers collect premiums from policyholders and use these funds to pay for enrollees' health care claims, as well as administer coverage, market products, and earn profits for investors. The Medical Loss Ratio provision of the ACA requires most insurance companies that cover individuals and small businesses to spend at least 80% of their premium income

---

[153] http://www.cms.gov/CCIIO/Programs-and-Initiatives/Health-Insurance-Market-Reforms/Medical-Loss-Ratio.html
[154] Self-funded employer sponsored health insurance plans are not considered insurance carriers and, therefore, not subject to the MLR rules.
[155] Kaiser Family Foundation, "Explaining Health Care Reform: Medical Loss Ratio (MLR), February 29, 2012, see http://kff.org/health-reform/fact-sheet/explaining-health-care-reform-medical-loss-ratio

on health care claims and quality improvement, leaving the remaining 20% for administration, marketing, and profit. The MLR threshold is higher for large group plans, which must spend at least 85 percent of premium dollars on health care and quality improvement.

A 2010 study by the *Government Accounting Office* (GAO) demonstrated that most US insurance companies were *not* meeting the MLR 80-85/20 standard and would be required to refund excessive profits to their subscribers once the regulations were in place. Congressman Pete Stark (D-Calif) compiled and published a list showing the profitability of investor-owned health insurance companies in 2010, the same year the ACA was signed into law[156] --

Table 4 – Profitability of For-Profit Insurance Companies: 9 Months in 2010

For-Profit Insurers - Profits for the First Nine Months of 2010

Company	2010 Profits (first nine months)	2009 Profits (first nine months)	Change in Profits (first nine months)	Percent Change in Profits
UnitedHealthcare	$3.59 billion	$2.88 billion	+$713 million	+24.8%
WellPoint	$2.34 billion	$2.00 billion	+334 million	+16.7%
Aetna	$1.55 billion	$1.11 billion	+441 million	+39.7%
Humana	$992 million	$789 million	+203 million	+25.7%
Coventry	$288 million	$133 million	+155 million	+116.4%
AmeriGroup	$194 million	$109 million	+84.6 million	+77.5%
HealthSpring	$143 million	$94.8 million	+48.6 million	+51.3%
HealthNet	$124 million	-$3.8 million	+127.6 million	---
Centene	$69.4 million	$60.0 million	+9.4 million	+15.7%
Molina	$37.3 million	$35.3 million	+2.0 million	+5.7%

Sources: Third quarter earnings reports for UnitedHealth Group, Inc.; WellPoint, Inc.; Aetna, Inc.; Humana, Inc., Coventry Health Care, Inc., Amerigroup Corporation; HealthSpring, Inc.; Health Net, Inc.; Centene Corporation; and Molina Healthcare, Inc.

Compiled by the Office of Congressman Pete Stark

The MLR regulations went into effect in 2011. HHS / CMS reported that a total of over $1 billion was returned to almost 13 million policy holders by insurance companies that year. The principal beneficiaries of the ACA health insurance reform are: (1) consumers, and (2) healthcare providers. Starting with the enrollment period at the end of 2013, the number of insured lives and patients increased substantially, resulting in a dramatic decline in the level of non-payment for services at healthcare facilities. Concurrently, insurers continued to revamp their operating practices while

---

[156] US Representative Pete Stark (D-CA), November 10, 2010, see https://www.healthinsurance.org/blog/2010/11/15/insurance-company-profits-up-41-percent/

employers expanded coverage to more full-time employees. The *American Hospital Association's* chart below shows aggregate hospital margins improved consistently following the implementation of the ACA, from a low of between 2% and 4% from 1994 - 2009 to about 6% from 2010 to 2014.[157]

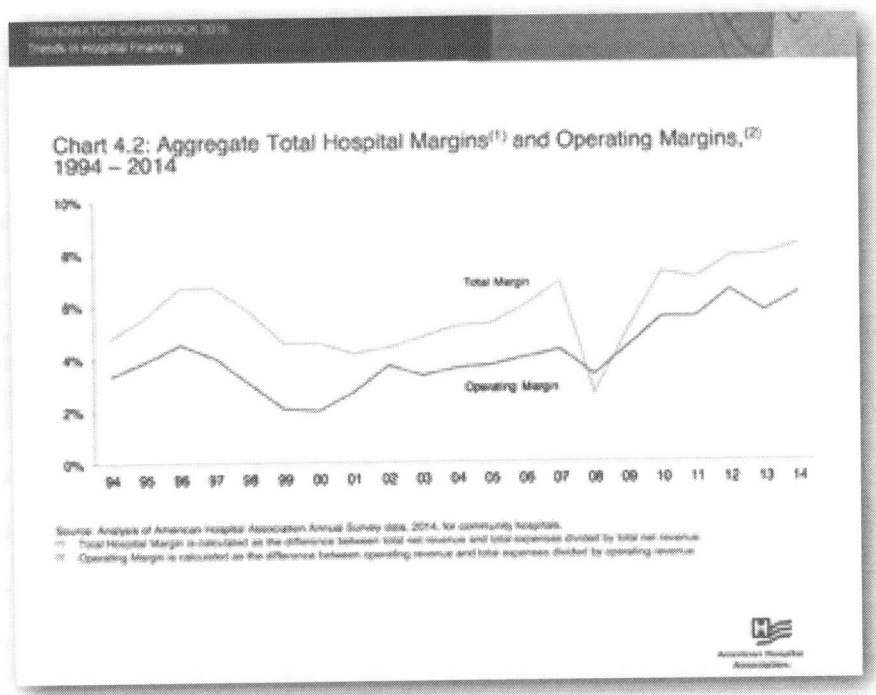

Graph 7 – Aggregate Hospital Margins: 1994-2014

The general sentiment of healthcare executives nation-wide is that healthcare reform *is working for both patients and providers* and should not be replaced without first having a definitive workable and viable alternative that is well vetted and remains *consumer-centric*. An unscientific survey reported in *Health Affairs Blog* December 2013 of hospital executives (74) from large academic health centers and referral hospitals (members of the University System Consortium and the National Association of Children's) were *favorable* about future changes resulting from the implementation of the ACA:[158]

- ✓ Fully 65 percent indicated that by 2020, they believe the healthcare system as a whole will be somewhat or significantly better than it is today
- ✓ Fully 93 percent predicted that the quality of care provided by their own system would improve [lower hospital acquired conditions, fewer medication errors, reduction of

---
157 American Hospital Association, see http://www.aha.org/research/reports/tw/chartbook/2016/table4-1.pdf
158 Andrew Steinmetz, et al., December 18, 2013, see http://healthaffairs.org/blog/2013/12/18/health-care-reform-views-from-the-hospital-executive-suite/

unnecessary re-admissions within 30 days of discharge, more appropriate ordering of tests, medications and procedures, etc.]
- ✓ 91 percent forecasted improvements on metrics of cost within their own health system by 2020 [shifting payment systems from fee-for-service to value-based incentives, bundled payments for high cost procedures, collaborative care systems, reducing unnecessary Emergency Room visits, population health management initiatives, efficiency strategies, enhanced use of EHR, expansion of ambulatory and home care, etc.]
- ✓ 31 percent anticipated savings from new payment methodologies within the Medicare and Medicaid programs

Health executives expressed reservations about the increasing complexity of administrative rules and regulations, more paperwork, and "lack of payment for coordination of services… and the lack of continuum-of-care reimbursement" as well as remuneration for preventive care and community health initiatives.[159] The graph [see original article URL] shows the cumulative healthcare executives' responses to the question: "If your organization's payers incentivized you [and your physicians] through some type of risk-based contract to reduce expenses, what do you believe are the three most likely ways your institution could reduce operating costs?"

The top three areas of hospital savings impacted by the ACA are: (1) reduction in the total number of hospitalizations, (2) reduction in the number of re-admissions within 30 days of discharge, and (3) reduction in the number of unnecessary ER visits (levels 1, 2, and 3). These executives estimated that the cumulative savings of these improvements across the entire US Health System could amount to $100 billion per year by 2020.

2.3 -- Transitioning from Volume to Value-Based Care

Our nation's leading hospitals have embarked on a momentous transformation, one that will benefit patients and improve our country's overall health. This process will take us from reliance on an outdated model – the hospital of today – to a state-of-the-art hospital of tomorrow.

The hospital of today is a stand-alone facility where services are provided mostly within its walls, and quality of care is too often measured by number of inpatient beds [for "sick-care"]. The number of inpatient beds in a hospital does not equate to better care in a community. This is an outdated metric, particularly in an era where numerous specialties, including pediatrics and HIV/AIDS, require mostly outpatient treatment. The hospital of tomorrow needs to be a large, integrated system providing extensive outpatient care beyond

---
[159] Ibid., p. 2.

> *its primary facility, dedicated to keeping community members healthy. A well-cared-for population should require less inpatient care, leading to lower demand for hospital beds.*
>
> *It's a matter of reactive versus proactive medicine.*
>
> Dr. Kenneth Davis, President and CEO of Mount Sinai Health System in New York City, Forbes, June 21, 2014.

Dr. Kenneth Davis, President and CEO of Mount Sinai Health System in New York City, exemplifies the "new" health leadership commitment to transform the way healthcare is delivered in America by supporting the ACA's goal of enhanced performance or **value-based care**.[160] Until the year 2000, the predominant provider-reimbursement approach by the government and commercial insurance companies was based on the number of procedures performed by providers on patients. This volume-based reimbursement system incentivizes overutilization of limited health resources; providers are financially rewarded for ordering more tests, admitting more patients, prescribing more medications, and referring more patients to specialists for additional high priced procedures. If a surgery is unintentionally botched, the insurer pays for the first procedure *and* the redo as well.

During the first decade of the 21st Century, HHS / CMS started several "innovation projects" involving Medicare and Medicaid patients focusing on *quality outcomes* and *cost-effectiveness of care* instead of just the intensity of treatment – they were encouraging *value-based* and *bundled-payment* systems. Large commercial insurance companies like United Healthcare, Aetna, Blue Cross Blue Shield, Cigna and others paid providers the regular fee-for-service rates **plus** bonuses for meeting specific care metrics that helped improve health status of their respective subscriber groups. *Advocate Health Partners* (a large integrated multi-hospital system with over 6,000 associated physicians) in Chicago, Illinois, were early adopters of value-based payment systems offered by government and private insurers receiving millions of dollars in bonus payments for their health improvement achievements year after year.[161]

ACA federal legislation incorporated value-based methodologies to foster measurable quality care indicators and "bend the cost curve." In a document entitled: *CMS Strategy: The Road Forward: 2013-2017*, the HHS Department charged with the responsibility of guiding the implementation of the healthcare reform program presented their strategic plan to transform the American health system from volume to value-based care.[162] Four central goals led CMS' efforts

---

160 See http://www.forbes.com/sites/robertlenzner/2014/05/21/the-hospital-of-tomorrow-redefining-hospitals-under-the-affordable-care-act/print/
161 *Advocate Health Partners 2009 Annual Value Report*, see https://www.advocatehealth.com/documents/app/value%20report.pdf
162 See https://www.cms.gov/About-CMS/Agency-Information/CMS-Strategy/Downloads/CMS-Strategy.pdf

and introduced a strong dependence on: (G1) better care and lower costs, (G2) prevention and population health, (G3) expanded health care coverage, and (G4) enterprise excellence.

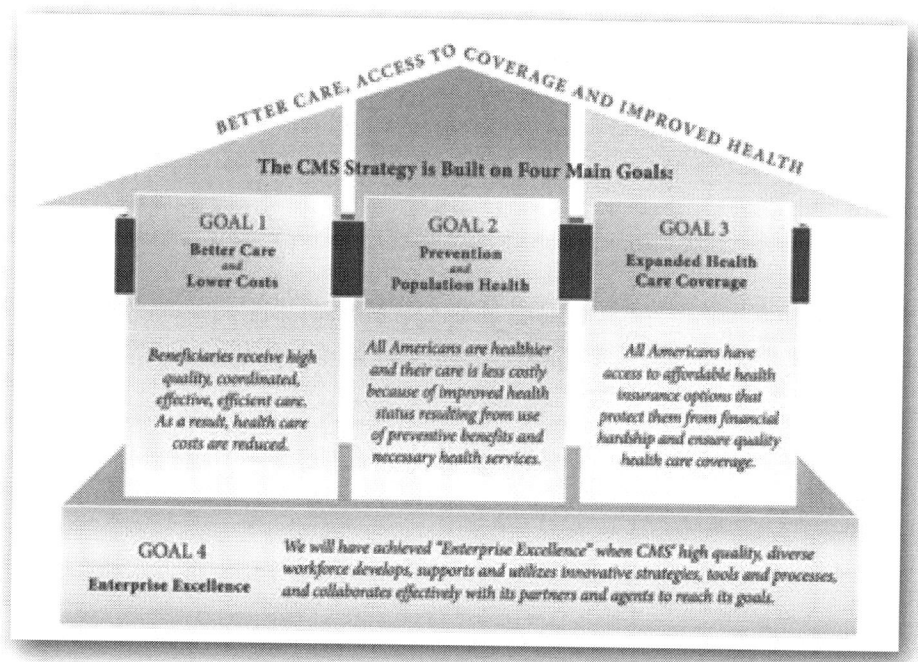

Figure 7 –CMS ACA Core Strategies and Goals: 2013-2017

Each of Ascension Health's *Goals* contain a series of implementation steps and associated measurable outcomes including, but not limited to:[163]

Improve Quality Care
- *Care is made safer by reducing harm caused in the delivery of care.*
- *Patients and families are engaged as informed, empowered partners in their care.*
- *Communication and care coordination across providers and health care facilities improves, leading to better health care quality at lower costs.*
- *A population-based approach to health care and preventive services improves health outcomes for all populations and helps individuals achieve their highest health-related quality of life [Population Health Management initiatives].*
- *The meaningful use of electronic health records results in better care, better coordination, and lower costs.*
- *Quality care is affordable for individuals, families, employers and governments.*

---
163 Ibid., for the complete list of CMS implementation steps and outcomes.

- *Integrated care models allow physicians and other providers to come together in new ways to better coordinate care.*

Improve Preventive Health Benefits
- *Use of evidence-based preventive services and primary care keeps individuals healthy, improves population health [status], and avoids adverse outcomes. CMS uses the latest scientific evidence to determine coverage.*
- *Disparities in the use of preventive benefits, community-based services, outreach, and education are identified and reduced.*

Strengthen Consumer Protections
- *Consumer protections in the private marketplace promote transparency into issuers' business operations and increases their accountability that results in cost savings for enrollees.*

Expand Coverage
- *Support to States as they create affordable insurance marketplaces reduce the number of uninsured and help ensure eligible individuals receive needed assistance.*

Strengthen Program Integrity
- *Compliance and oversight activities strengthen enforcement.*
- *Risk is managed and strategic investments provide high impact and rate of return.*
- *Decision makers and other key staff have necessary access to financial information related to Agency resources creating a more accountable, reliable, and transparent CMS.*

Improve Payment Models
- *Patient / provider incentives for better outcomes and more efficient care align payment with performance and provide new incentives that encourage care coordination, high quality, and efficient delivery. Value-based payment ensures providers are incentivized to provide high-quality, and efficient care.*
- *Claims processing accuracy and timeliness of payments to providers and States, through the use of electronic reporting tools and transparency; assure appropriate provision of care and services, and reduce the administrative burden for providers and States, while decreasing Agency administrative costs.*

Transform Business Operations
- *Regulatory burden decreases by reducing unnecessary, obsolete, or burdensome regulations, simplifying requirements of the public and private sectors, and enhancing net benefits of regulations.*

- *Efficiency and agility of "shared" and common support services promote timely access, transparency and communication, and improve service quality. The development of enterprise shared services, reduces costly redundancies and increases out effectiveness.*
- *Engagement with other public and private sector entities promote collaborative partnerships that enhance policy, operations, and other enterprise interests and initiatives. Partnerships extend the reach and impact of many programs aimed to improve the health and wellness of Americans.*
- *Investment in information systems expands the CMS knowledge base.*
- *New innovative technologies are adopted that enhance the availability, quality and delivery of information.*

CMS' strategies revolutionized the health delivery system in the United States throughout the progressive implementation of the ACA between 2013 to 2017, and facilitated radically new approaches to care throughout America. Key elements of the Plan driving the successful transformation of the US delivery of health services involved: sharing through communication and collaborative systems, emphasis on preventive services and primary care interventions, population health management initiatives, expanded application of EHR and sophisticated community health information networks, shared risk management arrangements, increased pricing transparency, exchange of patient clinical information, decision support systems, and regulation of private health insurance companies practices pertaining to policy subscribers and investor profits.

Mega health systems like the Catholic not-for-profit *Ascension Health* based in St. Louis, Missouri, quickly embraced CMS' new focus on *collaborative care* and *value-based reimbursement methodologies*.[164] Robert Henkel and Patricia Maryland, senior executives of Ascension Health, discuss their journey from the traditional volume-based payment system to value-based reimbursement including: "pay for performance (P4P), shared savings, bundled payments, shared risk, global capitation, and provider-sponsored health plans" in their article in the winter 2015 issue of the *Frontiers of Health Services Management Journal*.[165] Henkel and Maryland point to "today's fragmented delivery of care," as the culprit for ever increasing costs and less than satisfactory patient-centered quality care.[166] Ascension's leadership believe in the strategy of: "*Quadruple Aim*: improved health outcomes, enhanced patient experiences, and enhanced provider experiences at a lower overall cost of care." To achieve their goals, the authors stress:[167]

---

164 Ascension Health is the world's largest Catholic health system with 22,416 staffed beds and total operating revenue of $20.5 billion in 2015 (*Modern Healthcare*, 2016 hospital system survey based on 2015 figures).

165 Robert Henkel, FACHE, and Patricia Maryland, "The Risks and Rewards of Value-Based Reimbursement," *Frontiers of Health Services Management Journal*, ACHE, Winter 2015, 32:2, pp. 3-16, see http://journals.lww.com/frontiersonline/Fulltext/2015/10000/The_Risks_and_Rewards_of_Value_Based_Reimbursement.2.aspx

166 Ibid., p. 16.

167 Ibid., p. 6

Fundamental to our [Ascension Health] approach is the development of clinically integrated systems of care in each of our regions. A system of this scale requires collaboration among private-practice physicians, employed physicians, and other caregivers and health systems to develop a program of clinical initiatives that improves the quality and efficiency of care delivery. Clinically integrated systems of care are designed to collect and share data from all participating providers. This process fosters interdependence and collaboration among physicians and other clinicians that can lead to quality improvements and enhanced cost-effectiveness, as well as readily accessible health information for the people we serve. A fully developed clinically integrated system of care at Ascension includes evaluation, continuous clinical performance improvement, reduction of unnecessary services, and management and support for high-cost and high-risk patients.

The importance of *clinically integrated provider networks* (CIPN) can not be overemphasized. To be successful, CIPNs depend heavily on real-time health information systems that are available to providers at the time the patients present themselves at the points-of-care throughout the network. The intent of value-based initiatives is to improve the quality of care, reduce / eliminate unnecessary resource utilization, and ultimately bend the cost curve of health costs in America. Providers must efficiently share patient metrics and collaborate with each other in the delivery of care at all levels regardless of the type of value-based reimbursement methods.

Since 2011, Ascension Health has been evolving its integrated health delivery models using these strategic planning and implementation tools:[168]

- *Market Analysis* – assessing the degree of risk that is prevalent among cohorts in the communities that are served and insurance products that are available to the population.
- *Alignment* – fostering greater involvement of primary care physicians, specialists (employed and independent), and nurses in creating "high levels of positive patient experience and engagement" during the continuum of care contacts.
- *Infrastructure* – investing in sophisticated health information technology to supply necessary metrics to providers and decision-support managers that is timely and accurate to improve the quality of care and contain costs whenever appropriate.
- *Finances and Patient Volume* – managing the shift of business from inpatient, post-acute, outpatient, ambulatory, and wellbeing settings while maintaining financial solvency of the health system.
- *Payer Considerations* – forging win-win partnerships with government, private and commercial, and Marketplace insurers that are committed to "share the benefits" of performance improvement progress with providers that make value-based care possible.

---

168 Ibid., pp. 9-11.

The graphic representation below shows the multi-dimensional win-win relationships of Ascension Health's "Patients-First Approach" to the 21st Century health delivery system:[169]

Comparing *value-based incentive programs* with the *Health Maintenance Organization (HMO)*[170] *model* introduced in the US Congress in the early 1970s by Senator Edward Kennedy (D-Mass), the ultimate winners in HMO systems are the health insurance companies. The priority of HMOs is to curtail healthcare expenses. It is not surprising that HMOs had a short life span.

2.4 -- ACOs, Bundled Payments, Systems Consolidations, Population Health Management - Today's Collaborative Care Movement

"Only a few pages – four to be precise – of the Patient Protection and Affordable Care Act of 2010 (PPACA) are devoted to the development and deployment of the accountable care organization (ACO). Other than Medicare rate regulation, no other issue within the PPACA has stirred more interest, passion, and imagination among healthcare providers than the ACO."

MARC BARD AND MIKE NUGENT, (2011), ACCOUNTABLE CARE ORGANIZATIONS: YOUR GUIDE TO STRATEGY, DESIGN, AND IMPLEMENTATION, ACHE MANAGEMENT SERIES, HEALTH ADMINISTRATION PRESS, CHICAGO, P. 29

An obscure section buried in the 2,000 pages of the ACA permits providers and payers to collaborate and accelerate the transition from a *volume-based fee-for-service* (FFS) provider payment system to *patient-centered value-based* systems for Medicare patients and commercially insured non-seniors. Value-based systems financially reward stakeholders for significantly improving quality of care and controlling rising healthcare costs. The ACA collaborative care movement generated an array of innovative reimbursement and incentive payment schemes tied to exceeding pre-established performance metrics and improvement goals.

Leavitt Partners' Center for Accountable Care Intelligence summarized the extent that risk plays in value-based systems under the ACA in financial arrangements between providers and payers:[171] [172]

---

169 Ibid., p.13
170 HHS definition, see https://www.healthcare.gov/glossary/health-maintenance-organization-HMO/
171 See reports from Leavitt Partners, http://leavittpartners.com/category/white-papers/
172 Tianna Tu, et al., Accountable Care Organizations and Risk-Based Payment Arrangements: Strong Preference for Upside-Only Contracts, Leavitt Partners White Paper, November 30, 2016, p. 3, see http://leavittpartners.com/2016/11/accountable-care-organizations-and-risk-based-payment-arrangements-strong-preference-for-upside-only-contracts/

Figure 8 – Progression of Payment Arrangement Risk Models

episode-based → **INCREASING RISK** → population-based

POPULATION-BASED

[PRE-ACO]   FFS → CASE MGT → P4P →
[ACO]   SHARED SAVINGS → SHARED SAVINGS / LOSSES → PARTIAL CAPITATION → FULL CAPITATION

EPISODE-BASED

USUAL & CUSTOMARY → FEE SCHEDULE → PROSPECTIVE PAYM → BUNDLED PAYM

Accountable Care Organizations (ACOs) were authorized by Sec. 3022 Of PPACA that amends Title XVIII of the Social Security Act by adding Sec. 1899, the *Shared Savings Program.* [173] The essential requirements / criteria listed in the *Final Rules* for obtaining approval from the Secretary of Health and Human Services to operate as an ACO were published in the **Federal Register**, Vol. 76, No. 212, on November 2, 2011 (verbatim text):[174]

---

173 See detailed summary of the Shared Savings Program, https://www.ssa.gov/OP_Home/ssact/title18/1899.htm
174 See HHS FINAL RULES published in the **Federal Register**, Vol. 76, No. 212, November 2, 2011, p. 67822, at http://docplayer.net/1541331-Department-of-health-and-human-services-part-ii.html ; and updated June 9, 2015, FR Vol. 80, No. 110, pp. 32692-32845, at https://www.gpo.gov/fdsys/pkg/FR-2015-06-09/pdf/2015-14005.pdf

- *The ACO's operations would be managed by an executive, officer, manager, or general partner, whose appointment and removal are under the control of the organization's governing body and whose leadership team has demonstrated the ability to influence or direct clinical practice to improve efficiency processes and outcomes.*
- *Clinical management and oversight would be managed by a senior-level medical director who is a board-certified physician, licensed in the State in which the ACO operates, and physically present on a regular basis in an established location of the ACO.*
- *ACO participants and ACO providers / suppliers would have a meaningful commitment to the ACO's clinical integration program to ensure its likely success.*
- *The ACO would have a physician-directed quality assurance and process improvement committee that would oversee an ongoing quality assurance and improvement program.*
- *The ACO would develop and implement evidence-based medical practice or clinical guidelines and processes for delivering care consistent with the goals of better care for individuals, better health for populations, and lower growth in expenditures.*
- *The ACO would have an infrastructure, such as information technology, that enables the ACO to collect and evaluate data and provide feedback to the ACO providers/ suppliers across the entire organization, including providing information to influence care at the point of service.*

In order to determine an ACO's compliance with these requirements, as part of the application process we proposed that an ACO would submit all of the following:

- *ACO documents (for example, participation agreements, employment contracts, and operating policies) that describe the ACO participants' and ACO providers' / suppliers' rights and obligations in the ACO, how the opportunity to receive shared savings will encourage ACO participants and ACO providers/suppliers to adhere to the quality assurance and improvement program and the evidenced-based clinical guidelines.*
- *Documents that describe the scope and scale of the quality assurance and clinical integration program, including documents that describe all relevant clinical integration program systems and processes.*
- *Supporting materials documenting the ACO's organization and management structure, including an organizational chart, a list of committees (including the names of committee*

- *members) and their structures, and job descriptions for senior administrative and clinical leaders.*
- *Evidence that the ACO has a board-certified physician as its medical director who is licensed in the State in which the ACO resides and that a principal CMS liaison is identified in its leadership structure.*
- *Evidence that the governing body includes persons who represent the ACO participants, and that these ACO participants hold at least 75 percent control of the governing body. Additionally, upon request, the ACO would also be required to provide copies of the following documents:*
- *Documents effectuating the ACO's formation and operation, including charters, by-laws, articles of incorporation, and partnership, joint venture, management, or asset purchase agreements.*
- *Descriptions of the remedial processes that will apply when ACO participants and ACO providers/ suppliers fail to comply with the ACO's internal procedures and performance standards, including corrective action plans and the circumstances under which expulsion could occur.*

Once approved, ACOs (as a legal entity) can participate in financial incentives through MSSP and commercial programs contracted with insurers if they meet or exceed the HHS / CMS guidelines for specific quality and cost targets. The ACO quality measures are aimed at "improving beneficiary outcomes and increasing value of care," shown in the *example* below (issued March 2016, ICN 907407):[175]

The most prevalent **accountable care and incentive models** adopted by Accountable Care Organizations (ACOs) include: Pay-for-Performance, Shared Savings Programs, Bundled Payment Experiments, Shared Risk Arrangements, Hospital Readmission Reduction Program, Integrated Delivery Systems, Comprehensive Primary Care Initiatives, and Global Capitation for high-risk cohorts. We will explore these novel value-based reimbursement alternatives to traditional FFS.

1. **Pay-for-Performance (P4P)**

    The Centers for Medicare and Medicaid (CMS) have endorsed pay-for-performance incentive payments to selected provider / physician groups since 2005 as an effective method to encourage systematic changes in the healthcare delivery system. CMS explains that its goal for the P4P strategy is to "promote the 'right care for every patient every time.'" [176] Their definition of this goal includes care that is: (1) safe, (2) effective, (3) patient-centered, (4) timely, (5) efficient, and (6) equitable. P4P is often associated with *bundled payment demonstrations* contracts sponsored by CMS as an add-on payment for meeting or exceeding pre-established evidence-based measures of quality and cost targets. P4P incentives are considered both a part of the providers' practice revenue, and / or viewed as a performance bonus.

2. **Shared Savings Program (SSP)**

    The SSP was created by Section 3022 of the ACA. The program encourages providers and suppliers (paid on a FFS basis) to collaborate for the purpose of improving the quality and reduce unnecessary and duplicative costs of care. CMS rewards ACOs with a *portion* of the overall beneficiaries' savings realized through initiatives that enhance quality and "lower their [assigned group of Medicare beneficiaries] growth in health care costs,"[177] during the contracted period of a year.

    NOTE -- Participation of beneficiaries in an ACO is purely voluntary.

---

[175] See https://www.cms.gov/Medicare/Medicare-Fee-for-Service-Payment/sharedsavingsprogram/index.html?redirect=/sharedsavingsprogram and https://www.cms.gov/Medicare/Medicare-Fee-for-Service-Payment/sharedsavingsprogram/Downloads/ACO_Quality_Factsheet_ICN907407.pdf

[176] CMS PQRS / P4P guidelines, October 11, 2016, see https://www.cms.gov/Medicare/Quality-Initiatives-Patient-Assessment-Instruments/PQRS/index.html

[177] CMS.gov, *Shared Savings Program*, see https://www.cms.gov/Medicare/Medicare-Fee-for-Service-Payment/sharedsavingsprogram/index.html?redirect=sharedsavingsprogram and https://www.cms.gov/Medicare/Medicare-Fee-for-Service-Payment/sharedsavingsprogram/Downloads/ACO_Rural_Factsheet_ICN907408.pdf

3. **Bundled Payments for Care Improvement Initiative (BPCI)**

   According to CMS' Innovation Center (created by the ACA), the BPCI program is intended to contract with providers offering multiple services related to a specific *episode of care*. The BPCI motivates the full continuum of providers to actively collaborate on the entire treatment process from start to finish (instead of reimbursing individual providers separately at various stages of the continuum). The BPCI program started in 2013 and was updated in 2016 – four models were offered by CMS to providers:[178] High-cost patient groups were selected initially for the BPCI – cardiovascular surgery patients, orthopedic joint replacement surgery patients, endocrinology chronic disease patients, etc. Other patient cohorts were added to the program after January 2016.

   Model 1 – *Retrospective Acute Care Hospital Stay Only.* Hospitals are paid a discounted payment for an inpatient episode of care "consistent with rates established under the Inpatient Prospective Payment System used in the original Medicare program." Physicians are paid separately according to the Medicare fee schedule.

   Model 2 – *Retrospective Acute Care Hospital Stay Plus Post-Acute Care.* Bundled payments are made to Hospitals and / or a Physician Group for a patient's episode of care (up to 48 different clinical conditions) over a period of 30, 60, or 90 days after discharge from the hospital. The discounted bundled payment is made for provider facilities, physician services, and Medicare Part B services tied to the patient's episode of care.

   Model 3 – *Retrospective Post-Acute Care Only.* Bundled payments apply to post-acute care facilities after discharge from a hospital: skilled nursing facilities, inpatient rehabilitation facilities, long-term care hospitals, or home health agencies within 30 days of discharge from an inpatient hospital. The discounted bundled payment is made for provider facilities, physician services, and Medicare Part B services tied to the patient's episode of care.

   Model 4 – *Prospective Acute Care Hospital Stay Only.* Prospectively determined bundled payments are made to the hospital only for all related services an episode of care to inpatients during the entire duration of the stay. The hospital is responsible for paying all members of the contracted care team involved within 30 days of discharge from the hospital.

   NOTE: Beneficiaries retain the right to choose providers not participating in the CMS BPCI initiative. Readmissions of patients within 30 days of the original discharge from the hospital for an episode of care are considered an inclusive part of a single bundled payment.

---

178 CMS.gov, *Bundled Payments for Care Improvement Initiative*, see https://www.cms.gov/Newsroom/MediaReleaseDatabase/Fact-sheets/2016-Fact-sheets-items/2016-04-18.html

4. Shared Risk Arrangements (SRA)

The SRA program has similar participating criteria to CMS' SSP program, with higher *upside and downside risks* for providers caring for designated at-risk populations.[179] Essentially, the higher the provider risk, the higher the reward or loss.

Table 5 – CMS Parts A and B Shared Risk Arrangement Levels

Arrangement A – Increased Shared Risk
Parts A and B Shared Risk
- 80% shared rate (PY1-3, 2016-2018)
- 85% sharing rate (PY4-5, 2019-2020)
- 15% savings / losses cap

Arrangement B – Full Performance Risk
100% Risk for Parts A and B
- 15% savings / losses cap

5. Hospital Readmission Reduction Program (HRRP)

In 2012, HHS CMS published rules for the HRRP in response for escalating readmissions to Medicare contracted hospitals.[180] Participating hospitals receive financial incentives (or penalties) based on meeting quality of care performance benchmarks / criteria, reduction of unnecessary readmissions to any hospital within 30 days of the original hospitalization episode, and patient outcomes. The first patient groups considered by the HRRP include acute myocardial infarction (AMI), heart failure, and pneumonia cases. On May 7, 2014, CMS published very promising findings resulting from these and other ACA's initiatives to combat hospital acquired conditions and readmission rates of Medicare patients cared for at participating health facilities – showing an impressive drop from 19.5% in 2009 to 17.5% the end of 2013.[181]

The following additional high-cost patient groups were included at later dates to the list of participating hospitals with a minimum of 25 inpatient cases over a three-year period in each category:

---

[179] See CMS presentation, page 13, at https://innovation.cms.gov/Files/slides/nextgenaco-appprocessodf.pdf

[180] CMS Fact Sheet, Hospital Readmission Reduction Program, starting 2012, see https://www.cms.gov/medicare/medicare-fee-for-service-payment/acuteinpatientpps/readmissions-reduction-program.html; also see incentive / penalty computation formula in the fact sheet.

[181] CMS Office of Information Products and Data Analytics Report, see https://innovation.cms.gov/Files/reports/patient-safety-results.pdf; the readmissions trend through the end of 2013 fell to approximately 17.5% from a peak of 19.5% in January 2009, representing 150,000 fewer hospital readmissions and an 8 percent reduction in Medicare fee-for-service all-cause 30-day readmissions rate.

- ✓ Chronic obstructive pulmonary disease (COPD)
- ✓ Elective total hip and total knee replacement
- ✓ Coronary artery bypass graft (CABG) surgery
- ✓ Readmissions for pneumonia diagnosis with co-morbidities of (a) aspiration pneumonia, and (b) severe sepsis
- ✓ Selective other chronic diseases

6. **Integrated Delivery System (IDS)**

   HHS CMS recognizes that hospitals, health systems, and post-acute care facilities can not achieve progress toward the HRRP and other ACO initiatives without the commitment and active participation of physicians and other providers associated with the delivery of care to patients. The federal government health agency explains: "Section 646 of the Medicare Modernization Act (MMA) mandates 5-year demonstration programs under which the Centers for Medicare & Medicaid Services (CMS) will test major changes to improve quality of care while increasing efficiency across an entire health care system."[182] Approved CMS provider demonstration grants are supporting the establishment of Integrated Care Delivery Systems (IDS), Community-wide Health Information Exchanges (CHINs), Community Care Networks (CCN)s, Regional Health Care Consortia of providers, and other innovative arrangements for Medicare patient populations. Members of these arrangements can share in the financial rewards paid by Medicare for:

   - ✓ Improving patient safety
   - ✓ Enhancing quality care and patient outcomes
   - ✓ Increasing delivery of care efficiency and coordination
   - ✓ Reducing scientific uncertainty and the unwarranted variation in medical practice that results in both lower quality and higher costs (via Health Information Exchanges and Evidence-based Medicine systems)

   The future of the IDS is up in the air as ACOs have become the preferred quality / savings approach supported by CMS.

7. **Comprehensive Primary Care Initiatives (CPC)**

   The CPC program is an initiative of the CMS Center for Innovation launched in 2012 to advance "high-value primacy care" for contracted primary care physician groups (PCP).[183] The CPC program aims to accomplish:

---

[182] CMS Fact Sheet, Medicare Health Care Quality Demonstration, see https://innovation.cms.gov/initiatives/Medicare-Health-Care-Quality/

[183] CMS Fact Sheet, Comprehensive Primary Care Initiative, updated August 22, 2012, see https://innovation.cms.gov/Files/fact-sheet/Comprehensive-Primary-Care-Initiative-Fact-Sheet.pdf

- ✓ Managing Care for Patients with High Health Care Needs
- ✓ Ensuring Access to Care
- ✓ Delivering Preventive Care
- ✓ Engaging Patients and Caregivers
- ✓ Coordinating Care Across the Medical Neighborhood

NOTE -- The CMS Fact Sheet on the CPC program states: "Primary care is the first point of contact for many patients, and takes the lead in coordinating care as the center of patients' experiences with medical care. Under this initiative, primary care doctors and nurses will work together and with a patient's other health care providers and the patient to make decisions as a team. Access to and meaningful use of electronic health records should be used to support these efforts." In 2016, CMS authorized the second 5-year Comprehensive Primary Care Initiatives (CPC +) program expanding coordinated primary care to Americans starting January 2017.[184] CPC + is expected to encompass 5,000 primary care practices serving 3.5 million beneficiaries in 14 regions of the country. CPC + provider groups receive a monthly supplemental payment for CMS along with the customary fee-for-service compensation.

8. **Global Capitation**

Pure capitation arrangements (*payment per member per month* – PMPM) are most commonly associated with Health Maintenance Organizations (HMOs) tied to commercial health insurance companies, Global Capitation is a fixed amount allocated to provider networks on a per capita basis. HMOs can keep excess funds over cost of care, or may share the savings with insurers or larger self-insured employer groups. Controlling HMO utilization volume and costs are the main considerations for success.

Providers, insurers, and beneficiaries have generally embraced the ACO value-based reimbursement program throughout the United States. An important consideration by participants is the flexibility for attaining incentive payments and reliance on "real" quality indicators and cost improvements so that providers and payers can share in the savings realized by the collaborative networks. Hospitals and Health Systems are moving outside of the inpatient care walls into the communities they serve with resources for PHM preventive care and wellbeing initiatives for at-risk patients. Information compiled by the *Leavitt Partners* and published in the *HealthAffairs. org*[185] present evidence of the steady growth in the number of ACOs and lives covered by

---

[184] See CMS News Release at https://www.cms.gov/Newsroom/MediaReleaseDatabase/Press-releases/2016-Press-releases-items/2016-08-01.html

[185] See report http://healthaffairs.org/blog/2016/04/21/accountable-care-organizations-in-2016-private-and-public-sector-growth-and-dispersion/

the value-based program. By the end of the first quarter of 2016, and three years into the technical implementation of the ACA, the number of operational ACOs reached 838; a majority in the most populous states (California, Florida, Texas, Illinois, New York, Pennsylvania Michigan, Minnesota and Ohio).[186]

These ACOs had 28.3 million covered lives, with 17.2 million (61%) participating in commercial contractual arrangements, and 11.2 enrollees in Medicare and Medicaid contractual arrangements.

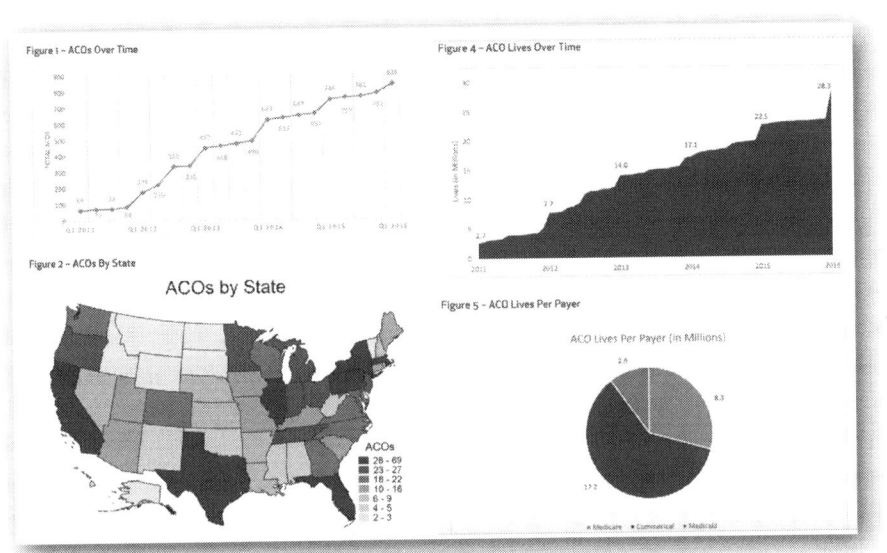

Graph 8 a, b, c, and d - ACO Activity from 2011 to 2016

These data reinforce the government's optimism about the long term success of of the ACA and Accountable Care Organizations along with financial incentives for performance improvement measures. ACOs have hastened the transition of national health care delivery systems from fee-for-service reimbursement (volume driven), to accountable and collaborative models driven by evidence-based medicine and quality / costs metrics in America. However, David Muhlestein and Mark McClellan caution, in their *Health Affairs Blog*, that the future of ACOs remains tenuous.[187] They state:

> *As accountable care payment mechanisms become more widespread and mature, we expect attention will shift to the challenges facing providers in adapting to such mechanisms. ACO leaders face many challenges in redesigning care, including achieving organizational buy-in, using technology to manage a population, and aligning intra-organizational incentives – all while making measurable progress on quality and cost.*

---

186 By the Numbers, "*States with the most ACOs: Ranked by number of ACOs*," *Modern Healthcare*, August 8, 2016, p.35; top 10 ranking states noted.
187 Ibid., p. 7 or 9.

> At the heart of becoming an ACO is changing how an organization operates. Organizational change is hard in any industry, but it is exacerbated in health care due to the fee-for-service infrastructure that has been designed over decades to focus organizations on volume. Shifting from that focus requires a significant amount of structural change, but more importantly, it requires individual providers to change how they practice medicine.

The flip side of the long standing healthcare reform debate is that the historical growth trend of overall costs in the United States is **not** sustainable beyond 2020 when expenditures are projected to be 20 percent of the US GDP. [My projection in the original 2009 thesis proposed an *economic break-point* close to $4 trillion per year – *the healthcare tab in 2016 topped $3.2 trillion*]. The consensus among healthcare leaders and providers is that ACOs represent another proactive step in the right direction to reform the American health delivery systems. Providers' mindset about value-based healthcare in this country has slowly improved.

The December 13, 2012 issue of *Health Policy Brief* from *Health Affairs* addressed the **upside opportunity** for substantial savings and cost reductions in the American health system estimated at 34 percent (midpoint estimate of 2011 spending) of the total annual expenditures.[188] A large portion of "wasteful" healthcare dollars paid out by government and commercial insurers identified by HHS CMS are due to six broad categories:[189]

1. Failures of care delivery – providers' poor execution of services clinical failures / adverse events and outcomes, unjustified regional variation in utilization and practice patterns, and minimal investment in preventive care
2. Failures of care coordination – fragmented and duplicative care practices, poor health information systems, and lack of shared patient data
3. Overtreatment – defensive medicine and outdated practice patterns
4. Administrative complexity – lack of standardization, billing / coding errors, excessive regulations and bureaucratic procedures / processes
5. Pricing failures – lack of transparency and market price competitiveness
6. Fraud and abuse – fake bills, unjustified surgeries, tests, and procedures, and costs related to inspections and regulatory enforcement

These *controllable waste factors* amounted to about $900 billion of the $2.7 trillion spent on healthcare in 2011. Accountable care and incentive models built into the ACA can make a serious dent in these unnecessary costs of healthcare in the United States in all these categories. In the

---

188 Health Policy Brief, "Reducing Waste in Health Care," December 13, 2013, see http://healthaffairs.org/healthpolicy-briefs/brief_pdfs/healthpolicybrief_82.pdf
189 Ibid., p. 2.

March 2012 article by Dr. Donald Berwick, MD, MPP and Andrew Hackbarth, MPhil, "Eliminating Waste in US Health Care," published in the *Journal of the American Medical Association* (JAMA), present the "% of GDP Wedges" graph below that shows the projected growth trend in spending reduction opportunities for the six healthcare categories of waste from 2011 to 2020:[190]

Henkel and Maryland (from *Ascension Health*, 2015)[191] caution providers that there are definitely *downside risk realities* to value-based P4P and shared-savings arrangements between ACOs and payers. Some of the most salient risks include: (1) the fact that there are no guarantees providers can actually offset the substantial upfront HIT and administrative investments necessary to create accountable care / savings initiatives with payer-rewards for bending the cost curve, (2) physicians are slow to change practice behaviors and adopt evidence-based best-practices that help reduce utilization and waste, (3) population cohorts and regional variability can have a huge impact on profits and losses under risk and capitation models, and (4) there is a finite cost reduction limitation over time even when excessive healthcare costs *start out* in the 20% to 40% in a particular health service area.

If the ACA were to be totally *repealed*, as Congressional Republican legislators have promised since 2010, I believe that the nation's providers and payers would likely migrate back to a predominantly fee-for-service reimbursement paradigm. This scenario rewards provider over-utilization, run away cost increases, less than optimal quality care, and perhaps over 25 million or more lower income Americans without access to *any* health insurance protection. Politicians must represent *everyone* in need of healthcare insurance coverage and be willing to continuously improve the ACA where it is not working satisfactorily, while strengthening regulations that offer *basic* access to quality healthcare for all citizens.

Chapters 4 and 5 of Section 2 attempt to address the crucial health policy question: *"What **are** the missing links in the current version of the ACA legislation that could dramatically enhance healthcare coverage for all Americans?"*

---

190 JAMA, *Special Communication* (online), March 14, 2012 p. E3, see http://www.christianacare.org/documents/valueinstitute/Berwick-Hackbarth%20-%20Eliminating%20Waste.pdf
191 Robert Henkel, FACHE, and Patricia Maryland, "The Risks and Rewards of Value-Based Reimbursement," *Frontiers of Health Services Management Journal*, ACHE, Winter 2015, 32:2, pp. 3-16, see http://journals.lww.com/frontiersonline/Fulltext/2015/10000/The_Risks_and_Rewards_of_Value_Based_Reimbursement.2.aspx

Three

Weathering of the Political Storm

3.1 -- The "Unprecedented" Presidential Election of 2016

The 2016 election has been characterized by political pundits as the most contentious in the past century in the United States. Republicans started out with a slate of 17 Presidential candidates and ended up with the nominating of Donald Trump for the Party's representative at the November 8th election. Democrats offered 3 candidates in the primary race – including former First Lady and US Secretary of State Hillary Rodham Clinton. She won the Democratic Party nomination. Without getting into the nitty-gritty of the Presidential race, the contrast between the two leading parties could not have been more salient. Clinton represented the status quo, supported by incumbent two-term President Barack Obama, and promised to support and enhance the ACA. Trump advocated radical change for the health policy direction of the country, vowing to "repeal and replace" ObamaCare.

On election day, the level of excitement and anticipation across America and the world was intense. I recall being glued to the television watching in amazement as the states reported their results late into the evening of Tuesday, November 8th. At 11:45 pm Hillary Clinton conceded the election to Donald Trump who had accumulated 289 Electoral College votes with 92% of the ballots counted nation-wide. Ultimately, Clinton and her VP running mate, US Senator (D – Virginia) Tim Kaine, captured the highest number of *popular votes* totaling 65.8 million, or 48.0 to 45.9 percent of all votes. The next morning, billionaire and business entrepreneur Trump and his Vice President candidate (VP) Mike Pence (R - Governor of Indiana) were declared winners of **304 Electoral College votes –** exceeding the 270 minimum necessary to assume the Presidency.

Republicans also gained control of the US Senate and retained a majority of seats in the US House of Representatives on November 8, 2016. During several weeks following the election, hundreds of thousands of citizens filled the streets of American cities chanting their convictions about Clinton or Trump. The media reported accusations of "massive" voter fraud, demonstrations, and claims by Federal Intelligence Agencies that foreign cyber-criminals had hacked the US election system to skew the results for Trump.[192] *Confusion reigned.*

Trump's principal campaign themes and slogans during the 2016 election campaign were:

- ✓ Need for wholesale changes in governmental leadership in Washington DC -- *"Drain the swamp."*
- ✓ Repeal and replace the ACA with a Republican version of healthcare reform – *"ObamaCare is a disaster."*
- ✓ Urgency of immigration reform and extending the border wall between Mexico and the United states – *"Mexico will pay for the wall."*
- ✓ Stimulating business expansion initiatives through tax and international trade pack reforms – *"Make America great again."*

Trump's call for repealing ObamaCare was *music to the ears* of at least 50 percent of adult Americans at rallies during his 16 months along the campaign trail. His disdain for Universal Health Insurance Coverage is indicated by these samplings of public statements and Internet tweets:

- *The ACA has "gotta go" and that he [Trump] would repeal the law and replace it with "something terrific."*[193]
- *According to Dan Diamond, contributor to Forbes Magazine, "Donald Trump has never supported socialized medicine. In 'The America We Deserve,' Mr. Trump called for health market reforms that would be 'affordable, well-administered, and provide freedom of choice'… The only solution is a free market oriented [sic.] plan that provides consumer choice, keeps plans portable and affordable and returns authority to the states. We also must break the insurance company monopolies and allow individuals to purchase health insurance across state lines."*[194]
- *"People must remember that ObamaCare just doesn't work, and it is not affordable. Bill Clinton called it 'CRAZY'"*[195]

---

192 Adam Goldman and Matt Apuzzo, December 15, 2016, "US Faces Tall Hurdles in Detaining or Deterring Russian Hackers," **The New York Times**, see https://www.nytimes.com/2016/12/15/us/politics/russian-hackers-election.html?_r=0

193 See Dan Diamond, Contributor, **Forbes**, see http://www.forbes.com/sites/dandiamond/2015/07/31/donald-trump-hates-obamacare-so-i-asked-him-how-hed-replace-it/#1578927b5d5e

194 Ibid.

195 See *Twitter Account*, https://twitter.com/realDonaldTrump/status/816264484629184513

Modern Healthcare reporter Bob Herman summed up the prevailing sentiment throughout the healthcare provider community in his November 9, 2016 article:[196]

> *That shift [in healthcare policies] will spill over to Americans with practically any type of health coverage -- Medicare, Medicaid, employer-based or individual -- which is creating anxiety for many in the industry and consumers alike. Among the most immediately affected were Medicaid-centric insurers, such as Centene Corp., Molina Healthcare and WellCare Health Plans, which took a beating in the stock markets Wednesday presuming the flood of Medicaid enrollees will come to a screeching halt.*
>
> *'We weren't expecting this. All the polling seemed to point to (Hillary) Clinton winning,' Molina Healthcare CEO Dr. J. Mario Molina told Modern Healthcare on Wednesday. 'I watched the returns last night, and all the political pundits, whether they were Democrats or Republicans, were surprised.'*
>
> *… With Republicans controlling the White House, Congress and a vast majority of statehouses, they're poised to shift Medicaid funding to block grants. Medicare premium support and the push toward more privatized Medicare Advantage plans also will be championed. Employer-based coverage has not oscillated much under the ACA, but even there the terrain will shift with the likely demise of the so-called Cadillac tax and employer mandate.*
>
> *Republicans are almost certain to eliminate the vital underpinnings of the ACA's coverage provisions: the individual mandate to buy health insurance, the premium and cost-sharing subsidies, and Medicaid expansion funding.*
>
> *One of the most popular provisions of the ACA is the prohibition against health plans charging more or denying coverage to people who have pre-existing health conditions. This policy is known as guaranteed issue. But the ACA included the individual mandate as a way to get healthier people to buy coverage and offset the higher costs of those sicker people. Removing the mandate but requiring insurers to cover all people isn't feasible from a policy perspective.*
>
> *'If you take one of those away, this doesn't work,' said Craig Garthwaite, a health economist at Northwestern University. "If you want to get rid of the mandate, you have to go back to underwriting."*

Trump was sworn in as the 45th President of the United States at noon on January 20, 2017.[197]

---

196 Bob Herman, November 9, 2016, "Trump, GOP sweep may disrupt every corner of health insurance market," Modern Healthcare, see http://www.modernhealthcare.com/article/20161109/NEWS/161109901?template=print

197 See **Huffington Post** article, at http://www.huffingtonpost.com/entry/2016-presidential-election-analysis-the-trump-cards_us_5845bdd3e4b0707e4c81715b

Republicans in the US Congress have proposed many alternatives to the ACA since March 2010 and none were successfully advanced. In the weeks prior to his being sworn in as President of the United States, Trump claimed he had a *replacement plan ready to go*, and that the repeal and replace process would be simultaneous. However, no definitive Republican-backed health plan had been shared with the public as of the inauguration celebration on January 20, 2010.

Thousands of Americans attended the inaugural celebrations for Donald Trump in the nation's Capitol. **The same afternoon shortly after the inauguration, President Trump made good on one of his key campaign promises by signing his first Executive Order directing the Congress to prepare legislation to "repeal and replace" ObamaCare**. According to CNN Wire:

> WASHINGTON — President Donald Trump on Friday night signed an executive order aimed at trying to fulfill one of his most impassioned campaign promises: Rolling back ObamaCare. The executive order signed in the Oval Office is designed "to ease the burden of ObamaCare as we transition from repeal and replace," White House press secretary Sean Spicer told reporters. Spicer did not respond when asked for further details.[198]

Although it takes an Act of Congress to repeal and replace all or parts of the ACA and enact new healthcare legislation, Trump's executive action on January 20th sent a loud and clear message that he meant business, and that millions covered by ObamaCare will have another insurance system to deal with in the near future. The Executive Order instructs government officials of agencies overseeing the implementation of the ACA regulations:

> Sec. 2. To the maximum extent permitted by law, the Secretary of Health and Human Services (Secretary) and the heads of all other executive departments and agencies (agencies) with authorities and responsibilities under the Act shall exercise all authority and discretion available to them to waive, defer, grant exemptions from, or delay the implementation of any provision or requirement of the Act that would impose a fiscal burden on any State or a cost, fee, tax, penalty, or regulatory burden on individuals, families, healthcare providers, health insurers, patients, recipients of healthcare services, purchasers of health insurance, or makers of medical devices, products, or medications.[199]

To carry out and oversee the replacement of ObamaCare, Trump quickly forwarded his nomination of US Representative Tom Price (R – Georgia) to the US Senate for confirmation to the post of Secretary of Health and Human Services. Dr. Price is a 63-year-old physician-politician (former

---

[198] See http://www.cnn.com/2017/01/20/politics/trump-signs-executive-order-on-ObamaCare/index.html
[199] See http://www.cnn.com/2017/01/20/politics/trump-ObamaCare-executive-order/index.html

practicing orthopedic surgeon) who has served in Congress since 2005 as the representative of Georgia's 6th congressional district, encompassing the northern portion of Atlanta's suburbs.

US Representative Price is on record opposing federal funding for elective abortion procedures. He sponsored the *Empowering Patients First Act* (EPFA) in 2009 – H.R. 3400 in the 111th Congress (July 30, 2009) as the Republican alternative to the Democratic bill that became the *Patient Protection and Affordable Care Act* (PPACA) of 2010 signed into law by President Obama March 23. 2010. The EPFA bill was reintroduced during the 112th (September 21, 2011) and 113th (June 6, 2013) Congressional Sessions, respectively as H.R.3000 and H.R. 2300. Senator John McCain (R – Arizona) introduced a *mirror healthcare bill* S. 1851 in the 113th Congressional Session. The EPFA failed to secure Congressional approval in all instance. An article in the *Washington Post*, October 7, 2009, by Ezra Klein, highlighted the main concerns over the proposed EPFA legislation:[200]

- No federal requirement for individual mandate under the universal health insurance coverage in order to spread risk among younger healthy persons and contribute revenue to cover sicker populations
- No federal requirement of insurers to accept *all* applicants regardless of pre-existing and catastrophic health conditions
- No federal mandate of insurer-guaranteed issuance of coverage or community rating
- Suggestion to move persons with pre-existing and high-risk conditions to "risk pools" operated by state-sponsored programs – typically these premiums are cost-prohibitive to subscribers

The 2015 version of the EPFA includes additional provisions summarized below by the *Kaiser Family Foundation*:[201]

- Repeal of the ACA in its entirety
- Promote tax exempt Health Saving Accounts (HSAs) as a way for subscribers to pay for health insurance costs
- Federal tax credits to assist to pay for health insurance coverage would be changed to be based on *age* and not *family income* as is the case with the ACA
- The ACA *Essential Health Benefits* (EHB) requirement for health insurance companies would be discarded resulting in much more limited coverage plans
- Elimination of the ACA requirement to include parental coverage of dependent children up to age 26

---

200 Ezra Klein, "Representative Tom Price's 'Empowering Patients First' Act," see http://voices.washingtonpost.com/ezra-klein/2009/10/rep_tom_prices_empower_patient.html
201 See http://kff.org/report-section/proposals-to-replace-the-affordable-care-act-rep-tom-price/

- Permission for insurers to sell plans across state lines
- Repeal of ACA support for expansion of state Medicaid programs

After lengthy confirmation hearings before the Senate Health, Education, Labor and Pensions Committee and vigorous opposition voiced by Democratic Senators, Tom Price's nomination to head up HHS was approved (52 *Aye*, 47 *Nay*) by the US Senate on February 10, 2017 (2:00 am) and a straight party-line simple majority vote. Vice President Pence swore Dr. Price into office Friday morning as the new Secretary of the US Department of Health and Human Services.

I concur with the prevailing sentiment expressed by the majority of American healthcare leaders. The bottom line impact of haphazardly repealing and replacing the ACA with a Republican variation of Representative Tom Price's proposed EPFA would be detrimental to providers and consumers. It would effectively return our country back to practices by insurance companies that prevailed in the years leading up to March 2010. Trump's anti-ObamaCare campaign rhetoric may have served him well as a political *call-to-arms* for garnering votes during his bid for the White House. However, as *President Trump*, he realizes the enormity of the challenge *how* to actually attain a "better and comprehensive plan" for healthcare reform for everyone. The leadership of the Republican controlled Congress has expressed they do not want to be blamed for hastily adopting a disastrous alternative to ObamaCare – that might affectionately be called "*TrumpCare.*"

Although President Trump and Republican legislators are politically motivated to repeal and replace the ACA early in 2017, it will likely take months, and perhaps years, to accomplish their *collective* healthcare reform objectives. This is particularly true because of complex parliamentarian rules in the US Senate that control the number of votes necessary to pass **budget resolution legislation** – requires a simple majority – compared to **unrelated non-budget repeal language** that takes 60 Senators voting in favor of the ACA's repeal (a super majority). A super majority approval means that at least *eight* Democratic Senators must join their Republican colleagues.[202] After all, it took Obama and Congress two difficult years to develop and approve the ACA.

Hopefully, both sides of the Congressional isles in the nation's Capitol will elect to collaborate with policy makers, providers, insurers, and consumers to continuously improve the Accountable Care Act for the benefit of all Americans. It is vitally important to the United States' future success that the Trump Administration and Congress succeed in leading America to its highest state of wellbeing in spite of political wrangling.

---

[202] Mary Clare Jalonick, December 31, 2016, "In 2017, GOP Congress sees mandate to Obama's agenda," *Associated Press*, see http://r.search.yahoo.com/_ylt=A0LEVicN3KBY1FAAUEYPxQt.;_ylu=X3oDMTBydWNmY2Mw BGNvbG8DYmYxBHBvcwM0BHZ0aWQDBHNlYwNzcg--/RV=2/RE=1486965901/RO=10/RU=https%3a%2f%2fwww. yahoo.com%2fnews%2f2017-gop-congress-sees-mandate-undo-obamas-agenda-163447989.html/RK=0/ RS=K42w3xBQFtrr4WL45uSOW_N0b7M-

3.2 -- The Proverbial Monetary Coin of America's Healthcare System Has Two Distinct Sides to the Argument

Where the Candidates Stand on Health Care, Housing

… Of course, for the optimist, there is always a chance that the combination of a new president and national fatigue over fighting the ACA for seven years would inspire a compromise, regardless of who wins. A possible bargain might consist of using Section 1332 of the ACA, which allows the federal government to grant waivers to states to leave the ACA exchanges and use their own methods to reach coverage and cost control goals. This would please conservatives as it takes power away from the federal government and gives it to states. In exchange, Democrats would likely ask for more cost-sharing subsidies for low-income enrollees.

Steve Kennedy, Senior Managing Director, The Capital Issue, Lancaster Pollard & Co., LLC, Columbus, Ohio, October-November 2016

I have reviewed vast amounts of material pertaining to health reform in the United States. This book attempts to provide a balanced perspective on this substantial issue that affects millions of Americans, even though my belief is that The United States Healthcare System Should be a Limited Human Right for All. It is possible, and even likely, that the two distinct sides of the argument about access to, and cost of quality health services are both partially correct. There are decidedly two sides to every coin, and the American healthcare tab reached $3.2 trillion in 2016. Experts agree that the nation will not turn its backs on those persons who truly need quality health services and can't afford to access them (that is part of our moral fiber). At the same time, these same experts know unequivocally that the rising cost of American healthcare system will soon become *unsustainable*, as the nation's overall healthcare tab approaches *20 percent of America's Gross Domestic Product* (GDP).

Clearly, no one yet has come up with the perfect solution. In this chapter I want to explore a *fair and balanced* discussion about where we as a nation have come from, and the principal alternatives our leaders face at this important fork in the road of our journey to achieve *accountable and affordable healthcare for all*.

An informative and balanced televised 90-minute debate put on by CNN **Town Hall** recently spotlighted "*the future of ObamaCare.*" This "friendly" debate was held at George Washington University, in Washington, DC, on Tuesday, February 7, 2017, 9:00 PM ET, between former Presidential candidates US Senator Bernie Sanders (D – Vermont) [considered one of the most liberal senators] and US Senator Ted Cruz (R -- Texas) [considered one of the most conservative senators].[203] Both

---

203 CNN Town Hall Debate, George Washington University, Washington, DC, February 7, 2017, see http://www.cnn.com/2017/02/07/politics/obamacare-cruz-sanders-highlights/index.html

Why The United States Healthcare System Should Be A Limited Human Right For All

Senators are strong advocates of their party's positions on the future of healthcare reform in the United States. The audience was invited to share comments and questions with these Senators and the resulting discussion was enlightening and productive. Let's review some of the *highlights* (taken from my personal recording of the CNN session – **paraphrased excerpts**).

Senator Bernie Sanders delivered his opening statement by asserting:

- *Republicans are in a panic over ObamaCare. If you are one of 20 million Americans who finally has received health insurance, forget about it – you're gone. Repealing ObamaCare means when you get sick, you aren't going to be able to go to the doctor. And when you end up in the hospital, you'll be paying for those bills for the rest of your life, or maybe you'll go bankrupt.*
- *If you have a preexisting condition like cancer, mental illness, etc., you will be rejected by insurance companies. Having a baby is a preexisting condition.*
- *The ACA is not perfect. But the debate is that Republicans want to get rid of it altogether.*
- *The majority of Americans say the ACA should not be repealed.*
- *The United States is the only country in the world that does not guarantee healthcare as a right. I believe that we should join the rest of the countries around the world and improve the ACA; If you are an American you should have healthcare as a right, not a privilege.*
- *The ACA has been a step forward.*

Senator Ted Cruz gave his opening remarks by restating the Republican Party position:

- *Healthcare is different than most other political issues. It affects our families. It can be the difference quite literally between whether we live or die.*
- *This is an issue where Bernie and I have fundamentally different approaches on this point – Bernie and the Democrats believe the government should control healthcare. I trust you, and I trust your doctor. I think healthcare works better when you are in charge and decide what is best for you. Without government setting rules, setting wait periods, and without rationing.*
- *Six years ago, former President Barack Obama made a series of promises that were broken – Obama said "If you like your plan, you can keep your plan. If you like your doctor, you can keep your doctor." Millions discovered that was not true.*
- *There were promises that the ACA would not raise premiums… "The average family's premiums would drop $2,500." Not only was this not true, but premiums have risen $5,000. Its reduced your choice, reduced your freedom, and that's why this last election was a referendum on ObamaCare. Voters decided this plan is not working.*

The CNN moderator presented a question from the audience after discussion about health insurance company profits and outrageous prices for medicines sold by Big Pharma (national and internationally):

- A woman (NP) told the Senators about her medical battle with breast cancer – she is undergoing radiation treatment now. She is fearful that without ObamaCare, she would not be able to afford health insurance.
- How can the GOP protect those who rely on the ACA?

Senator Cruz:

- *My mom had breast cancer, our prayers and thoughts are with you… Every proposal by Republicans lawmakers to replace ObamaCare supports the prohibition for insurance companies to be able to cancel coverage just because someone is sick. Cruz said: replacement legislation for ObamaCare by the Republicans prohibits companies from jacking up the insurance rates because they got sick or injured… Absolutely, we've got to fix it. And I am confident that we will!*

Senator Sanders:

- *Sanders quipped: I can't believe you just said. It is a contradiction to everything you just said… you wanted to get rid of every word of ObamaCare [and its mandates]. The only way that we are going to make sure that you and … can get health insurance with a pre-existing condition. The only way is to make sure that any insurance company can't say no to you or any other person in this country. Ted says it [ObamaCare] is a terrible a government intrusion. I say it is the moral and the right thing to do. So when you hear Ted and other Republicans say they are going to get rid of all of ObamaCare and leave it up to the states. What do you think the states will do? Will they maintain the ability to protect people with pre-existing conditions? We will go back to the obscenity the way we were before ObamaCare was passed.*

Senator Cruz:

- *… I said hundreds of times on the campaign trail [for President] that we should repeal every word of ObamaCare. But we are not done yet with healthcare reform … we need healthcare reform and the principles of healthcare reform. I talked about a lot of common sense ideas that were part of every Republican proposal so far –*
  - *We should expand competition*
  - *We should empower patients*
  - *We should keep government from getting between between you and your doctor*

  … I talked about all sorts of common sense ideas to accomplish just that. A requirement that is included in every piece of GOP legislation is a prohibition for insurance companies

- *cancelling people because they got sick. Bernie, it is easy to say to people "gosh you will loose your coverage..."*
- *Virtually all the Republican legislation that have been filed, and Democrats have opposed, maintains continuity of insurance coverage... There are people across this country that can't afford insurance because their deductibles are so high, the premiums are so high, they say my family can't make it on this... And here is a fact that most people don't know – most of the people covered by ObamaCare are on Medicaid. They jammed a bunch of people on Medicaid and their outcomes are markedly worse than people with private insurance ...*

Senator Sanders:

- *Sanders pointed out -- listen carefully to what Senator Cruz said, "I you go to the doctor tomorrow and are diagnosed with a terrible illness, the insurance companies don't have to provide you with insurance [coverage]. You just discovered the cancer. Insurance companies could say we can't make money off of you so we won't cover you." And, "If you [already] have insurance and get an illness, coverage must be kept." We are moving into an era where millions of people will develop terrible illnesses and they'll not be able to get insurance, "and God only knows how many of them will die."*

The CNN moderator introduced another woman from the audience that is five-months pregnant and her concerns about being able to afford health insurance:

- *(MB) said she had been a nurse practitioner from Florida for 25 years and has a family of four [and husband], but under ObamaCare I am not able to get the insurance coverage I need for myself and my family of four because of a $13,000 annual deductible. Last year I had a very abnormal PAP smear, and could not get additional tests because she had not met her $13,000 out-of-pocket deductible, before it will cover anything, and now fears she may have undiagnosed cancer. [I pay $25,000 per year in premiums for basic preventative coverage].*
- *Why should my family be forced to pay so much money for a plan that is essentially useless?*

Senator Sanders:

- *... The real question is why Americans, as a nation, pay nearly twice as much per capita on healthcare than other industrialized nations. If you were in Canada or the UK, France, Germany, and Scandinavia, you would get the care you need as a right of being a citizen in those countries.*

- A policy like the one you described is clearly outrageous, and we should tell every American that we should join the rest of the industrialized world and guarantee healthcare as a right. And If we do that right away their family incomes will go up right away.

Senator Cruz:

- I am sorry for the challenges you are facing. There are vast amounts of people in the United States exactly in the same way you are in the wreckages of ObamaCare, with skyrocketing premiums and deductibles that are unaffordable and with really limited care.
- Cruz commended Bernie for his candor, his view all along is that we need government run and government controlled healthcare for everyone. He says we pay more than many other countries and points to Canada and UK – he asks why? I was born in Canada and I can tell you how it really is.
- The reason we pay more is that we get a lot more and a lot better healthcare than other countries. Let me tell you about some basic statistics... I noticed that during the debates Democrats don't like to talk about the facts on the other side.
- The United States, population controlled, delivers three times as many mammograms than Europe; two and a half times as many MRI scans; and 31 percent more C-sections... we provide more healthcare. The wait times are a lot less; ... there are 3.7 million persons on a list in the UK waiting for healthcare.
- Whenever you put the government in charge of healthcare, they will ration...
- I don't think the government has any business telling you are not entitled to healthcare.
- The answer is not to create more government regulations under ObamaCare, the solution it is to empower people. Give them more choices, lower prices, lower deductibles, and put them back in charge of their own healthcare.

Senator Sanders (adding to this dialogue):

- Ted talks about the problems of rationing in other countries. In America we do rationing in a different way. If you are very rich, you can buy the best care in the world. We should be proud of that. But if you are working class you are having a very difficult time affording the outrageous cost of healthcare.
- Every single year tens of thousands of our fellow Americans die because they don't go to the doctor when they should.
- Let me give you some examples...Doctors all over this country they explain patients come to their offices very sick, and they say to the patients – why didn't you come sooner... and they say I didn't have any insurance; or my deductible was so high; some of those people die and others end up in the hospital with outrageous costs for illnesses that could have been treated for far less a while ago.

Why The United States Healthcare System Should Be A Limited Human Right For All

- *This country has more rationing than any industrialized country on earth. Except the rationing is done by income. Working people and poor people are suffering as a result of that practice.*

The CNN moderator shifted the debate to the topic of the employer mandate:

- *A small business owner (LH), who owns five hair salons in Fort Worth, Texas, stated she can't afford to provide health insurance for herself and her employees due to low profit margins. LH mentioned that ObamaCare is getting in the way of growing her business. The burden of having to offer healthcare coverage to her employees if she exceeds the regulatory limit of 49 employees is unfair.*
- *My question is to you, Senator Sanders, is how do I employ more Americans without raising my prices to customers or lowering wages to my employees?*

Senator Sanders:

- *I'm going to give you an answer you won't like. Given the nature of our healthcare insurance system right now, where most people get their insurance through their places of employment, "I'm sorry, I think that in America today, everybody should have health care, and if you [the business owner] have more than 50 people... I'm afraid to tell you I think that you will have to provide health insurance."*
- *Yes, you should be providing health insurance for your employees [once you hit the 50 employees minimum].*
- *This is why I want you to join me and help me to pass a "Medicare-for-all" universal health care program for Americans of all ages – a good single-payer affordable plan funded by the government.*

Senator Cruz:

- *I have to say that my view is very different than Bernie's. Bernie and the Democrats would say that you the small business are a "bad actor," because you are not allowed to manufacture money.*
- *Let me introduce you to two [Obamacare] terms – 29ers and 49ers. ObamaCare kicks in after an employee works over 29 hours per week so they remain part timers; 49ers are millions of small businesses that are in the same situation you are that limit their growth because they can't afford to pay health insurance when they exceed 50 employees...*
- *Democrats are telling millions of businesses – "tough luck." This [employer mandate] is one of the most damaging things about ObamaCare.*

The CNN moderator posed the question about ACA's push for Medicaid expansion:

- *A woman afflicted with multiple sclerosis (CH) told her story about moving from Texas [one of the Republican states which did not expand Medicaid under the ACA and US Supreme Court decision in 2012[204]] to Maryland [where Medicaid expansion took place] after the ACA became law so she could qualify for the expanded Medicaid and receive treatment for her illnesses.*
- *She posed a question to Senator Cruz and Republicans against ObamaCare can assure her that she will continue to receive Medicaid health insurance coverage if the law is repealed?*
- *"I like my coverage, can I keep it?"*

Senator Cruz:

- *Congratulations on your success dealing with MS. It is a terrible disease. More than half of the former uninsured that have received coverage under the ACA are part of the Medicaid expansion efforts. The problem is that Medicaid is a profoundly troubled program. The outcomes are very poor among Medicaid patients. Nationally, 54% of doctors won't take new Medicaid patients. Dental care appointments are denied at a 63% rate for Medicaid… Medicaid patients are twice as likely to die that patients covered by private insurance.*
- *The solution is to have a system that allows as many people as possible to be on the private insurance of their choice, because ObamaCare expansion of the Medicaid program is not working… The wait times for Medicaid patients are increasing, in fact in Illinois over 742 people have died while on the waiting list for care for Medicaid. Why? Because Medicaid is "rationed care" for all…*
- *I would much rather have a system where we can have millions who are on Medicaid getting private insurance, and the only way they can is if we have competition so the rates are lower and patients can afford to have health insurance.*

Senator Cruz:

- *The stories we have heard today … my friends you are living, I know you don't know this by these stories, in the wealthiest country in the history of the world… These stories are obscene and should not be taking place in the United States.*
- *Are the problems with Medicaid? Of course there are. I will tell you that for the governors of the Republican states that did not expand their Medicaid programs – and they were not*

---

204 The first challenge reviewed by the highest court in America known as the 2012 NFIB v Sebelius *(no. 11-392)* ruled in favor in part, and reversed in part, of the ACA -- https://www.supremecourt.gov/opinions/11pdf/11-393c3a2.pdf

able to go to a doctor for the first time in years -- even though the federal government was paying 100% of the additional cost for three years, I hope they can sleep well at night.
- *We are looking at a dysfunctional system, we spend more and get less...*
- *I do believe healthcare is a human right, and I believe that this country must join every other major country and say you can stay home and get quality care because you are an American; you can run your small business well and get care because you are an American.*

The Senators were in *broad agreement* about the exorbitant prices of drugs in America compared to the cost abroad and the need to work together [all political parties and officials] to go after big Pharma (pharmaceutical *re-importation*):

- *Cruz – we need to work together to go after big Pharma... though he emphasized to the audience that the Food and Drug Administration is enforcing the importation ban from other nations into the United States.*
- *Sanders – I am asking Senator Cruz to support legislation that allows Medicare prices with the pharmaceutical industry...*

The debate that took place at George Washington University on February 7th at the CNN Town Hall meeting characterizes the fundamental differences between the two dominant political parties in the United States Congress and other levels of government. The chart below attempts to identify the main ideological and philosophical positions held by the present Congressional body toward healthcare reform under the new Trump Administration leadership:

Table 6 – 2017 Push in the US Congress to Address Changes to PPACA

2017 Push in the US Congress to Address Changes to PPACA

*Main **Republican Positions** Regarding ObamaCare Reform*

- *Repeal and Replace the PPACA*
- *Expand health savings accounts*
- *Offer refundable tax credits to help buy private health insurance coverage*
- *Eliminate the individual mandate*
- *Decrease dependence on employer-sponsored plans*
- *Maintain the requirement that insurers permit subscriber-parents to keep their adult children on their policies up to age 26*
- *Maintain the ACA ban on discrimination by insurers for persons with pre-existing conditions and catastrophic illnesses*

- *Provide $25 billion over 10 years to help fund high-risk pools*
- *Devolve Medicaid to the states on a block grant and / or per capita basis (with some 70 million enrollees)*
- *Partially privatize Medicare beginning in 2024 through "premium support" option*
- *Address the re-importation of drugs into the US*
- *reducing government regulation of health insurance marketplaces*
- *Reduce healthcare spending by giving subscribers incentives to purchase less costly insurance and more "skin in the game"*
- *Allow purchase of health insurance plans across all states*
- *Cap tax exclusion for employer-provided health insurance*

Main **Democratic Positions** Regarding ObamaCare Reform

- *Revise and Enhance the PPACA*
- *Modification of the Essential Health Benefits requirements (EHB)*
- *Re-affirm the Individual Mandate and Employer Mandate*
- *Protect the ACA coverage of some 25 million people who have secured health insurance on the Marketplaces and Medicaid Expansion*
- *Address the re-importation of drugs into the US and give authority to Medicare to negotiate prices*
- *Expand coverage and strengthen consumer protections in the health insurance marketplace through government regulation*
- *Regulate the annual increases in Marketplace premiums to the single-digit range*
- *Create a "public option" health insurance product similar to Medicare and the Federal Employees Benefit Program to compete with commercial insurance plans operating on the exchanges*
- *Provide more freedom to patients and more flexibility to states over insurance products on the Marketplaces*
- *Expand funding to Community and Rural Health Centers programs*
- *Explore taxation schemes to control foods that promote diabetes and obesity*
- *Increase funding for preventive care, Pop Health Management and ACOs*

Note: Mark Tozzio, Multiple sources were used to develop this list.[205] [206] [207]

---

[205] Daniel McLaughlin, Editor, (2015), *Guide to Healthcare Reform: Readings and Commentary*, ACHE Health Administration Press, Chicago, Illinois, Chapters 8 and 9.

[206] Drew Altman, *The Fundamentally Different Goals of the Affordable Care Act and Republican Plans*, Wall Street Journal, June 7, 2016, see http://blogs.wsj.com/washwire/2016/06/07/the-fundamentally-different-goals-of-the-affordable-care-act-and-republican-replacement-plans/

[207] Russell Berman, Republicans Offer a Plan to Replace Obamacare, The Atlantic, June, 22,2016, Politics, see https://www.theatlantic.com/politics/archive/2016/06/house-gop-obamacare/488168/

Why The United States Healthcare System Should Be A Limited Human Right For All

In his *Guide to Healthcare Reform*, Daniel McLaughlin [editor] notes that health policymaking is primarily motivated by the "traditional economic market."[208] In the United States, this translates into a commitment to the free market model where government interference is held to a minimum between sellers and buyers of products and services.[209] According to Beaufort Long Est's [included in McLaughlin, 2015] article entitled "The Context and Process of Health Policymaking," he points out that (McLaughlin, 2015, p. 360):

> *Health policies – indeed, all public policies – are made in the context of political markets, which in many ways operate like traditional economic markets. However, are notable differences [with access healthcare]. The most fundamental is that buyers or demanders in economic markets express their preferences by spending their own money. That is, they reap the benefits of their choices, and they directly bear the costs of those choices. In political markets, on the other hand, the link between who receives benefits and who bears the cost is less direct. Feldstein (2006), for example, observes that public policies that impose costs on future generations are routinely established. The nature of the political marketplace dictates that many decisions made by contemporary policymakers are influenced by the preferences of current voters, perhaps to the detriment of future generations. Such allocative policies as Medicare and Social Security are examples of this phenomenon. In the care Social Security, outlays are projected to exceed revenues in the future; it is currently projected that this could occur first in 2019 (Congressional Budget Office 2008b).*

Perhaps this same argument holds true concerning the appropriateness and viability of the *Patient Protection and Affordable Care Act of 2010*. My take on Longest's statement above is that "fair and equitable" healthcare policies can not be developed along traditional party-line votes in Congress. This is especially true regarding healthcare legislation that affects the future of the entire nation. Unfortunately, this has been the case when *either* political party controls both the Congress and White House (i.e. 2009 and 2017 terms).

In Section One of this book, I presented a growth projection that anticipates the total costs associated with the United States healthcare system may not be sustainable beyond $4.0 trillion per year. Serious economic challenges could materialize as early as 2020 according to the projections by the CMS National Health Expenditure Data (NHE).[210] [211] It was also asserted in

---

208 Ibid. p.358-359.
209 Ibid., p. 359.
210 CMS, National Health Expenditure (NHE) Amounts by Type of Expenditure and Source of Funds: Historical and Projections CY 1960-2025; the projections are based on the 2014 version of the NHE released in December 2015, see https://www.cms.gov/Research-Statistics-Data-and-Systems/Statistics-Trends-and-Reports/NationalHealthExpendData/Downloads/NHE60-25.zip
211 CMS NHE, CY 2000 actual = $1,369,679; 2019 projected = $3,958,611; and 2025 projected = $5,631,016.

Section One that healthcare should be a limited human right for all American because it directly impacts the health and wellbeing of citizens. We must reconcile these two critical factors as the nation pursues the future of healthcare reform in the United States. This is particularly notable, because as the nation's population ages and the *Boomers* retire by the millions, the dependency ratio of seniors' to the workforce increases dramatically. Fewer tax paying employees (20 to 64 years of age; declining from 1960 = 5.5:1.0 to 2040 = 2.5:1.0) will support funding for Social Security, Medicare, Medicaid, and other beneficial / entitlement programs (Graph 15 shows a declining ratio of working-age Americans to those 65 and older).[212]

This puts more pressure on the population 20 to 64 years old to: (1) stay healthy, (2) become better educated, and (3) be more productive, in order to boost the economic wellbeing of the United States. Consider the economic burden of 25 to 30 million persons losing their health insurance that are less than optimally healthy and productive citizens (recall Senator Bernie Sanders' comment at the CNN Town Hall, February 7, 2017).

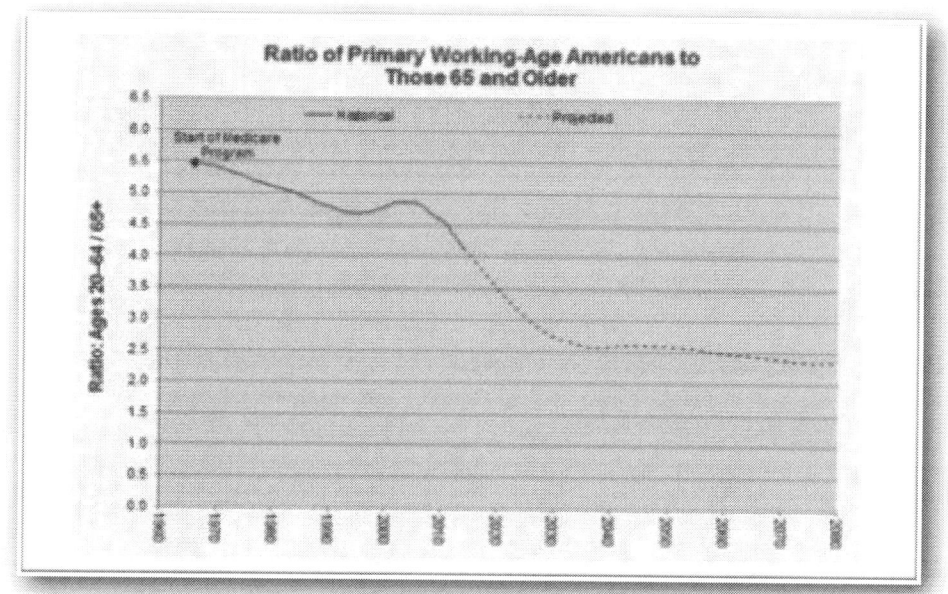

Graph 9 – Ratio of Primary Working-Age Americans to Those 65 and Older

How do healthcare insurance reform's guiding principles identified in Chapter 3 relate to the American *value system* of providing (*and paying for*) quality and affordable *preventive and healthcare services for all as a limited human right*? I believed the dichotomy between the *economics* and *human rights* (ethical stance) of healthcare is the crux of polarization of the political parties in Congress. *How do we (the American people and their representatives in Congress)* **collaborate** *to achieve a balance between efforts to foster universal access to cost-effective and*

---

212 CMS actuarial projections, trend from 1960 (estimates) to 2080 (projections).

value-based healthcare in the United States? Perhaps Republicans and Democrats are BOTH correct in their stances, thus a cooperative negotiating approach where neither party is "right" or "wrong" and factual information leads to compromising legislative reform.

3.3 -- Do Politics Trump Logic?

> *[Dr.] Price promises access, but not insurance for everyone*
>
> *President-elect Donald Trump's HHS secretary nominee repeatedly and pointedly said on Wednesday [January 18, 2017] that all Americans should have access to healthcare coverage --but he stopped short of saying all Americans should be covered by credible health insurance coverage, despite Trump's recent statement that the replacement for the Affordable Care Act would include "insurance for everyone."*
>
> *Rep. Tom Price (R-Ga.) answered questions for nearly four hours at a courtesy hearing before the Senate Health, Education, Labor and Pensions Committee. His official confirmation will be before the Senate Finance Committee, which has scheduled a hearing for Tuesday.*
>
> *Republicans referenced the replacement plan Trump alluded to over the weekend but offered no new details, and some in the party reportedly are not sure Trump's plan actually exists.*
>
> By Shannon Muchmore, Modern Healthcare, January 18, 2017, http://www.modernhealthcare.com/article/20170118/NEWS/170119903

From mid-2015 to election day on November 8, 2016, political candidates exchanged heated campaign barbs on numerous topics including healthcare insurance reform (ObamaCare). The healthcare industry was caught *off-guard* by the Electoral College win by Donald Trump as the new President. After six years of getting accustomed to the federal regulatory shift from fee-for-service reimbursement to value-based purchasing for care, health system leaders are adapting to innovative ways to improve the quality of care and enhance cost-containment strategies and incentives. By getting rid of ObamaCare, particularly if there is not a reasonable replacement law, healthcare executives of health systems, "especially those in rural areas, could be tremendously hard hit if the replacement rolls back the progress made under the ACA to insure patients and the incentives for providers to make sure patients get care before their illnesses require emergency room visits or hospitalization," according to Robert Annas, private equity senior managing director of Solic Capital.[213] The consequences of an ACA repeal translate to real losses in the numbers of insured subscribers and billions of dollars of increased cost to Americans, as predicted in January 2017 by the *Congressional Budget Office*:[214]

- *The number of people who are uninsured would increase by 18 million in the first new plan year following enactment of the bill [the latest substantial Republican proposal to repeal the ACA, H.R. 3762, Restoring American's Healthcare Freedom Reconciliation Act of 2015]. Later after the elimination of the ACA's expansion of Medicaid eligibility and of subsidies for insurance purchased through the ACA marketplaces, that number would increase to 27 million, and then to 32 million in 2026.*
- *Premiums in the non-group market (for individual policies purchased through the marketplaces or directly from insurers) would increase by 20 percent to 25 percent – relative to projections under current law – in the first new plan year following enactment. The increase would reach about 50 percent in the year following elimination of the Medicaid expansion and the marketplace subsidies, and premiums would double by 2026.*

The myriad of issues associated with healthcare reform legislation are complex – a great review of the complexities and economic levers that drive healthcare costs and population health status is presented in the article by Anne Martin, et al., in *Health Affairs*, December 2, 2016. It is rich with valuable information for policymakers, politicians, providers and consumers for charting the future of health insurance reform. The link to this article is:

http://content.healthaffairs.org/content/36/1/166.abstract[215]

On *Inauguration Day*, January 20, 2017, President Donald Trump signed one of his first Executive Orders in the Oval Office declaring that the PPACA would be repealed and replaced with a new law.[216] The Executive Order sets in motion the process in the US Congress to alter the health insurance coverage legislation known as ObamaCare and fulfills a key campaign promise by declaring – "By the authority vested in me as President by the constitution and the

---

213 Dave Barkholz and Bob Herman, "Threat of ACA repeal fuels angst at hospitals," *Modern Healthcare*, November 14, 2016, p. 19.
214 Congressional Budget Office, (January 2017), "How Repealing Portions of the Affordable Care Act Would Affect Health Insurance Coverage and Premiums, p. 1, see https://www.cbo.gov/sites/default/files/115th-congress-2017-2018/reports/52371-coverageandpremiums.pdf
215 Anne Martin et al., (January 2017), "*National Health Spending: Faster Growth in 2015 as Coverage Expands and Utilization Increases*," Health Affairs, vol. 36, no. 1, pp. 166-176; see https://www.thelundreport.org/content/national-health-spending-grows-faster-2015-coverage-expands-and-utilization-increases
216 See full text of the Executive Order on repealing and replacing PPACA at http://www.cnn.com/2017/01/20/politics/trump-obamacare-executive-order/

laws of the United States of America, it is herby ordered and follows: 'Section 1. It is the policy of my Administration to seek the prompt repeal of the Patient Protection and Affordable Care Act (Public Law 111-148), as amended (the "Act").'"

In the early weeks of the Trump Administration, the tone about the ACA "repeal" evolved into a sobering realization that it could take some time to get rid of ObamaCare without a reasonable replacement law that most Republicans embraced. Fox News political commentator Bill O'Reilly interviewed President Trump during half-time of the *Super Bowl LI* game in Houston where Trump commented briefly on his views on repealing ObamaCare, Sunday, February 5, 2017:[217]

> **Bill O'Reilly:** *Can Americans in 2017 expect a new healthcare plan rolled out by the Trump Administration? This year?*
>
> **President Trump:** *Yeah–in the process, and maybe it'll take 'til sometime into next year, but we are certainly going to be in the process–very complicated. Obamacare is a disaster. You have to remember–Obamacare doesn't work, so we are putting in a wonderful plan–it's statutorily–takes a while to get–we're going to be putting it in fairly soon–I think that, yes–uh–I would like say by the end of the year–uh–at least the rudiments, but we should have something within the year and the following year.*

It is encouraging to learn that President Trump is willing to admit to the nation on national TV that finding an alternative to the PPACA legislation is not going to be an overnight process as originally asserted on the campaign trail. Particularly since Trump's "wonderful plan" does not exist yet. Republicans in Congress can't agree on which of many versions of a repeal and replacement Bill put forth by many Republican Senators is *the* acceptable replacement for ObamaCare. Democrats presently have vowed to oppose any plan to repeal the ACA, but they do not have the votes in the Senate to block a Republican assault since they hold a minority 48 of the 100 seats. This kind of political gridlock has been ongoing in the US Congress for decades and has fueled frustration and anxiety of the American public and healthcare providers.

As Secretary Dr. Tom Price assumed the helm of the Department of Health and Human Services (HHS) after confirmation by the full US Senate on February 10, 2017, it is anticipated that he will champion the "dismantling of the [ACA] law through Administrative measures" on behalf of President Trump.[218] Politically, Dr. Price is a staunch conservative Republican Congressman from Georgia and the co-architect of legislation to eliminate ObamaCare in 2015. Dr. Price's priorities, in keeping with his track record in the US House of Representatives, include:[219]

---

217 YouTube, February 5, 2017, See https://www.youtube.com/watch?v=tszQS7PcNdU
218 Virgil Dickson and Harris Meyer, "New HHS Secretary Price faces crushing inbox," *Modern Healthcare*, February 13, 2017, p. 6.
219 Ibid., p. 7.

- ✓ Continue the shift of Medicare payment from fee-for-service to value-based incentives reimbursement
- ✓ Consideration of converting Medicare for a defined-benefit program to a defined-contribution with premium support (vouchers) from the federal government to buy private insurance.
- ✓ Matching the coverage start date for Medicare beneficiaries with Social Security's enrollment at age 67, instead of the current 65 years old (currently there are 57 million people enrolled in the Medicare program)
- ✓ Evaluation of mandatory hospital bundled-payment programs for joint replacements and cardiac care
- ✓ Slowing the rise of chronic diseases through population health management initiatives
- ✓ Use of "big data" to direct processes for healthcare quality improvements
- ✓ Shift to Medicaid waivers and federal block grants to states to handle their lower income citizens' health needs
- ✓ Revision of federal regulations and subsidies for existing mandated women's services
- ✓ Reforms to the FDA drug approval processes

During his confirmation hearings before the Democrats expressed concern that Dr. Price's appoints to Secretary of HHS would politicize the Department and move further away from the ACA's goal of affordable quality healthcare for all Americans.

Another critical health-related Trump appointee is Seema Verma, a Medicaid consultant (founder of SVC Inc.) that worked under contract with Vice President Mike Pence while he was Indiana's Governor of that state, for the post of Administrator of the Centers for Medicare and Medicaid Services (CMS) with a budget of over $1 trillion annually. CMS also regulates the insurers' EHB requirements offered on the Marketplaces nation-wide. Joanne Finnegan and Illene MacDonald with the *FiercePracticeManagement*, who attended Verma's confirmation hearing on February 16, 2017 conducted by the US Senate Finance Committee reported:[220]

> *For her part, Verma said she favored policies that result in better health outcomes and lower costs. She said she would support efforts to make drug costs more affordable and favor offering people more choices when it comes to healthcare.*

Verma told the Senate Finance Committee on February 16th, ""I want to be part of the solution making the system work for all Americans. I want to be able to look my children in the eye and tell them I did my part to serve my country and make things better for people who often do not

---

[220] For information about Seema Verma, see http://www.fiercehealthcare.com/healthcare/seema-verma-questioned-future-medicare-medicaid-programs-during-confirmation-hearing-for and http://healthaffairs.org/blog/2016/08/29/healthy-indiana-2-0-is-challenging-medicaid-norms/ and Senate hearing video https://www.c-span.org/video/?423823-1/cms-administrator-nominee-seema-verma-testifies-confirmation-hearing

have a voice."[221] She was officially confirmed by the entire US Senate on March 13, 2017 (by a vote of 55-43).

Back in November 2016, President-Elect Trump announced: "Together, Chairman Price and Seema Verma are the dream team that will transform our healthcare system for the benefit of all Americans."[222] The alignment of a Republican White House, Republican controlled House of Representatives and Senate, supported by Dr. Price and Seema Verma over the Department of Health and Human Services is likely to ensure that **politics will trump logic** when it comes to the fate of PPACA under the Trump Administration, in my opinion. Although, it may be at a much slower pace than President Trump originally promised during the Presidential campaign.

President Trump has consistently promised that **every** American would have access to *affordable and quality care* following the repeal and replacement of ObamaCare, and for a *lot less money*. The President emphasized that If the US Congress approves the replacement to ObamaCare – with the **American Health Care Act** (AHCA) – **everyone** will have the coverage they want without the Federal Government's interference.

On Monday, March 13, 2017, the *Congressional Budget Office* (CBO) published their "scoring" of the proposed AHCA stating: "The proposed bill would reduce the federal deficit by $337 billion over the 2017 to 2026 period." This amounts to a reduction of approximately $33 billion annually over the next ten years of the current $3.5 trillion of healthcare expenditures projected for 2017.

Additionally, the CBO predicted that the proposed Republican AHCA legislation would result in the loss of health insurance for *24 million* Americans presently covered by the ACA, in the short term. As many as *54 million* would become uninsured by the end of ten years. The groups most affected would include lower income individuals (primarily adults on Medicaid), as well as the senior population age 50 to 64 years due to excessively high premium costs for older Americans. Congressional and Senate Democrats vehemently oppose the proposed AHCA.

In a live radio interview with Eddie Andelman of the Boston Herald Radio show, March 17, 2017, Dr. Donald Berwick, former Administrator for the CMS and co-founder and president emeritus of the Institute of Health Improvement, predicted:

> *If you want to see disaster, pass this bill, because we know now, from analysis over and over again, that if this affordable care act replacement bill were to pass, then insurance markets would really implode; premiums would skyrocket, and even more than that, costs would soar.*

President Trump's claim and the CBO projection can't both be right!

---

221 See video of live testimony of Seema Verma before the Senate Finance Committee, February 16, 2017, at the Capitol in DC, https://www.finance.senate.gov/hearings/hearing-to-consider-the-nomination-of-

222 Henry Powderly, "Tom Price to lead HHS, Seema Verma to lead CMS, Donald Trump announces," *Healthcare Finance*, November 29, 2016, see http://www.healthcarefinancenews.com/news/tom-price-lead-hhs-seema-verma-lead-cms-donald-trump-announces

Four

Going Forward in a New Post-ObamaCare Era

4.1 -- Revisiting Why the United States Healthcare System Should be a Limited Human Right for All in 2017 and Beyond

Congress remains in the dark on Trump healthcare plan
CNN/ORC Poll shows last-minute love for ObamaCare

Washington (CNN) Americans views of ObamaCare tilt narrowly positive, according to a new CNN/ORC poll, marking the first time more have favored than opposed the law since its passage in 2010. The shift comes at the same time more than 8-in-10 say the law is likely to be repealed and replaced by incoming president Donald Trump.

Overall, 49% say they favor the 2010 health care law, more formally known as the Patient Protection and Affordable Care Act, while 47% oppose it. Though a mostly mixed review overall, that's a sharp improvement compared with previous polling on the law.

More have opposed than favored the law in every CNN/ORC poll on this question from March 2010 until now. The shift in the law's favor stems largely from Democrats and independents, while views among Republicans haven't moved much.

By Jennifer Agiesta, CNN Polling Director
CNN Updated 11:10 AM ET, Thu January 19, 2017

Why The United States Healthcare System Should Be A Limited Human Right For All

Hindsight of the past six years with the ACA's implementation prove history is *20: 20 vision* of the successes and failures of the healthcare reform legislation signed by President Obama in March 2010. The authoritative *evidence* gathered for writing Section 2 of my book leads me to conclude that the US Healthcare System *has* in fact improved. According to a poll by *Kaiser Family Foundation* released December 2016, most Americans support retaining and tweaking the ACA, instead of a total repeal of the healthcare law.[223] Republicans determined to terminate ObamaCare should take notice of the feedback from their constituents before acting on healthcare reform alternatives.

No doubt, there is still a long way to go before we perfect the "weak and broken links" of the current iteration of the ACA. Furthermore, providers have come to accept and adapt to *evidence-based value-driven payer incentives* that foster better quality / outcomes and cost-effective delivery of care to **all** Americans. I believe that an important and practical question that should be answered for our nation early in 2017 is:

> *Do Americans really want to rekindle the heated debates that transpired in 2009 over healthcare reform being a limited human right for all, or a purchased commodity for those who can afford the price of health insurance coverage in competitive markets across America?*

Hopefully, political leaders and policymakers under the new Trump Administration will see the wisdom of **"revising and enhancing"** the current ACA legislation instead of **"repealing and replacing"** the law. I perceive that a larger issue to be addressed is how to initiate a *collaborative* discussion among the stakeholders. As long as the parties insist on remaining in their own political corners, little if any progress can be achieved.

To initiate this critical dialogue, we need to objectively examine the various elements of the ACA that *are working and are palatable* to all sides at the negotiating table. Some areas of *general* agreement articulated by the President and Congressional Republicans are:

1. Maintain coverage of basic health insurance for all Americans with subsidies for lower income individuals and families
2. Retain the ability of parents to keep their dependent children on their health insurance policies until age 26
3. No annual or lifetime limits on health insurance coverage for beneficiaries
4. Non discrimination of pre-existing conditions and exclusions for getting insurance
5. Control the rising drug prices and allow importation of qualified products from other nations to foster competition

---

[223] Richard Gonzales, December 2, 2016, "Only 26 Percent of Americans Support Full Repeal of Obamacare, Poll Finds," NPR, see http://www.npr.org/sections/thetwo-way/2016/12/02/504068263/kaiser-poll-only-26-of-americans-support-full-repeal-of-obamacare

6. Continue quality and outcomes incentives by payers to improve provider performance
7. Maintain / expand pricing transparency of provider services and insurer coverage
8. Support preventive care coverage at low or no cost to subscribers of health insurance plans
9. Encourage population health management and wellness initiatives by providers
10. Encourage collaborative care delivery systems that improve continuity, quality, and cost containment of health care services
11. Include catastrophic coverage in all health insurance plans
12. Address rising incidence of chronic diseases with preventive care strategies
13. Reward value-based outcomes and move away from fee-for-volume reimbursement
14. Integrate social services programs and funding with health prevention initiatives
15. Facilitate more flexibility at the state levels to innovate delivery systems for the poor
16. Support the expansion of primary care providers and services
17. Resist a *single-payer* health system in the United States
18. Explore an "opt-out" rather than the present "opt-in" health insurance enrollment system
19. Control high-deductible plan limits
20. Tighten federal fraud and abuse and Stark Law provisions and penalties

This is a *healthy* list of important priorities to work on *before* proceeding with plans to repeal the ACA. These items should keep policy-makers, legislators, providers, insurers, employers, and the public-at-large busy for quite a while, maybe until at least the end of 2017. At that time, a more informed decision about the future of healthcare reform could be made with reasonable support from a majority of stakeholders.

It seems to me that President Trump is proposing to *"having his cake and eating it to,"* when it comes to reforming ObamaCare legislation. In a phone interview with *The Washington Post*, the President was quoted as saying to reporters according to a story in the newspaper on January 15, 2017:[224]

> ... "It's very much formulated down to the final strokes. We haven't put it in quite yet but we're going to be doing it soon," Trump said. He noted that he is waiting for his nominee for secretary of health and human services, Rep. Tom Price (R-Ga.), to be confirmed. That decision rests with the Senate Finance Committee, which hasn't scheduled a hearing.
> ... "We're going to have insurance for everybody," Trump said. "There was a philosophy in some circles that if you can't pay for it, you don't get it. That's not going to happen

---
[224] Robert Costa and Amy Goldstein, January 15, 2017, "Trump vows insurance for everybody in Obamacare replacement plan," *The Washington Post*, p. , see https://www.washingtonpost.com/politics/trump-vows-insurance-for-everybody-in-obamacare-replacement-plan/2017/01/15/5f2b1e18-db5d-11e6-ad42-f3375f271c9c_story.html?utm_term=.a621aa2ae3e6

with us." People covered under the law "can expect to have great health care. It will be in a much simplified form. Much less expensive and much better."

... "It's not going to be their plan," he said of people covered under the current law. "It'll be another plan. But they'll be beautifully covered. I don't want single-payer. What I do want is to be able to take care of people," he said Saturday.

The President's goals certainly echo what the majority of Americans want to hear as discussions about the repeal and replacement of Obama's landmark health legislation circulate in Washington DC. Realistically, *universal healthcare* that is better and cheaper than the current version of the PPACA will be a *tall order to fill*. It will definitely demand give and take from all sides of the negotiating table. [A televised interview with healthcare expert Ezekiel Emanuel and Juliet Eiliet, reporter with *The Washington Post*, February 16, 2017, can be seen at https://www.washingtonpost.com/video/politics/obamacare-architect-health-care-reform-is-difficult/2017/02/16/e0a6be52-f48a-11e6-9fb1-2d8f3fc9c0ed_video.html]

Regarding healthcare being a perceived limited human right for all in the United States, I asserted in 2009 that: "a *healthier* nation enables its citizens to achieve increasing social and economic progress that is the result of a rational methodology for promoting and restoring normal individual functioning relative to one's circumstances along the continuum of life," (Fisk, 2000).[225] The principal tenet outlined in Section One of my book continues to hold true at this time in history. It will foster economic growth and development in America.

How should Americans proceed with healthcare reform over the next decade?

4.2 -- Conclusions and Recommendations

Applying the foundational principles of limited healthcare human rights for all explored in the original book, I suggested specific steps that could further *moralize* healthcare reform in the United States, beginning in 2010:

---

[225] Mark Tozzio, (2009), *Why the United States Healthcare System Should Be A Limited Human Right For All*, Printed by CreateSpace, An Amazon.com Company, p. 4.

Table 7 – Tozzio's [original] Prescription for Healthcare Reform: 2009

Tozzio's Prescription for Healthcare Reform in the United States Based on the Principles of Justice for Healthcare (2009)

CRITICAL SUCCESS FACTORS /
Key Action Steps

1. **Implement aggressive health promotion and prevention programs instead of pouring more money into the "sick care" system**
Shift payment from traditional medical care to prevention by requiring that all providers prove to the IRS and HHS that they are spending real dollars on demonstrable community health promotion programs – at least 30% of all patient care revenue received from all sources (commercial, government, and other)

2. **Limit overall healthcare expenditures to a maximum of 18% of the GDP – statutorily**
Cap national health expenditures at around $4.8 trillion annually by 2028

3. **Create a government-sponsored, universal health insurance program for uninsured, underinsured and small employers – enact federal legislation requiring universal health care for all Americans by 2010**
Through regionally developed / managed cooperatives supported and sanctioned by the federal government, create a competitively priced (and perhaps subsidized) national insurance program, in addition to existing Medicare, Medicaid, Federal Employees, and Military plans

4. **Renew and enhance support for primary care services**
Increase payment to primary care providers substantially, with higher differentials paid to rural providers (physicians, NP, PA, allied health providers) to encourage growth in this sector of healthcare

5. **Implement government regulation of profit levels for proprietary providers (hospital corporations, pharmaceutical companies, etc.) and non-profit healthcare entities**
Limit profit margins (EBITDA) to a three-year average of 6.0% to 8.0%, which will allow reasonable growth and ROI without creating a windfall for providers, commercial insurers, or suppliers of healthcare services (pharmaceutical, equipment manufacturers, etc.)

6. **Motivate health care providers to implement innovative provider-patient health information systems by 2012**

Provide federal grants and subsidies to collaborative healthcare groups and facilitate the development of Community Health Information Networks (CHINs), electronic medical record systems and other proven information management systems

Evaluation of the Healthcare Reform Principles proposed in 2009 and enumerated above:

1. This recommendation was supported by the ACA and investment in preventive care rose substantially. We have not reached the recommended 30% level, but progress has been made since 2010.
2. No caps have been set by HHS or Congress; 2016 the total expenditures reached $3.2 trillion and are projected to grow to $4.5 trillion in 2021[226]
3. Universal health care was implemented with the individual and employer mandates in place; no government-sponsored insurance plan alternative provided
4. Primary care services were improved in Medicare and Medicaid programs; reimbursement for PCP services increased substantially with ACA
5. No commercial insurance limitation on profit levels; Marketplace-insurance participants must invest 80 and 85 percent of premiums to care for subscribers
6. Implemented through CMS Center for Innovation; grants for CHINs were piloted nationally

A paradigm-shift in government and commercial reimbursement approaches has gradually moved providers in the direction of performance related incentives and *value-based purchasing*, gradually replacing volume-driven payment systems by 2016 as a result of the ACA. Larry Sobal, Executive Vice President and a Senior Consultant at *MedAxiom* shared an excellent graphic representation of the shift taking place in health systems across the United States in his weekly blog:[227]

---

226 CMS, National Health Expenditure (NHE) Amounts by Type of Expenditure and Source of Funds: Historical and Projections CY 1960-2025; the projections are based on the 2014 version of the NHE released in December 2015, see https://www.cms.gov/Research-Statistics-Data-and-Systems/Statistics-Trends-and-Reports/NationalHealthExpendData/Downloads/NHE60-25.zip

227 See https://www.medaxiom.com/blog/has-value-reached-the-tipping-point

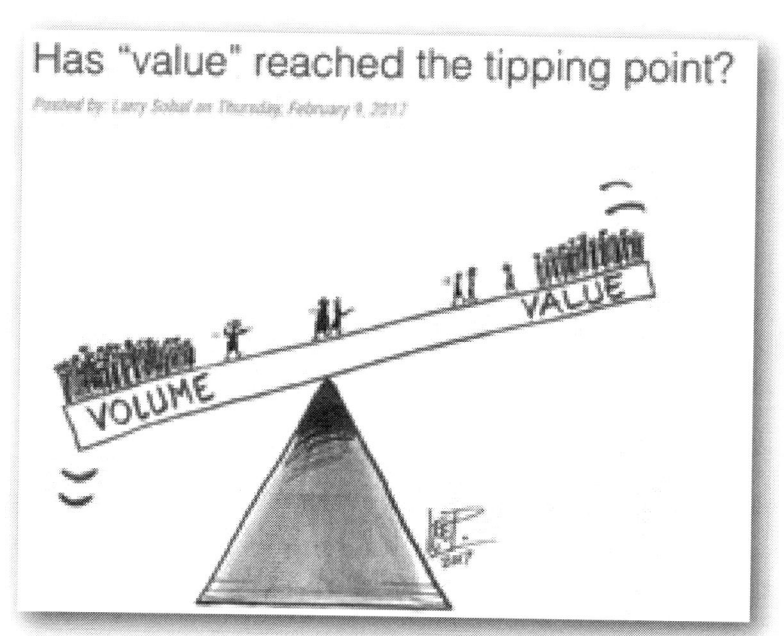

Graph 10 – Larry Sobal's "Value" Tipping Point

Large health systems have adopted the value-based payment systems and assumed more risk for populations they care for. A guestimate of the magnitude of adoption of incentive / risk-based payment systems tied to to overall revenue at the end of 2016 is approximately 35 percent. One of the largest single purchasers of health services in the United States, the Centers for Medicare and Medicaid, declared in 2015 an ambitious goal of shifting 50 percent of its provider payments tied to bundled and value-based methodologies by 2018 that promote quality and cost containment.[228] As President Trump and the Republican controlled Congress considers changes to the ACA, it is critical that we do not back-slide to an era when fee-for-service payment schemes prevailed. Careful consideration should be given to revising the present health insurance reform legislation (PPACA) and adding features that will enhance the wellbeing and productivity of Americans. My new *prescription* for healthcare reform in 2017 includes the remaining recommendations listed in 2009 that have not been adopted, plus requirements that will support the progress made during the ACA period since 2010:

---

[228] Marilyn Tavenner, former Administrator of CMS (2010-2015), see https://www.cms.gov/Newsroom/MediaReleaseDatabase/Fact-sheets/2015-Fact-sheets-items/2015-01-26-3.html

Table 8 –Tozzio's Updated Prescription for Healthcare Reform: 2017

IMPLEMENT REMAINING ORIGINAL 2009 RECOMMENDATIONS PLUS ADDITIONAL STRATEGIES TO REVISE AND ENHANCE PPACA FOR 2017

1. Limit overall healthcare expenditures to a maximum of 18% of the GDP – statutorily cap national health expenditures at around $4.8 trillion
2. **Implement government regulation over profits of proprietary providers (hospital corporations, pharmaceutical companies, insurers, etc.) and non-profit healthcare entities; limit profit margins (EBITDA) to a three-year average of 6.0% to 8.0%, which will allow reasonable growth and ROI without creating a windfall for providers, commercial insurers, or suppliers of healthcare services (pharmaceutical, equipment manufacturers, etc.)**
3. Shift payment approaches from traditional medical care to emphasize preventive health measures by requiring that all providers to demonstrate to the IRS and HHS / CMS that they are spending real dollars on demonstrable community health promotion programs – at least 30% of all revenue received from all sources (commercial, government, and other)
4. **Revise current version of ACA; do not repeal**
5. Award tax exemptions only to hospitals and health systems that demonstrate meaningful and measurable community health status improvement according to pre-established targets for health service areas; equal eligibility for both non-profit and for-profit facilities
6. **Establish a public health insurance option for under-65 individuals akin to Medicare systems; beneficiaries pay into a fund similar to Medicare**
7. Continue Federal Tax Credit subsidies for up to 400% of FFPL
8. **Continue Fed / State / Combined Marketplace exchanges with revisions**
9. Allow dependent children to remain on parent's policy up to age 26
10. **Maintain individual and employer mandates**
11. Expand preventive and wellness funding and local initiatives
12. **Expand Population Health Improvement funding for data integration, interoperability, community engagement, and targeted intervention programs**
13. Limit insurance companies' out-of-pocket / deductibles to a maximum of $5,000 for a family of four per annum
14. **Continue prohibition of exclusion due to preexisting policy**
15. Refine EHB requirements for insurers selling on the Marketplaces
16. **Integrate social services into ACOs**

17. Maintain unlimited annual and lifetime coverage
18. **Expand provider and insurer price transparency requirements**
19. Maintain commercial insurers' requirement to reinvest 85 / 80 percent of premium revenue back into subscribers' health care services
20. **Expand value-based incentives and ACO arrangements to improve quality and control cost increases of participating providers**
21. Establish specific health initiatives to help reduce preventable Tort-related legal cases and unnecessary defensive medicine practices.
22. **Community-based chronic health intervention; integrate with existing social and educational outreach programs using social indicators to target high-risk adult and early childhood populations.**

In conclusion, the future of America's health system, without rationalizing the limits of healthcare costs and refocusing on value and not quantity of health services, *appears bleak*. The objective data outlined in this book indicates that the healthcare tab in this nation may not be sustainable beyond $4.5 trillion, or 20% of the GDP.

If the 114th US Congress is willing to accept that unlimited growth in healthcare expenditures is not viable over 20 percent of the nation's GDP, and chooses to establishes an overall national *cap on healthcare expenditures, then the prospects of a thriving health system are much stronger. Simply funding the continual growth of healthcare costs at any rate is not realistic*, as was the case when the prospective payment system of Diagnosis Related Groups (DRGs) was instituted nation-wide for Medicare patients in the 1980s to limit the run-a-way cost for the Medicare program, the healthcare industry *did* adjust and survived.

It seems highly improbable that President Trump's claim he will sign a *"fantastic* replacement health [insurance] plan," covering the 20 million lower income citizens recently insured by ObamaCare, that is "much less expensive and far better" than the "*disastrous*" ObamaCare program *[paraphrased]. As the saying goes:* "You can't have your cake, and eat it too." The nation is forecasted to exceed the $4.5 trillion threshold of total healthcare dollars before the year 2020.[229]

I am encouraged by the slight overall increase of Government Public Health, Home Care, and Non-Commercial Research investments before the ACA (2006 and 2008) and post-ACA (2012 and 2014). In 2014, these three combined categories represent $208 billion of the $3.1 Trillion spent on healthcare related activities nationally, or about 7 percent of the grand total. From 2006 to 2014, we experienced a 39 percent growth in Public Health / Home Care / Research.

---

[229] Sean Keehan, et al., "National Health Expenditure Projections, 2016-25: Price Increases, Aging Push Sector to 20 Percent of the Economy," Health Affairs (online version), February 2017, see http://pnhp.org/blog/2017/02/16/dismal-projections-for-national-health-expenditures-and-the-numbers-of-uninsured/

However, $208 billion is a small fraction of the proposed target of 30 percent presented in this thesis that could help bend the cost curve over time.

Table 9 – Trend of US Healthcare Expenditures: 2006 to 2014

Trend of US Healthcare Expenditures: 2006, 2008, 2012, and 2014

	Pre ACA - Billions		Post ACA - Billions	
	2006	2008 (Crash)	2012	2014
Total National HC Exp	**2.1**	**2.4**	**2.8**	**3.1 Trillion**
Prescription Drugs	217	237	290	298 Billion
Physician/Clinical Svc	450	487	543	604
Hospital Care	649	722	873	972
Dental Svc	91	102	110	114
Net Cost Private Health Ins (Premiums Less Benefits Paid)	150	135	162	195
Homecare Svc	**53**	**62**	**80**	**83**
Gov Public Health Exp	**60**	**73**	**91**	**79**
Non-Comm Research	**41**	**43**	**57**	**46**

Source: CMS' Office of the Actuary, National Health Statistics Group, various years.

I feel strongly that the answer lies with a foundational shift in health policy emphasis of simply funding *sick care*, for a greater commitment to a real *healthcare orientation*. At least *30 percent of the current expenditures* on healthcare (about $1 trillion) should be refocused on *prevention and wellbeing initiatives* in order to stimulate the maturation of **Population Health Management** for our nation. Together, we can devote significant resources to promote value and evidence-based **health care initiatives** starting in 2018. This strategy promises to "bend the cost curve," and improve the health status of Americans and strengthen the economy of the United States during the 21st Century.

Thank you for joining this *healthy* discussion regarding healthcare reform in the United States.

Appendix A (2017)

Obama Signs Historic Health Care Bill: 'It Is the Law of the Land'

The $938 Billion Bill, Facing Fire from Republicans, Brings Significant Changes to American Health Care

ABC NEWS BY HUMA KHAN

After more than a year of negotiations, debate and political drama, President Obama today signed the historic health care bill that could reshape care for millions of Americans while setting up a divisive battle with Republicans that's expected to spill into the November elections and beyond.

"After a century of striving, after a year of debate, after a historic vote, health care reform is no longer an unmet promise," Obama said at an event after the signing ceremony at the Department of Interior. "It is the law of the land."

The president took a direct stab at critics of health care overhaul, saying they are "still making a lot of noise" about what the new law means. "I heard one of the Republican leaders say this was going to be Armageddon. Well, two months from now, six months from now, you can check it out. We'll look around and we'll see," Obama said to applause.

The president signed the health care bill into law at the White House this morning. He was joined by Americans whose stories have touched the president, and Democrats who voted for the health care bill.

"Today, after almost a century of trying, today, after over a year of debate, today, after all the votes have been tallied, health insurance reform becomes law in the United States of America," Obama said to a standing ovation.

"It's easy to succumb to the sense of cynicism about what's possible in this country. But today, we are affirming that essential truth, a truth every generation is called to rediscover for itself: That we are not a nation that scales back its aspirations. We are not a nation that falls prey to doubt or mistrust," the president added. "We are a nation that faces its challenges and accepts its responsibilities."

The attendees chanted "Fired up, ready to go" -- Obama's campaign slogan -- as the president and Vice President Joe Biden arrived at the East Room. "Ladies and gentleman, to state the obvious, this is a historic day," Biden said to a cheering crowd before the president took the podium.

As Biden finished his remarks and shook Obama's hand, he was heard on the microphone whispering, "This is a big f-ing deal." White House Press Secretary Robert Gibbs tweeted soon afterward, "And yes Mr. Vice President, you're right..."

Appendix B (2017)

Supreme Court Allows Nationwide Health Care Subsidies

By ADAM LIPTAK JUNE 25, 2015

President Obama and Vice President Joseph R. Biden Jr. in the White House on Thursday after the Supreme Court's decision. Credit Stephen Crowley/The New York Times

WASHINGTON — The Supreme Court ruled on Thursday that President Obama's health care law allows the federal government to provide nationwide tax subsidies to help poor and middle-class people buy health insurance, a sweeping vindication that endorsed the larger purpose of Mr. Obama's signature legislative achievement.

The 6-to-3 ruling means that it is all but certain that the Affordable Care Act will survive after Mr. Obama leaves office in 2017. For the second time in three years, the law survived an encounter with the Supreme Court. But the court's tone was different this time. The first decision, in 2012, was fractured and grudging, while Thursday's ruling was more assertive.

"Congress passed the Affordable Care Act to improve health insurance markets, not to destroy them," Chief Justice John G. Roberts Jr. wrote for a united six-justice majority. In 2012's closely divided decision, Chief Justice Roberts also wrote the controlling opinion, but that time no other justice joined it in full.

In dissent on Thursday, Justice Antonin Scalia called the majority's reasoning "quite absurd" and "interpretive jiggery-pokery."

Demonstrators expressed their support for the Affordable Care Act outside of the Supreme Court on Thursday. Credit Doug Mills/The New York Times

He announced his dissent from the bench, a sign of bitter disagreement. His summary was laced with notes of incredulity and sarcasm, sometimes drawing amused murmurs in the courtroom as he described the "interpretive somersaults" he said the majority had performed to reach the decision.

"We really should start calling this law Scotus-care," Justice Scalia said, to laughter from the audience.

In a hastily arranged appearance in the Rose Garden on Thursday morning, a triumphant Mr. Obama praised the ruling. "After multiple challenges to this law before the Supreme Court, the Affordable Care Act is here to stay," he said, adding: "What we're not going to do is unravel what has now been woven into the fabric of America."

The ruling was a blow to Republicans, who have been trying to gut the law since it was enacted. But House Speaker John A. Boehner vowed that the political fight against it would continue.

"The problem with Obamacare is still fundamentally the same: The law is broken," Mr. Boehner said. "It's raising costs for American families, it's raising costs for small businesses and it's just fundamentally broken. And we're going to continue our efforts to do everything we can to put the American people back in charge of their health care and not the federal government."

The case concerned a central part of the Affordable Care Act that created marketplaces, known as exchanges, to allow people who lack insurance to shop for individual health plans. Some states set up their own exchanges, but about three dozen allowed the federal government to step in to run them. Across the nation, about 85 percent of customers using the exchanges qualify for subsidies to help pay for coverage, based on their income.

The question in the case, King v. Burwell, No. 14-114, was what to make of a phrase in the law that seems to say the subsidies are available only to people buying insurance on "an exchange established by the state."

A legal victory for the plaintiffs, lawyers for the administration said, would have affected more than six million people and created havoc in the insurance markets and undermined the law.

Chief Justice Roberts acknowledged that the plaintiffs had strong arguments about the plain meaning of the contested words. But he wrote that the words must be understood as part of a larger statutory plan. "In this instance," he wrote, "the context and structure of the act compel us to depart from what would otherwise be the most natural reading of the pertinent statutory phrase."

This was challenging, he said, in light of the law's "more than a few examples of in-artful drafting," a consequence of rushed work behind closed doors that "does not reflect the type of care and deliberation that one might expect of such significant legislation."

But he said the law's interlocking parts supported a ruling in favor of the subsidies, particularly given that a contrary decision could have given rise to chaos in the insurance markets. A ruling rejecting subsidies in most of the nation would have left in place other parts of the law, including its guarantee of coverage regardless of pre-existing conditions, its requirement that most Americans obtain insurance or pay a penalty, and its expansion of Medicaid.

Without the subsidies, many people would be unable to afford insurance, and healthier consumers would go without coverage, leaving insurers with a sicker, more expensive pool of customers. That would raise prices for everyone, leading to what supporters of the law called death spirals.

Copies of the court's ruling in favor of nationwide health insurance subsidies were rushed to television news reporters. Credit Doug Mills/The New York Times

"The statutory scheme compels us to reject petitioners' interpretation," Chief Justice Roberts wrote, referring to the challengers, "because it would destabilize the individual insurance market in any state with a federal exchange, and likely create the very 'death spirals' that Congress designed the act to avoid."

In dissent, Justice Scalia wrote that the majority had stretched the statutory text too far.

"I wholeheartedly agree with the court that sound interpretation requires paying attention to the whole law, not homing in on isolated words or even isolated sections," Justice Scalia wrote. "Context always matters. Let us not forget, however, why context matters: It is a tool for understanding the terms of the law, not an excuse for rewriting them."

"Reading the act as a whole leaves no doubt about the matter," he wrote. " 'Exchange established by the state' means what it looks like it means."

Justice Scalia said the decision had damaged the court's reputation for "honest jurisprudence."

The court, he said, had taken into its own hands a matter involving tens of billions of dollars that should have been left to Congress.

"The court's decision reflects the philosophy that judges should endure whatever interpretive distortions it takes in order to correct a supposed flaw in the statutory machinery," Justice Scalia wrote.

"It is up to Congress to design its laws with care," he added, "and it is up to the people to hold them to account if they fail to carry out that responsibility."

Justices Clarence Thomas and Samuel A. Alito Jr. joined Justice Scalia's dissenting opinion.

Chief Justice Roberts rejected the argument that Congress had limited the availability of subsidies in order to encourage states to create their own exchanges, a notion that had occurred to almost no one at the time the law was enacted.

Highlights: The Times collected reaction to the Supreme Court's decision.

Sixteen states and the District of Columbia have established their own exchanges. Under the law, the federal government has stepped in to run exchanges in the rest of the states.

"The whole point of that provision," Chief Justice Roberts wrote, "is to create a federal fallback in case a state chooses not to establish its own exchange. Contrary to petitioners' argument, Congress did not believe it was offering states a deal they would not refuse — it expressly addressed what would happen if a state did refuse the deal.

Justices Anthony M. Kennedy, Ruth Bader Ginsburg, Stephen G. Breyer, Sonia Sotomayor and Elena Kagan joined the majority opinion. In the 2012 case, Justice Kennedy was in dissent.

The case started when four plaintiffs, all from Virginia, sued the Obama administration, saying the phrase meant that the law forbids the federal government to provide subsidies in states that do not have their own exchanges.

The plaintiffs challenged an Internal Revenue Service regulation that said subsidies were allowed whether the exchange was run by a state or by the federal government. They said the regulation was at odds with the Affordable Care Act.

In July, the United States Court of Appeals for the Fourth Circuit, in Richmond, Va., ruled against the challengers.

Judge Roger L. Gregory, writing for a three-judge panel of the court, said the contested phrase was "ambiguous and subject to multiple interpretations." That meant, he said, that the I.R.S. interpretation was entitled to deference.

The Supreme Court's ruling was more forceful. "This is not a case for the I.R.S.," Chief Justice Roberts wrote. "It is instead our task to determine the correct reading."

Julie Hirschfeld Davis and Michael D. Shear contributed reporting.

Follow The New York Times Politics and Washington on Facebook and Twitter, and sign up for the First Draft politics newsletter.

Appendix C (2017)

Kaiser Health Tracking Poll: Future Directions for the ACA and Medicaid

Feb 24, 2017 | Ashley Kirzinger, Elise Sugarman, and Mollyann Brodie

[To view charts and graphs, click on the URL to the source site at the end of article]

KEY FINDINGS:

- **The latest Kaiser Health Tracking Poll finds attitudes towards the Affordable Care Act (ACA) have shifted with a larger share reporting a favorable opinion towards the law (48 percent) than reporting an unfavorable opinion (42 percent). This is the highest level of favorability of the ACA measured in more than 60 Kaiser Health Tracking Polls since 2010 and is largely driven by a change in the views of independents, among which 50 percent now view the law favorably.**
- **Despite this shift in overall favorability, the public remains divided on what they would like lawmakers to do when it comes to the 2010 health care law with 47 percent wanting lawmakers to vote to repeal the law compared to 48 percent who say they should not vote to repeal it. Of those who want to see Congress vote to repeal the law, a larger share say they want lawmakers to wait to vote to repeal the law until the details of a replacement plan have been announced (28 percent) than say Congress should vote to repeal the law immediately and work out the details of a replacement plan later (18 percent).**
- **Republican lawmakers have also discussed possible changes to Medicaid – to either a per capita allotment program or to giving states the option to receive federal Medicaid funding in the form of a block grant. When examining these two proposed changes to Medicaid, more Americans (65 percent) would prefer to see Medicaid continue as it is today than either of the offered alternatives to the current federal funding structure.**
- **The vast majority of Americans say it is either "very important" (55 percent) or "somewhat important" (29 percent) for ACA replacement plans to ensure that states that have received federal funds to expand Medicaid continue to receive those funds, with majorities of Democrats (95 percent), independents (84 percent), and Republicans (69 percent) saying it is important.**

The February 2017 Kaiser Health Tracking Poll finds that Americans have concerns about the shifting landscape of health care in this country. Six in ten (62 percent) Americans say that when it comes to health care, things in this country have pretty seriously gotten off on the wrong track, compared to three in ten who say things are generally going in the right direction.

Figure 1: Six in Ten Say When It Comes to Health Care, Things in US Have Gotten Off on the Wrong Track *[see source]*

These results are consistent across demographic groups with roughly twice as many individuals – regardless of party identification or health status – saying things are on the wrong track as saying things are headed in the right direction. This month's survey examines two specific policy areas that may be driving these concerns: the future of the Affordable Care Act and Medicaid.

FUTURE DIRECTIONS FOR THE AFFORDABLE CARE ACT
With lawmakers debating the future of the Affordable Care Act (ACA), the latest Kaiser Health Tracking survey finds that more Americans now have a favorable view of the health care law (48 percent) than have an unfavorable opinion (42 percent).

Figure 2: More Americans Now Have a Favorable View of the Health Care Law than Have an Unfavorable View *[see source]*

Attitudes towards the ACA are largely viewed through a partisan lens with about seven in ten Republicans and about seven in ten of those who approve (either somewhat or strongly) of the way President Trump is handling his job reporting an *unfavorable* opinion towards the law (74 percent and 69 percent, respectively). This compares to a majority of both Democrats and those who disapprove of President Trump reporting a *favorable* view of the law (73 percent and 71 percent).

Figure 3: View of Affordable Care Act Varies by Party Affiliation and Trump Approval

The Shifting Attitudes of Independents *[see source]*

The latest shift in favorability of the law is largely driven by the views of independents, among whom a larger share now say they have a favorable opinion (50 percent) of the law than an unfavorable opinion (39 percent). This is the first survey since 2010 that has found a larger share of independents reporting a favorable view than an unfavorable view. *[On average, individuals who identify as political independents have accounted for about one-third of the total sample in Kaiser Health Tracking Polls].*

Figure 4: A Larger Share of Independents Now Say They Have Favorable Opinion of the ACA *[see source]*

Repealing and Replacing the Affordable Care Act

As lawmakers debate replacement plans for the ACA, Americans are divided on what they want to see lawmakers do with the health care law, with 48 percent saying they do not want Congress to vote to repeal the law and 47 percent saying they want Congress to vote to repeal it. Of those who want to see Congress vote to repeal the law, a larger share say they want lawmakers to wait to vote on repeal until the details of a replacement plan have been announced (28 percent) than say Congress should vote to repeal the law immediately and work out the details of a replacement plan later (18 percent). These findings are similar to the results from the December 2016 Kaiser Health Tracking Poll. [A Kirzinger, B Wu, M Brodie, Kaiser Health Tracking Poll: Health Care Priorities for 2017. http://kff.org/health-costs/poll-finding/kaiser-health-tracking-poll-health-care-priorities-for-2017/]

Figure 5: Americans Divided on ACA Repeal and Replacement *[see source]*

Attitudes on the ACA's next steps are largely partisan with the vast majority of Democrats (78 percent) saying they do not want Congress to vote to repeal the health care law compared to about half of independents and 16 percent of Republicans who say the same. On the other hand, while the majority of Republicans want to see Congress vote to repeal the law, fewer want them to vote to repeal the law immediately (31 percent) than want them to wait until they have the details of a replacement plan announced (48 percent). With more than half of Republicans (64 percent) wanting lawmakers to do something other than immediate repeal of the ACA, this is a clear indication of the challenge facing Republican lawmakers.

Table 1: Next Steps for the ACA *[see source]*

How ACA Repeal Efforts Are Affecting Americans

As Americans watch their elected leaders debate repeal and replacement plans for the ACA, more feel worried (56 percent) and hopeful (53 percent) than confused (45 percent), angry (38 percent), or enthusiastic (33 percent).

Figure 6: More Americans Are "Worried" and "Hopeful" About Current Plans to Repeal Health Care Law than "Angry" or "Enthusiastic" *[see source]*

Related to the partisan nature of the health care law and current repeal efforts, Democrats (81 percent) are more likely to say they feel "worried" about current plans than independents (57 percent) and Republicans (26 percent). Republicans, on the other hand, are more likely to report feeling "hopeful" than independents and Democrats (78 percent compared to 55 percent and 30 percent, respectively). An equal share of independents report feeling "worried" (57 percent) as report feeling "hopeful" (55 percent).

Underscoring that perceptions sometimes exceeds the impact of what policies may or may not be, half of Americans (48 percent) are either "very worried" (26 percent) or "somewhat worried" (22 percent) that they or someone in their family will lose their health insurance coverage if the health care law is repealed and replaced, compared to 51 percent of those who are not worried. A larger share of Democrats and independents report being worried about losing their health insurance than Republicans (70 percent, 51 percent, and 17 percent, respectively). In addition, 67 percent of those who disapprove of President Trump say they are worried about losing their coverage under an ACA replacement plan, as do one-fourth of those who approve of President Trump.

Figure 7: Worries over Losing Coverage Vary by Party Affiliation and Trump Approval *[see source]*

Individuals in families with ongoing health needs and individuals who report being in fair or poor health are more likely to be worried about losing their health insurance coverage if the ACA is repealed and replaced. Among those who report being in fair or poor health, 64 percent say they are either "very" or "somewhat" worried about losing their health insurance coverage compared to 44 percent of those in excellent, very good, or good health. About half (55 percent) of individuals with a chronic health condition that requires ongoing medical treatment also report being worried about losing their coverage compared to 41 percent of those without ongoing health needs.

Table 2: Health Status Affects How Worried Individuals Are About Losing Coverage *[see source]*

FUTURE DIRECTIONS FOR MEDICAID

Republican lawmakers' plans to repeal and replace the 2010 health care law also include proposed changes to Medicaid – the program that provides coverage for medical care and long-term care services to low-income people. Overall, nearly six in ten Americans (56 percent) say Medicaid is either "very" or "somewhat" important to them and their family; however, this does vary by party identification with larger shares of Democrats (62 percent) and independents (57 percent) reporting that the program is important than Republicans (43 percent).

Figure 8: More than Half of Americans Say Medicaid Is Important for Their Family; Fewer Republicans Say So *[see source]*

In addition, over half of Americans report some connection to the Medicaid program, either because they personally have received some assistance from Medicaid (26 percent) or they have close friends or family who have (31 percent).

Figure 9: Over Half Report Some Connection to Medicaid *[see source]*

Proposed Changes to Federal Funding for Medicaid

Currently, Medicaid is jointly financed by federal and state governments, with each state deciding how to structure benefits, eligibility, and care delivery within guidelines set by the federal government. The federal government matches state spending on an open-ended basis but Republican lawmakers are proposing two alternatives to this current structure: per capita allotments and block grants.

Medicaid Per Capita Allotment vs. Block Grant Proposal

Under a Medicaid per capita cap, the federal government would set a limit on how much to reimburse states per enrollee. When provided with the option of keeping Medicaid largely as it is today or changing to a per capita allotment program, Americans largely prefer the status quo with two-thirds saying the program should continue as it is today with the federal government guaranteeing coverage, setting standards and benefits, and matching state spending. About a third (31 percent) say, instead, Medicaid should be changed to a per capita allotment structure rather than matching state Medicaid spending.

Another option that has been proposed by Republican lawmakers calls for giving states the option to receive federal Medicaid funding in the form of a block grant. Under a block grant structure, the federal government would limit the amount it gives states to help pay for Medicaid coverage but could allow states more flexibility in determining which groups of people and what services are covered under the program. Here again, most Americans prefer the status quo, with 63 percent saying the program should continue as it is today while 32 percent say Medicaid should be changed to a block grant structure.

When examining these two proposed changes to Medicaid, more Americans (65 percent) would prefer to see Medicaid continue as it is today than either of the offered alternatives to the current federal funding structure.

Figure 10: Two-Thirds of Americans Say Medicaid Should Continue Largely as It Is Today *[see source]*

Six in ten Republicans support the per capita allotment proposal while about half of Republicans support changing Medicaid to a block grant program.

Table 3: Proposed Changes to Medicaid *[see source]*

VAST MAJORITY OF AMERICANS THINK CONTINUING FEDERAL FUNDING FOR MEDICAID EXPANSION IS IMPORTANT

Medicaid is also one of the primary ways the Affordable Care Act expanded coverage to millions more low-income, uninsured adults. The vast majority of Americans say it is either "very important" (55 percent) or "somewhat important" (29 percent) for ACA replacement plans to make sure that states that have received federal funds to expand Medicaid continue to receive those funds – with majorities of Democrats (95 percent), independents (84 percent), and Republicans (69 percent) saying it is important.

Table 4: Majorities of Democrats, Independents, and Republicans Say Continued Federal Funding for Medicaid Expansion Is Important [see source]

The vast majority (87 percent) of individuals living in the 16 states that have expanded Medicaid and have a Republican governor say it is either "very" or "somewhat" important that a replacement plan makes sure states that received federal funds to expand Medicaid continue to receive those funds. This is similar to the share of those living in Medicaid expansion states with Democratic governors (85 percent) and more than those living in states without Medicaid expansion (80 percent).

Figure 11: Large Majorities Say Continued Funding for Medicaid Expansion Is Important

Medicaid Spending Compared to Other National Priorities [see source]

Reflecting the high regard the public holds for Medicaid, Americans are generally opposed to cutting back federal spending on the program. Overall, about half of Americans want to keep federal spending on Medicaid the same, while 36 percent want to increase spending and 12 percent want to decrease spending.

With the exception of increased spending on education, partisans have largely different spending priorities. Majorities of Democrats (81 percent), independents (66 percent), and Republicans (57 percent) would like to see the president and Congress increase spending on education; yet, that is where the consensus ends with a majority of Republicans calling for increased spending on national defense and about half of Democrats calling for increased spending on each of the three major entitlement programs – Medicare, Social Security, and Medicaid.

Table 5: Partisans Differ on Spending Priorities [see source]

Which Sources Does the Public Trust?

President Trump's administration has frequently lamented the accuracy of news from major news organizations. Therefore, this month's Tracking Poll aims to find out if there are sources that Americans trust when it comes to news about proposed changes to the US health care system. Overall, six in ten (59 percent) Americans say there is a source in the news media that they trust compared to 39 percent who say there is no source that they trust for information about proposed changes to the health care system. One-fifth of all Americans say they most trust a cable news network for information about proposed changes to the US health care system, with 10 percent of those saying they trust Fox News, 8 percent saying they trust CNN, and 3 percent saying they trust MSNBC. Smaller shares of Americans say they most trust national broadcast news (6 percent), national newspapers (5 percent), public television or radio (4 percent), local television or radio news (4 percent), and the internet (4 percent).

When it Comes to Health Care News, Americans Are Divided on What Sources They Trust

When it comes to information about proposed changes to the US health care system, Americans are more likely to say they trust their Congressional representative (55 percent), their friends and family (51 percent), and local (53 percent) and national news organizations (51 percent) than say the same about information from President Trump (42 percent) or social networking sites, such as Facebook and Twitter (16 percent). While fewer than half of Americans say they trust information about proposed changes to the US health care system from President Trump "a lot" or "some," about one-fourth of Americans do say they trust information from the President "a lot" (23 percent) which may be an indication of the current divisive political environment. In fact, about half of Republicans say they trust information from President Trump "a lot" compared to 19 percent of independents and 4 percent of Democrats.

Source: For complete narrative and tables / figures referenced in the Kaiser Family Foundation article, see http://kff.org/health-reform/poll-finding/kaiser-health-tracking-poll-future-directions-for-the-aca-and-medicaid/

Supplemental Resources for Section Two (2010-2017)

Altman, Stuart H., Reinhardt, Uwe E., & Shields, Alexandra E. (Eds.). (1998). *The future US healthcare system: Who will care for the poor and uninsured?* Chicago: Health Administration Press.

Arinola, Olajumoke K., Aula, Mercy E, and Tozzio, Mark G. "Africa's Changing Disease Patterns: The Need to Pay More Attention and Strategies to Improve," Medical Records Institute, *The African Journal of Health Information Systems*, October 4, 2016, Vol. 1, Number 1, Special Edition, pp. 28-33,

Engstrom, Timothy H. and Robinson, Wade L. (2006). *Health Care Reform: Ethics and Politics*, Rochester: University of Rochester Press.

Feldstein, Paul J. (2006, 3rd Ed.). *The Politics of Health Legislation: An Economic Perspective*, Chicago: Health Administration Press.

Flareau, Bruce MD, Yale, Ken DDS JD, Bohn, J.M., and Konschak. (2011, 2nd Ed.). *Clinical Integration: A Roadmap to Accountable Care*, Virginia Beach, Virginia: Convergent Publishing, LLC.

Harris, Dean M. (2014, 4th Ed.). *Contemporary Issues in Healthcare Law & Ethics*, Chicago: Health Administration Press.

Joshi, Maulik S., Ransom, Elizabeth R., Nash, David B., and Ransom, Scott B., Editors. (2014, 3rd Ed.). *The Quality Healthcare Book: Vision, Strategy, and Tools*, Chicago: Health Administration Press.

Longest, Beaufort B. Jr. (2006 4th Ed.). *Health Policymaking in the United States*, Chicago: Health Administration Press.

McLaughlin, Daniel B., Editor. (2015). The Guide to Healthcare Reform: Readings and Commentary, Chicago: Health Administration Press.

Nugent, Mike and Bard, Marc. (2011). *Accountable Care Organizations: Your Guide to Strategy, Design, and Implementation*, Chicago: Health Administration Press.

Tozzio, Mark G. (2009). *Why The United States Healthcare System Should Be A Limited Human Right For All*, original thesis material, *Section One Only*, Printed by *CreateSpace*, An Amazon.com Company (paperback and e-book versions).

Made in the USA
San Bernardino, CA
15 April 2017